Contents

Assessment Scales in Old Age Psychiatry

Alistair Burns MD FRCP FRCPsych

Professor of Old Age Psychiatry

University of Manchester, UK

Brian Lawlor MD FRCPI MRCPsych

Professor of Old Age Psychiatry

St Patrick's Psychiatric Hospital

Dublin, Ireland

Sarah Craig MB MSc MRCPsych

Consultant in Old Age Psychiatry

The Royal Bolton Hospitals NHS Trust

Bolton, UK

MARTIN DUNITZ

© Martin Dunitz Ltd 1999

First published in the United Kingdom in 1999 by
Martin Dunitz Ltd
The Livery House
7–9 Pratt Street
London NW1 0AE

A CIP catalogue record for this book is available from the British Library

ISBN 1-85317-562-5

Distributed in the United States by:
Blackwell Science Inc.
Commerce Place, 350 Main Street
Malden, MA 02148, USA
Tel: 1-800-215-1000

Distributed in Canada by:
Login Brothers Book Company
324 Salteaux Crescent
Winnipeg, Manitoba, R3J 3T2
Canada
Tel: 204-224-4068

Distributed in Brazil by:
Ernesto Reichmann Distribuidora de Livros, Ltda
Rue Coronel Marques 335, Tatuape 03440-000
São Paulo,
Brazil

Composition by Scribe Design, Gillingham, Kent, UK
Printed and bound in Italy

Foreword

I am delighted to be able to write a foreword for this book. Old age psychiatry is an area of medical practice where there are exciting developments, particularly in therapy. The ageing population has increased the need for effective use of resources, and it is becoming more important to make accurate diagnosis so that proper treatment can be initiated, progress monitored and outcome evaluated. When dealing with old people, assessment scales are necessary for these aspirations to be achieved.

This book contains a comprehensive collection of scales relevant to old age psychiatry. The very fact that there are around 150 included, points to the complexity of the subject. To have brought so many diverse instruments together represents a considerable achievement. The authors have classified them in a sensible manner and commented on their usefulness.

The various measures are set out in an orderly form and the book will act as a reference guide for those who are searching for an appropriate assessment tool. Anyone constructing a scale will be helped by using the book to determine whether earlier work is relevant.

The assessment of old people is becoming a complex process. There are many different situations where assessment is needed – in primary care, in the community, in hospital, or prior to movement from one environment to another. Assessment may be for the person as a whole or concentrate on one aspect: physical, mental, functional or social. Not only the patient needs assessing, often the needs of the carers, social background and home conditions require examination. Research, audit and evaluation of progress also need assessment tools. The advantage of

reliable instruments is that a baseline can be established and referred back to when progress is being monitored.

By its comprehensiveness the book takes note of this complexity. Quite rightly, prominence is given to scales associated with depression and dementia; but activities of daily living, physical examination, caregiver assessment and measurement of function are also included. I am impressed with the fact that each individual scale is commented upon and the main indications included. Full references and the addresses for correspondence are given. Although some of the instruments date back several years, their inclusion gives a sense of a developing technology.

Particularly helpful will be the 'what to use and when' appendix. It neatly puts into perspective the range of circumstances requiring assessment.

Who therefore will find this book useful? It is essentially a book of reference for those presented with clinical problems which require analysis, and where a particular assessment tool which is appropriate needs to be found. Researchers will want to consult the book when planning projects with the elderly. All the major assessment scales in common use appear in the book. For everyone working with old people, the book will be interesting in that it sets in perspective the place of the well-known scales and demonstrates the wide range of possible measures which are needed in modern old age psychiatry.

Professor E Idris Williams OBE
Emeritus Professor of General Practice, University of Nottingham
Chairman, Morecambe Bay Hospitals NHS Trust

Preface

There are a large number of scales used to measure the various manifestations of mental and physical diseases affecting older people. It was in an attempt to put some form of order into these myriad scales that the idea of creating this book originated. We have attempted to list a large number of scales in some form of order which we hope makes sense to the reader. Where possible, we have reproduced the scale in full. Literature subsequent to the original publication has been added in some cases, but we have not done this in a structured or formal way and it is therefore not extensive. It has sometimes been a salutary lesson to look back at the original papers and see how the scales were devised and validated.

A few warnings. The book is meant as a map rather than a guidebook, and we recommend that if you are using a scale seriously, you should check the original publication. The permission given by the copyright holder is for this publication only. The time taken to complete the scales varies, and in the majority of cases we have used our own estimate as an approximation. In some instances, a scale can be completed in a matter of a minute or so by someone who knows the patient, but takes longer if the information has to be gathered de novo. The majority of the scales have appeared in peer-reviewed journals and so have passed that particular academic hurdle. We have tried to give as standardized a description as possible for the reliability and validity of the scales, but this has not always been possible. The choice of instrument depends primari-ly on the question to be answered, as well as on a number of other factors, and we have been circumspect in recommending any particular scale in individual circumstances. We realize we risk accusations of being over-inclusive – we did this simply to allow the reader to choose for himself or herself. By including some older scales we hope the reader will be able to judge them in their historical perspective, and while perhaps not choosing them directly, might use them to inform a judgement about a later scale.

We have been as complete as possible in gaining permission to reproduce scales, and if in error we have done so inappropriately we apologize and would ask the injured parties to contact us so we may put it right.

We thank Ruth Dunitz and her colleagues at the publishers for their gentle and appropriate persuasion to all the authors and publishers who agreed that their scales could be included, to Professor Idris Williams for his generous foreword, and to Donna Wright our librarian at Withington Hospital, who conducted a literature search for us. However, the biggest thanks go to Barbara Dignan, without whose secretarial skill and patience this project would never have been completed, let alone on time.

Alistair Burns
Brian Lawlor
Sarah Craig

Introduction

There were several aims behind producing this compendium of scales. The first was simply to bring together in one volume as many scales as was practical for ease of reference. Other publications have expertly summarized smaller numbers of scales, but not since the book by Israel et al of 1984,[1] and the *Psychopharmacology Bulletin* supplement of 1988 (Vol. 24, no. 4), has there been an attempt to synthesize the whole field. Also, a great number of scales have been published in the last decade and a half, and an update seemed appropriate. Presenting them in an ordered form with information about the completion of the instrument would be convenient and allow the reader to see at a glance the scope of the scale and its application. The compendium may also act as a reference guide and allow readers to interpret the use of scales they may read about in journal articles. We have concentrated on scales available in the English language literature and on those which can be completed relatively easily. We have not, therefore, attempted to include detailed neuropsychological tests, which are the remit of specialist neuropsychology. The scales are approximately in the order of their annualized citation index.

The second aim was to provide the reader with a document allowing them to pick whichever scale was appropriate to the question being asked. Care protocols and clinical guidelines with an emphasis on outcomes are now commonly adopted in clinical practice, and it is important for clinicians to be aware of ways in which performance can be measured. Formal documentation of clinical variables allows individual patients (and thereby a service) to be evaluated. This must obviously be carried out carefully using valid and appropriate instruments, and should be led by clinicians of any discipline (ideally the process should be multidisciplinary). Awareness of the range of measures available is essential to this process. We have therefore included in each chapter a short summary of the main scales which, from reading the literature and from knowledge of the field, we feel would be the most appropriate for the researcher, hospital specialist or general practitioner. A caveat is that the best scale depends on the question being asked and not the clinical discipline of the inquirer. The characteristics of an ideal scale can easily be summarized in terms of reliability (test retest, inter-rater) and validity (content, face and construct validity). However, in practice, this can seldom be interpreted with clarity – it is comparatively easy to document reliability in any clinically based scale, and validity can usually be demonstrated by comparison with an existing instrument, especially if the two are similar. Clever statistical manipulation can prove most things (or at least cannot disprove them). Information enabling one to recommend the ideal scale (in terms of psychometric characteristics, ease of administration and predictive in terms of outcomes) is simply not available. We would have liked to present a standardized account of each scale, with reliability, validity, cut-off points, sensitivity and specificity measurements, drawbacks, advantages and disadvantages, but this information is simply not available. To have confined ourselves to scales which provide that level of detail would have resulted in a very different book. We have preferred to be inclusive (we will be accused of being overinclusive) and allow the reader to make up his or her own mind. There are now more scales than there are measurable facets of illness, and so duplication is inevitable. For instance, there are only a limited number of ways in which to test for disorientation in time by direct questioning (i.e. what time, date, year, day and season is it?). Variations occur in terms of the individual characteristics of a scale such as adaptation to a particular environment (e.g. a scale specifically for nursing homes) or brevity (reductionism facilitates ease of administration).

The third aim was to inform anyone considering constructing a scale of the large number available and that referring back to a previous scale, perhaps with modification, would be more cost-effective than starting from scratch.

The fourth, and most indulgent, aim was to put together a collection of scales, many of which have been used only occasionally but which form a body of work supporting the concept of accurate, reliable and valid measurement of signs and symptoms of disease in older people. Some of these are only of historical interest and have not stood the test of time, but many have been adapted to inform the development of later, more commonly used scales.

---

[1]Israel L, Kozarevic D, Sartorius N (1984) *Source book of geriatric assessment,* Vols I & II. Basel: S Karger AG.

Chapter 1

Depression

Depression can mean either a mild feeling of lowered mood which is transient and may reflect an individual response to life circumstances or a major illness with biological features (e.g. weight loss, diurnal variation in mood, sleep disturbance). It also covers anything in between. Scales which measure depressed mood do so at a symptomatic level with the general assumption that there is a linear relationship between the score and the severity of the illness. Particular difficulties with the measurement of depression unique to older people include the tendency of older people to deny feelings of depression, the atypical presentation of depression (more somatic complaints) and the coexistence of depression and cognitive impairment. The symptoms of depression, however, are sufficiently commonly recognized that there is general agreement about what should be asked. Some questions have to be addressed carefully – many a centenarian has roared with laughter when asked by a nervous interviewer what they feel about the future. In practice, this demonstrates a valuable point of amending what is said to the situation: asking that question to a younger person conjures up thoughts of months and perhaps years in the future; in a centenarian, the time scale should be adapted, at least when trying to elucidate depression, to the next day or so. DSM IV criteria for major depressive illness include five or more of the following symptoms, present during the same two-week period and representing a change from previous function:

- Depressed mood most of the day, nearly every day;
- Markedly diminished interest or pleasure in all, or almost all activities;
- Significant weight loss, or decrease or increase in appetite nearly every day;
- Insomnia or hypersomnia;
- Psychomotor agitation or retardation;
- Fatigue or loss of energy;
- Feelings of worthlessness or excessive or inappropriate guilt;
- Diminished ability to think or concentrate, or indecisiveness;
- Recurrent thoughts of death, suicidal ideation with or without a plan.

Scales can be self reports, interviews by trained or non-trained staff and informant-based measures. The Hamilton Depression Rating Scale (page 4) is probably the gold standard of depression scales and in general psychiatry probably has yet to be beaten. It is often used in studies of older people to act as an anchor by which to measure new instruments, although it was not designated for use with elderly people. This is because the psychometric properties have not been well established for that age group and some of the questions are not really appropriate for older people. For example, it has a number of questions relating to somatic symptoms and therefore depression in the elderly may be overdiagnosed. Another disadvantage is that it is based on a skilled interview procedure by a competent clinician. The Montgomery and Åsberg Depression Rating Scale (MADRS; page 7) taps ten domains of depression and has been used in a number of drug studies, having been shown to be sensitive to change. It can be used by any trained interviewer. The Geriatric Depression Scale (GDS; page2) is essentially a self-reported inventory with a simple yes/no format which lends itself to ease

of administration by the older person or by an interviewer. It is the most widely used in old age psychiatry and has several versions, going from a 30-item to a 15-item (the most commonly used) to a 4-item test. Self-report questionnaires like the Beck Depression Inventory (BDI; page 6) have been used with older people, and contain a severity rating and a suicide item. The SELFCARE (D) (page 12) is adapted from a larger rating scale and has been used in general practice, as has the Center for Epidemiological Studies – Depression Scale (CES-D; page14), which has been validated in epidemiological samples. The Mood Scales – Elderly (MS-E; page 20) and the Carroll Rating Scale (CRS; page 18) are more lengthy interviews and could not be used for screening (the latter has not been used specifically in elderly people but is validated against the dexamethasone depression test). The OARS Depressive Scale (ODS; page 15) can be used by trained interviewers where a diagnosis of depression against DSM criteria is required.

Depression in special settings

In medical inpatients, the necessity of interviewing in a noisy atmosphere makes a sensitive and private interview problematic. This led to the development of the Brief Assessment Schedule Depression Cards (BASDEC; page 10), adapted by using a set of cards which the patient simply puts into piles (true/false or don't know). The CRS is essentially a self-rated version of the Hamilton Depression Rating Scale with many of the advantages. It has been used in neuroendocrine studies with the dexamethasone test, but data relating to its use in the elderly are lacking.

The assessment of depression in dementia is an important clinical issue, and a number of scales reflect this. The special circumstances of interviewing a patient with cognitive impairment have been addressed in scale design, particularly emphasizing the need for direct observation of the patient and the difficulties of an informant answering on behalf of the patient. The elucidation of depressive symptomatology in patients with severe cognitive impairment is problematic. There is some evidence that there are two situations where depression occurs in dementia. In the early stages there is a reactive, almost understandable, reaction to loss of cognitive powers and fears for the future, whereas in the later stages the depression is more related to biological changes in the disease. The level of cognitive loss below which the communication of complex depressive ideation cannot be expressed by the patient (or captured by the interviewer) is not known (although guessed at by many), but there is general agreement that as the severity of dementia increases, determination of depressive symptoms direct from the patient becomes less reliable and proxy measures become necessary. The Cornell Scale for Depression in Dementia (page 8) set the standard for assessment in this area. Other scales (e.g. the Hamilton Depression Rating Scale) can be used if adapted appropriately for the clinical situation. Care must be taken in these circumstances to ensure that phenomena are assessed accurately, perhaps by checking with an informant after the examination rather than having them interrupt during an interview (Schneider, personal communication). The Depressive Signs Scale (DSS; page 16) has been less used in the rating of depressive symptoms, but has been validated against the dexamethasone suppression test.

Geriatric Depression Scale (GDS)

Reference Yesavage JA, Brink TL, Rose TL, Lum O, Huang V, Adey M, Leirer O (1983) Development and validation of a geriatric depression screening scale: a preliminary report. *Journal of Psychiatric Research* 17: 37–49

Time taken 5–10 minutes (reviewer's estimate)
Rating self-administered

Main indications

To rate depression in elderly people, the emphasis being on a scale that was simple to administer and did not require the skills of a trained interviewer.

Commentary

The Geriatric Depression Scale (GDS) was devised by gathering 100 questions relating to depression in older people, then selecting the 30 which correlated best with the total score. Each question has a yes/no answer, with the scoring dependent on the answer given. Some 100 subjects took part in the validation study, using the Hamilton Depression Rating Scale (page 4) and the Zung Self-Rating Depression Scale (page 252). Internal consistency was assessed in four ways and found to be higher for the GDS than for the other two scales. Test/retest reliability was assessed by 20 subjects completing the questionnaire twice, one week apart, with a correlation of 0.85. The GDS correlated well with the number of research diagnostic criteria symptoms for depression. Sensitivity and specificity of the GDS had been shown in a previous study (Brink et al, 1982), and a cut-off of 11 had an 84% sensitivity and 95% specificity rate whereas a cut-off of 14 decreased the sensitivity rate to 80% but increased the specificity rate to 100%.

A 15-item version of the GDS has been described by Shiekh and Yesavage (1986). This has a cut-off of between 6 and 7 and correlates significantly with the parent scale. Logistic regression analysis has been used to derive a four-point item of the GDS with specificity of up to 88% with a cut-off of 1/2 and sensitivity of 93% with a cut-off of 0/1 (Katona, 1994). Shah et al (1997) have reported that both the 4- and 10-item versions can be used for screen-ing successfully. The GDS has also been used to assess depression in dementia of the Alzheimer type, the results suggesting it does not maintain validity in that population (Burke et al, 1989).

Additional references

Brink T, Yesavage J, Lum O et al (1982) Screening tests for geriatric depression. *Clinical Gerontologist* 1: 37–43.

Burke WJ, Houston MJ, Boust SJ et al (1989) Use of the Geriatric Depression Scale in dementia of the Alzheimer type. *Journal of the American Geriatrics Society* 37: 856–60.

Katona C (1994) *Depression in old age.* Chichester: John Wiley & Sons.

Shah A, Herbert R, Lewis S et al (1997) Screening for depression among acutely ill geriatric inpatients with a short geriatric depression scale. *Age and Ageing* 26: 217–21.

Shiekh J, Yesavage J (1986) Geriatric Depression Scale; recent findings and development of a short version. In Brink T, ed. *Clinical gerontology: a guide to assessment and intervention.* New York: Howarth Press.

Address for correspondence

JA Yesavage
Department of Psychiatry and Behavioral Sciences
Stanford University Medical Center
Stanford
CA 94395
USA

Geriatric Depression Scale (GDS)

Choose the best answer for how you felt the past week

1. Are you basically satisfied with your life?
2. Have you dropped many of your activities and interests?
3. Do you feel that your life is empty?
4. Do you often get bored?
5. Are you hopeful about the future?
6. Are you bothered by thoughts you can't get out of your head?
7. Are you in good spirits most of the time?
8. Are you afraid that something bad is going to happen to you?
9. Do you feel happy most of the time?
10. Do you often feel helpless?
11. Do you often get restless and fidgety?
12. Do you prefer to stay at home, rather than going out and doing new things?
13. Do you frequently worry about the future?
14. Do you feel you have more problems with memory than most?
15. Do you think it is wonderful to be alive now?
16. Do you often feel downhearted and blue?
17. Do you feel pretty worthless the way you are now?
18. Do you worry a lot about the past?
19. Do you find life very exciting?
20. Is it hard for you to get started on new projects?
21. Do you feel full of energy?
22. Do you feel that your situation is hopeless?
23. Do you think that most people are better off than you are?
24. Do you frequently get upset over little things?
25. Do frequently feel like crying?
26. Do you have trouble concentrating?
27. Do you enjoy getting up in the morning?
28. Do you prefer to avoid social gatherings?
29. Is it easy for you to make decisions?
30. Is your mind as clear as it used to be?

Code answers as Yes or No

Score 1 for Yes on: 2–4,6,8,10–14,16–18,20,22–26,28
Score 1 for No on: 1,5,7,9,15,19,21,27,29,30

0–10 = Not depressed
11–20 = Mild depression
21–30 = Severe depression
GDS 15: 1,2,3,4,7,8,9,10,12,14,15,17,21,22,23 (cut-off of 5/6 indicates depression)
GDS 10: 1,2,3,8,9,10,14,21,22,23
GDS 4: 1,3,8,9 (cut-off of 1/2 indicates depression)

Reprinted from *Journal of Psychiatric Research*, Vol. 17, Yesavage JA, Brink TL, Rose TL, Lum O, Huang V, Adey M, Leirer O, Development and validation of a geriatric depression scale: a preliminary report, 1983, with permission from Elsevier Science.

Hamilton Depression Rating Scale

Reference   Hamilton M (1960) A rating scale for depression. *Journal of Neurology, Neurosurgery and Psychiatry* 23: 56–62

Time taken 20–30 minutes
Rating by semi-structured interview with trained interviewer

Main indications

To assess the severity of depression for clinical research purposes, in patients of any age.

Commentary

This is a widely used and reliable scale. Although not specific to the elderly, it is the most commonly used depression scale. Nine items are scored 0–4, and a further eight items are scored 0–2 as they represent variables which cannot be expressed quantatively. The last four items do not measure intensity of depression, and are commonly omitted to give the 17-item version. The scale has been devised primarily for use on patients already diagnosed as suffering from affective disorders, and is used for quantifying results of interviews. Its value depends on the skill of the interviewer in eliciting the necessary information. A cut-off of 10/11 is generally regarded as appropriate for the diagnosis of depression.

Additional reference

Hamilton M (1967) Development of a rating scale for primary depressive illness. *British Journal of Social and Clinical Psychology* **6**: 278–96.

Hamilton Depression Rating Scale

1.	DEPRESSION (MOOD)	0–4		12.	SOMATIC SYMPTOMS (GASTRO INTESTINAL)	0–2
2.	DEPRESSION (GUILT)	0–4		13.	GENERAL SOMATIC SYMPTOMS	0–2
3.	DEPRESSION (SUICIDE)	0–4		14.	SOMATIC SYMPTOMS (GENITAL SYMPTOMS)	0–2
4.	INSOMNIA (INITIAL)	0–2		15.	HYPOCHONDRIASIS	0–4
5.	INSOMNIA (MIDDLE)	0–2		16.	LOSS OF INSIGHT	0–2
6.	INSOMNIA (DELAYED)	0–2		17.	LOSS OF WEIGHT	0–2
7.	WORK AND INTERESTS	0–4		18.	DIURNAL VARIATION	0–2
8.	RETARDATION	0–4		19.	DEPERSONALISATION ETC.	0–4
9.	AGITATION	0–4		20.	PARANOID SYMPTOMS	0–4
10.	ANXIETY (PSYCHIC SYMPTOMS)	0–4		21.	OBSESSIONAL SYMPTOMS	0–2
11.	ANXIETY (SOMATIC SYMPTOMS)	0–4				

(0–4):

0 = Absent
1 = Doubtful or slight (trivial)
2 = Mild
3 = Moderate
4 = Severe

(0–2):

0 = Absent
1 = Doubtful or slight (trivial)
2 = Clearly present

Reproduced with permission of the BMJ Publishing Group, BMA House, Tavistock Square, London WC1H 9JR.

Beck Depression Inventory (BDI)

Reference   Beck AT, Ward CH, Mendelson M, Mock J, Erbaugh J (1961) An inventory for measuring depression. *Archives of General Psychiatry* 4: 53–63

Time taken 20 minutes (reviewer's estimate)
Rating self-rating

Main indications

Self-rating scale for depression.

Commentary

The Beck Depression Inventory (BDI) like the Zung Self-Rating Depression Scale (page 252) is not used specifically for older people but, along with the Zung Scale, is included here because of its widespead use. It represents the gold standard for self-rating depression scales and is often used in assessing depression in carers of patients with dementia, many of whom are younger. The original paper described the administration of the scale to two groups or subject (409 in total) showing excellent external consistency and validation as scored by independent ratings by psychiatrists. A cut-off of 12/13 is taken to indicate the presence of depression.

Address for correspondence

Center for Cognitive Therapy
Room 602
133 South 36th Street
Philadelphia
PA 19104
USA

Beck Depression Inventory (BDI) – summary

The BDI is a 21-item scale with a series of statements rated 0, 1, 2 and 3 denoting increasing severity of symptoms. The person completing the questionnaire is asked to read each group of symptoms and then pick the one that best describes the way that they have felt in the past week. Examples of questions include feelings of sadness, concerns about the future, suicidal ideation, tearfulnesss, sleep, fatigue, interests, worries about health, sexual interest, appetite, weight loss and general enjoyment.

Montgomery and Åsberg Depression Rating Scale (MADRS)

Reference Montgomery SA, Åsberg M (1979) A new depression scale designed to be sensitive to change. *British Journal of Psychiatry* 134: 382–9

Time taken 20 minutes
Rating by trained interviewer

Main indications

The scale is designed as a sensitive measure of change in the treatment of depression. The scale may be used for any time interval between ratings, be it weekly or otherwise, but this must be recorded.

Commentary

The Montgomery and Åsberg Depression Rating Scale (MADRS) was developed from 65 original items from the Comprehensive Psychopathological Rating Scale (CPRS; page 190) (Asberg et al, 1978). The 17 most common items were reduced to 10. These 10 variables specifically deal with the treatment of depression, apparent sadness, reported sadness, inner tension, reduced sleep, reduced appetite, concentration difficulties, lassitude, an ability to feel pessimistic thoughts and suicidal thoughts. Inter-rater reliability was >0.90. Validation studies were carried out on inpatients and outpatients in England and Sweden with concurrent validity tested by the Hamilton Depression

Scale (page 4) and shown to be satisfactory. The scale is now probably the most widely used in drug treatment trials, in young and older patients.

Additional references

Åsberg M, Montgomery S, Perris C et al (1978) A comprehensive psychopathological rating scale. *Acta Psychiatrica Scandinavica, Supplement* 271: 5–27.

Montgomery S, Åsberg M, Jörnestedt L et al (1978) Reliability of the CPRS between the disciplines of psychiatry, general practice, nursing and psychology in depressed patients. *Acta Psychiatrica Scandinavica, Supplement* 271: 29–32.

Address for correspondence

Stuart A Montgomery
Academic Department of Psychiatry
St Mary's Hospital Medical School
London W9 3RL
UK

Montgomery and Åsberg Depression Rating Scale (MADRS)

1.	Apparent sadness	6.	Concentration difficulties
2.	Reported sadness	7.	Lassitude
3.	Inner tension	8.	Inability to feel
4.	Reduced sleep	9.	Pessimistic thoughts
5.	Reduced appetite	10.	Suicidal thoughts

Score:
0 = No difficulties/normal
2 = Fluctuating/fleeting difficulties or feelings
4 = Continuous/pervasive feelings or thoughts
6 = Unrelenting/overwhelming feelings or thoughts

Cornell Scale for Depression in Dementia

Reference   Alexopoulos GS, Abrams RC, Young RC, Shamoian CA (1988) Cornell Scale for Depression in Dementia. *Biological Psychiatry* 23: 271–84

Time taken 20 minutes with the carer, 10 with the patient
Rating by clinician interview

Main indications

The diagnosis of depression in patients with a dementia syndrome.

Commentary

The importance of diagnosing depression in the setting of dementia is self-evident in terms of improved diagnosis and recognition of a potentially treatable condition. The authors state that most other depression scales are completed with information provided by the patient – something not always possible in dementia – hence the combination of observed and informant-based questions. The difference from other scales is therefore mainly in the method of administration rather than based on an analysis of the different phenomenology of depression in the set-ting of dementia. The 19-item scale is rated on a three-point score of absent, mild or intermittent and severe, with a note when the score was unevaluable. Twenty-six subjects were examined, with an inter-rater reliability kappa of 0.67, satisfactory internal consistency (0.84) and validity when measured against research diagnostic criteria and the Hamilton Depression Rating Scale (page 4). A score of 8 or more suggests significant depressive symp-toms.

Address for correspondence

GS Alexopoulos
Department of Psychiatry
Cornell University Medical College
New York Hospital – Westchester Division
21 Bloomingdale Road
White Plains
NY 10605
USA

Cornell Scale for Depression in Dementia

A. Mood-Related Signs
1. Anxiety
   anxious expression, ruminations, worrying
2. Sadness
   sad expression, sad voice, tearfulness
3. Lack of reactivity to pleasant events
4. Irritability
   easily annoyed, short tempered

B. Behavioral Disturbance
5. Agitation
   restlessness, handwringing, hairpulling
6. Retardation
   slow movements, slow speech, slow reactions
7. Multiple physical complaints
   (score 0 if GI symptoms only)
8. Loss of interest
   less involved in usual activities (score only if change
   occurred acutely, i.e. in less than 1 month)

C. Physical Signs
9. Appetite loss
   eating less than usual
10. Weight loss
    (score 2 if greater than 5 lb in 1 month)

11. Lack of energy
    fatigues easily, unable to sustain activities
    (score only if change occurred acutely, i.e. in less than
    1 month)

D. Cyclic Functions
12. Diurnal variation of mood
    symptoms worse in the morning
13. Difficulty falling asleep
    later than usual for this individual
14. Multiple awakenings during sleep
15. Early morning awakening
    earlier than usual for this individual

E. Ideational Disturbance
16. Suicide
    feels life is not worth living, has suicidal wishes, or
    makes suicide attempt
17. Poor self-esteem
    self-blame, self-depreciation, feelings of failure
18. Pessimism
    anticipation of the worst
19. Mood-congruent delusions
    delusions of poverty, illness, or loss

Rating:
a = Unable to evaluate; 0 = Absent; 1 = Mild or intermittent; 2 = Severe
All based on week prior to interview

Brief Assessment Schedule Depression Cards (BASDEC)

Reference   Adshead F, Day Cody D, Pitt B (1992) BASDEC: a novel screening instrument for depression in elderly medical inpatients. *British Medical Journal* 305: 397

Time taken 3½ minutes (range 2–8 minutes)
Rating the patient choses the response prompted by an interviewer

Main indications
Screening for depression in geriatric inpatients.

Commentary
The Brief Assessment Schedule Depression Cards (BASDEC) is based on the Brief Assessment Schedule (Macdonald et al, 1982), with the novel development that, because of the difficulties of questions being overhead on geriatric wards, the patients themselves would choose from a deck of cards the answers to particular questions. The BASDEC comprises 19 cards with enlarged black print on a white background. The cards are presented one at a time. Every response of "true" gains 1 point except "I have given up hope" and "I seriously con-sidered suicide", which score 2. The maximum score available is 21 and answers of "don't know" score half a point. A validation study was carried out on 79 subjects comparing the responses with the 30-item Geriatric Depression Scale (GDS; page 2) and the BASDEC (using a cut-off score of less than 7 as a non-case and 7 or greater as a case of depression). Both the GDS and the BASDEC performed identically well with a sensitivity of 71%, specificity of 78%, positive predictive value of 74% and negative predictive value of 86% against a psychiatric diagnosis.

Additional reference
Macdonald A, Mann A, Jenkins R et al (1982) An attempt to determine the impact of 4 types of care upon the elderly in London by the study of matched groups. *Psychological Medicine* 12: 193–200.

Brief Assessment Schedule Depression Cards (BASDEC)

BASDEC (BRIEF ASSESSMENT SCHEDULE DEPRESSION CARDS)

Each item in this scale is reproduced on a separate large-print card. The instructions for its administration are as follows

1   Remove TRUE and FALSE cards from pack
2   Shuffle pack of cards
3   Hand the cards, one by one, to the patient
4   Ask the patient to place the cards in one of two piles 'TRUE' or 'FALSE'
5   Any cards which cause confusion or doubt should be placed in a 'don't know' pile (these may form a useful focal point for discussion)

The cards

I've been depressed for weeks at a time in the past
I am a nuisance to others being ill
I'm not happy at all
I seem to have lost my appetite
I have regrets about my past life
I'm kept awake by worry and unhappy thoughts
I've felt very low lately
I've seriously considered suicide
I feel anxious all the time
I feel life is hardly worth living
I feel worst at the beginning of the day
I'm too miserable to enjoy anything
I'm so lonely
I can't recall feeling happy in the past month
I suffer headaches
I'm not sleeping well
I've lost interest in things
I've cried in the past month
I've given up hope
True
False

Scoring

Each 'TRUE' card has a value of ONE POINT. Each 'DON'T KNOW' card has a value of HALF A POINT. The cards in the 'FALSE' pile do not score. The exceptions to this are the cards

   I've given up hope
   I've seriously considered suicide
which have value of TWO POINTS if 'TRUE' and 'ONE POINT if 'DON'T KNOW'.
   A patient scoring a total of SEVEN or more points may well be suffering from a depressive disorder

This table was first published in the *BMJ* [Adshead F, Day Cody D, Pitt B, BASDEC: a novel screening instrument for depression in elderly medical inpatients, 1992, Vol. 305, p. 397] and is reproduced with kind permission of the *BMJ*.

SELFCARE (D)

Reference   Bird AS, MacDonald AJD, Mann AH, Philpot MP (1987) Preliminary experience with the SELFCARE (D): a self-rating depression questionnaire for use in elderly, non-institutionalized subjects. *International Journal of Geriatric Psychiatry* 2: 31–8

Time taken 15 minutes (reviewer's estimate)
Rating self-rating

Main indications

A self-rating depression scale for use with elderly subjects in general practice.

Commentary

The SELFCARE (D) was devised from the larger Comprehensive Assessment and referral Evaluation (CARE) schedule (Gurland et al, 1977). The items were chosen as the ones previously known to discriminate subjects with and without depression. The results were compared with an independent assessment in 75 patients, using a cut-off of 5/6, attending their general practitioners in London. The sensitivity of the scale at detecting depression was 77% and specificity 98% with a positive predictive value of 96%. Kappa reliability scores were 0.77.

Additional references

Beck AT, Ward CH, Mendelson M et al (1961) An inventory for measuring depression. *Archives of General Psychiatry* 4: 53–63.

Gurland B, Kuriansky J, Sharpe L et al (1977) The Comprehensive Assessment and Referral Evaluation (CARE) – rationale, development and reliability. *International Journal of Ageing in Human Development* 8: 9–42.

Address for correspondence

MP Philpot
Section of Old Age Psychiatry
Institute of Psychiatry
Denmark Hill
London SE5 8AF
UK

SELFCARE (D)

(1) In general, how is your health compared with others of your age?
    Excellent ☐
    Good ☐
   * Fair ☐
    Don't know what is meant by question ☐

(2) How quick are you in your physical movements compared with a year ago?
    Quicker than usual ☐
    About as quick as usual ☐
   * Less quick than usual ☐
   * Considerably slower than usual ☐
    Don't know what is meant by question ☐

(3) How much energy do you have, compared to a year ago?
    More than usual ☐
    About the same as usual ☐
   * Less than usual ☐
   * Hardly any at all ☐
    Don't know what is meant by question ☐

(4) In the last month, have you had any headaches?
    Not at all ☐
    About the same as usual ☐
   * Some of the time ☐
   * A lot of the time ☐
   * All of the time ☐
    Don't know what is meant by question ☐

(5) Have you worried about things this past month?
    Not at all ☐
    Only now and then ☐
   * Some of the time ☐
   * A lot of the time ☐
   * All of the time ☐
    Don't know what is meant by question ☐

(6) Have you been sad, unhappy (depressed) or weepy this past month?
    Not at all ☐
    Only now and then ☐
   * Some of the time ☐
   * A lot of the time ☐
   * All of the time ☐
    Don't know what is meant by question ☐

(7) In the past month, have you been lying awake at night feeling uneasy or unhappy?
    Not at all ☐
    Once or twice ☐
   * Quite often ☐
   * Very often ☐
    Don't know what is meant by question ☐

(8) Do you blame yourself for unpleasant things that have happened to you in the past?
    Not at all ☐
    About one thing ☐
   * About a few things ☐
   * About everything ☐
    Don't know what is meant by question ☐

(9) How do you feel about your future?
    Very happy ☐
    Quite happy ☐
    All right ☐
   * Unsure ☐
   * Don't care ☐
   * Worried ☐
   * Frightened ☐
   * Hopeless ☐
    Don't know what is meant by question ☐

(10) What have you enjoyed doing lately?
    Everything ☐
    Most things ☐
    Some things ☐
   * One or two things ☐
   * Nothing ☐
    Don't know what is meant by question ☐

(11) In the past month, have there been times when you've felt quite happy?
    Often ☐
    Sometimes ☐
   * Now and then ☐
   * Never ☐
    Don't know what is meant by question ☐

(12) In general, how happy are you?
    Very happy ☐
    Fairly happy ☐
   * Not very happy ☐
   * Not happy at all ☐
    Don't know what is meant by question ☐

Score 1 for each asterixed item ticked; scoring is made with reference to symptoms experienced over the past month.
Non-case/case cut point = 5–6
Don't know >4 = unreliable

Reproduced from Bird AS, MacDonald AJD, Mann AH, Philpot MP (1987) Preliminary experience with the SELFCARE (D): a self-rating depression questionnaire for use in elderly, non-institutionalized subjects. *International Journal of Geriatric Psychiatry* **2**: 31–8. Copyright John Wiley & Sons Limited. Reproduced with permission.

Center for Epidemiological Studies – Depression Scale (CES-D)

Reference Radloff LS, Teri L (1986) Use of the Center for Epidemiological Studies – depression scale with older adults. *Clinical Gerontologist* 5: 119–37

Time taken 5 minutes
Rating self-administered

Main indications

To detect depressive symptoms, particularly for research purposes or screening.

Commentary

The sensitivity and specificity of the Center for Epidemiological Studies – Depression Scale (CES-D) compare favourably with scales such as the Beck Depression Inventory (BDI; page 6) and Zung Self-Rating Depression Scale (page 252). Although originally developed for a large general population study of depressive symptoms the instrument has been found to be particularly useful in older adults. The scale should be used cautiously in visually or cognitively impaired elderly individuals.

The CES-D was developed from a large community study reporting depression symptoms (Radloff, 1977) and consists of 20 items. Scores range from 0 to 60.

Test/retest reliability over weeks averaged 0.57 and interval consistency was high (0.92). Validity was satisfactorily assessed by correlation with other depression rating studies. A cut-off of 16 has been suggested to differentiate patients with mild depression from normal controls and 23 and over to indicate significant depression.

Additional reference

Radloff L (1977) The Centre for Epidemiological Studies Depression Scale. A self-report depression scale for research in the general population. *Applied Psychological Measurements* 3: 385–401.

Centre for Epidemiological Studies – Depression Scale (CES-D)

During the past week:

1. I was bothered by things that usually don't bother me. (S)
2. I did not feel like eating; my appetite was poor. (S)
3. I felt that I could not shake off the blues even with help from my family or friends. (D)
4. I felt that I was just as good as other people. (P)
5. I had trouble keeping my mind on what I was doing. (S)
6. I felt depressed. (D)
7. I felt that everything I did was an effort. (S)
8. I felt hopeful about the future. (P)
9. I thought my life had been a failure.
10. I felt fearful.
11. My sleep was restless. (S)
12. I was happy. (P)
13. I talked less than usual.
14. I felt lonely. (D)
15. People were unfriendly. (I)
16. I enjoyed life. (P)
17. I had crying spells. (D)
18. I felt sad. (D)
19. I felt that people disliked me. (I)
20. I could not get "going." (S)

Rating:
Rarely/None of the time (< 1 day)
Some/Little of the time (1–2 days)
Occasionally/moderate amount of time (3–4 days)
Most/All of the time (5–7 days)
D = Depressed affect
P = Positive affect
S = Somatic/vegetative signs
I = Inbterpersonal distress

OARS Depressive Scale (ODS)

Reference   Blazer D (1980) The diagnosis of depression in the elderly. *Journal of the American Geriatrics Society* **28**: 52–8

Time taken 20 minutes (reviewer's estimate)
Rating by trained interviewer

Main indications

Indentification of elderly people with depressive symptomatology, based on DSM-III.

Commentary

For the OARS Depressive Scale (ODS), Blazer described 18 items derived from DSM-III indicators of depressive symptomatology and assessed internal reliability and construct validity, and compared this scale with the Zung Self-Rating Depression Scale (page 252). The ODS was assessed on a random sample of 997 people over the age of 65. Split half reliability was 0.74 and the coefficient alpha was 0.801, confirming the reliability of the instrument. Factor analysis revealed three factors – factor 1 relating to the symptoms of dysphoria, factor 2 items assessing the criteria for assessing diagnosis of depressive disorder and factor 3 around items assessing general pessimism for the future. When compared with clinical diagnosis, it was found that the ODS was specific but not quite as sensitive as other assessment instruments. People scoring at least four of the DSM-III symptoms for depression (poor appetite, weight loss, sleep disturbance, fatigue, agitation/retardation, loss of interest, guilt, poor concentration and suicidal ideas) were rated as positive on the ODS scale.

Factors: feelings of uselessness, can't get going, mind works slower, feelings of guilt, decreased self-confidence, decreased life satisfaction, loss of interest, weakness, poor appetite, difficulty concentrating, sadness, frequent worry, restlessness, pessimism about the future.

Additional references

Micro D (1978) Revision in the diagnostic criteria of DSM-III 1/15/78 draft. Prepared by the Task Force on Nomenclature and Statistics of the American Psychiatric Association. Washington DC.

Zung WWK (1965) A Self-Rating Depression Scale. *Archives of General Psychiatry* **12**: 63–70.

Address for correspondence

Dan Blazer
Duke University Medical Center
Box 3173
Duke Medical Center
Durham
NC 27710
USA

OARS Depressive Scale (ODS)

Do you have a good appetite?
Is your daily life full of things that keep you interested?
Do you find it hard to keep your mind on a task or job?
Have you had periods of days, weeks or months when you couldn't take care of things because you couldn't get going?
Much of the time, do you feel you have done somthing wrong or evil?
Are you happy most of the time?
Do you feel useless at times?
Do you feel weak all over much of the time?
Do you feel your sins are unpardonable?
Do you frequently find yourself worrying about something?

Do you have periods of such great restlessness that you cannot sit long in a chair?
Does your mind seem to work more slowly than usual at times?
Do you usually expect things will turn out well for you?
Do you sometimes feel unhappy because you think you are not useful?
In general, how happy would you say you are – very happy, fairly happy or not happy?
Taking everything into consideration, how would you describe your satisfaction with life in general at the present time – good, fair or poor?

The above items are all rated yes or no, except the last two, where a three-point choice is given.

Depressive Signs Scale (DSS)

Reference Katona CLE, Aldridge CR (1985) The Dexamethasone Suppression Test and depressive signs in dementia. *Journal of Affective Disorders* 8: 83–9

Time taken 10 minutes (reviewer's estimate)
Rating by interview with subject followed by interview with informant

Main indications
Depressive symptoms in patients with dementia.

Commentary
The authors were initially looking at the characteristics of patients with dementia who were non-suppressors on the Dexamethasone Depression Test (DST) (Carroll, 1982). The Depressive Signs Scale (DSS) aims to detect depressive signs in people with severe dementia. Failure of suppression was found in 10 out of 20 patients with dementia, who scored higher on the DSS. Inter-rater reliability was 0.98.

Additional reference
Carroll BJ (1982) The Dexamethasone Suppression Test for melancholia. *British Journal of Psychiatry* **140**: 292–304.

Address for correspondence
Cornelius Katona
Univesity College London Medical School
2nd floor
Wolfson Building
48 Riding House Street
London W1N 8AA
UK

Depressive Signs Scale (DSS)

1. Sad appearance
1.1 Reactivity of sad appearance
2. Agitation by day
3. Slowness of movement
4. Slowness of speech

5. Early waking
6. Loss of appetite
7. Diurnal variation in mood (mornings worst)
8. Interest in surroundings

Score:
2 = Marked/consistent or persistent
1 = Intermediate/mild or intermittent
0 = Absent

Except:
8–2 = Never, 1 = Occasional, 0 = Equally
and
1.1–1 = Absent, 0 = Present

Carroll Rating Scale (CRS)

Reference   Carroll BJ, Feinberg M, Smouse PE, Rawson SG, Greden JF (1981) The Carroll Rating Scale for Depression. I. Development, reliability and validation. *British Journal of Psychiatry* 138: 194–200

Time taken 15 minutes (reviewer's estimate)
Rating self-rating

Main indications
Screening for depressive illness.

Commentary
The Carroll Rating Scale (CRS) was developed from the 17-item Hamilton Depression Rating Scale (page 4). Concurrent validity was measured against other scales of depression, e.g. the Hamilton Depression Rating Scale and the Beck Depression Inventory (BDI; page 6). External validity was measured using a clinical rating of the severity of depression. A cut-off score of 10 or above indicates the presence of at least mild depression. Reliability was assessed using a test/retest and split half reliability, and sensitivity was measured in its ability to discriminate depressed and non-depressed subjects. All were satisfactory. The same authors in companion papers assessed the factor structure of the CRS and compared it to other available scales.

The CRS has not been used specifically in elderly people, but it is included here as a very well validated and reliable instrument.

Additional references
Feinberg M, Carroll B, Smouse P et al (1981) The Carroll Rating Scale for Depression. III. Comparison with other rating instruments. *British Journal of Psychiatry* 138: 205–9.

Smouse P, Feinberg M, Carroll B et al (1981) The Carroll Rating Scale for Depression. II. Factor analyses of the feature profiles. *British Journal of Psychiatry* 138: 201–4.

Carroll Rating Scale (CRS)

1. I feel just as energetic as always
2. I am losing weight
3. I have dropped many of my interests and activities
4. Since my illness I have completely lost interest in sex
5. I am especially concerned about how my body is functioning
6. It must be obvious that I am disturbed and agitated
7. It am still able to carry on doing the work I am supposed to do
8. I can concentrate easily when reading the papers
9. Getting to sleep takes me more than half an hour
10. I am restless and fidgety
11. I wake up much earlier than I need to in the morning
12. Dying is the best solution for me
13. I have a lot of trouble with dizzy and faint feelings
14. I am being punished for something bad in my past
15. My sexual interest is the same as before I got sick
16. I am miserable or often feel like crying
17. I often wish I were dead
18. I am having trouble with indigestion
19. I wake up often in the middle of the night
20. I feel worthless and ashamed about myself
21. I am so slowed down that I need help with bathing and dressing
22. I take longer than usual to fall asleep at night
23. Much of the time I am very afraid but don't know the reason
24. Things which I regret about my life are bothering me
25. I get pleasure and satisfaction from what I do
26. All I need is a good rest to be perfectly well again
27. My sleep is restless and disturbed
28. My mind is as fast and alert as always
29. I feel that life is still worth living
30. My voice is dull and lifeless
31. I feel irritable or jittery
32. I feel in good spirits
33. My heart sometimes beats faster than usual
34. I think my case is hopeless
35. I wake up before my usual time in the morning
36. I still enjoy my meals as much as usual
37. I have to keep pacing around most of the time
38. I am terrified and near panic
39. My body is bad and rotten inside
40. I got sick because of the bad weather we have been having
41. My hands shake so much that people can easily notice
42. I still like to go out and meet people
43. I think I appear calm on the outside
44. I think I am as good a person as anybody else
45. My trouble is the result of some serious internal disease
46. I have been thinking about trying to kill myself
47. I get hardly anything done lately
48. There is only misery in the future for me
49. I worry a lot about my bodily symptoms
50. I have to force myself to eat even a little
51. I am exhausted much of the time
52. I can tell that I have lost a lot of weight

Code: Yes or No on all

In addition, Visual Analogue Scale of how patient feels on day of test from worst ever to best ever

Depression – 32,16,34,48
Guilt – 14,20,24,44
Suicide – 12,17,29,46
Initial insom – 9,22
Middle insom – 19,27
Delayed insom – 11,35
Work and interests – 3,7,25,42
Retardation – 21,28,30,47
Agitation – 6,10,37,43
Psychological anxiety – 8,23,31,38
Somatic anxiety – 13,18,33,41
Gastrointestinal – 36,50
General somatic – 1,51
Libido – 4,15
Hypochondriasis – 5,39,45,49
Loss of insight – 26,40
Loss of weight – 2,52

Mood Scales – Elderly (MS-E)

Reference   Raskin A, Crook T (1988) Mood Scales – Elderly (MS-E). *Psychopharmacology Bulletin* **24**: 727–32

Time taken 25 minutes (reviewer's estimate)
Rating self-rating

Main indications
Assessment of depression in elderly people.

Commentary
The Mood Scales – Elderly (MS-E) consists of 50 adjectives taken from a number of sources. The individual is asked to complete the scale on a five-point choice from "not at all" through to "extremely". The validity of the scale was assessed using a factor analysis – seven factors were described: tense/irritable; considerate; cognitive disturbances; inept/helpless; depressed; fatigued and energetic/capable. Internal consistency was good, with a Cronbach's alpha of 0.8 or higher for the factors. Validity was asssessed by the scale's ability to differentiate between diagnostic groups and a high correlation was found between the MS-E and that of other ratings of psychopathology. Good sensitivity is reported with regard to the ability of the MS-E to detect change with treatment.

Additional references
Raskin A, Crook T (1976) Sensitivity rating scales completed by psychiatrists, nurses and patients to antidepressant drug effect. *Journal of Psychiatric Research* **13**: 31–41.

Zuckerman M (1960) The development of an affect adjective checklist for the measurement of anxiety. *Journal of Consulting Psychology* **24**: 457–62.

Address for correspondence
Allen Raskin
7658 Water Oak Point Road
Pasedena
MD 21122
USA

Mood Scales – Elderly (MS-E)

1.	Sad	26.	Worn out
2.	Tense	27.	Lively
3.	Angry	28.	Efficient
4.	Happy	29.	Depressed
5.	Warmhearted	30.	Restless
6.	Tired	31.	Annoyed
7.	Full of pep	32.	Considerate
8.	Confused	33.	Weary
9.	Able to think clearly	34.	Alert
10.	Downhearted	35.	Blue
11.	On edge	36.	Nervous
12.	Irritable	37.	Rude
13.	Sluggish	38.	Awkward
14.	Relaxed	39.	Troubled
15.	Good natured	40.	Jittery
16.	Worthless	41.	Sarcastic
17.	Sleepy	42.	Kind
18.	Active	43.	Absent-minded
19.	Forgetful	44.	Lonely
20.	Able to concentrate	45.	Able to work
21.	Unhappy	46.	Clumsy
22.	Friendly	47.	Bewildered
23.	Cheerful	48.	Energetic
24.	Capable	49.	Helpless
25.	Useless	50.	Carefree

Score: 1 = Not at all
2 = A little
3 = Moderately
4 = Quite a bit
5 = Extremely

Reproduced from Raskin A, Crook T (1988) Mood Scales – Elderly (MS-E). *Psychopharmacology Bulletin* **24**: 727–32.

Mania Rating Scale

Reference   Bech P, Rafaelsen OJ, Kramp P, Bolwig TG (1978) The Mania Rating Scale: scale construction and inter-observer agreement. *Neuropharmacology* 17: 430–1

Time taken 15–30 minutes
Rating by clinician

Main indications

To quantify the severity of manic states, and said to be useful in clinical trials in patients of all ages.

Commentary

The Mania Rating Scale was developed to measure manic symptomatology based on a previous attempt to devise a scale (Petterson et al, 1973). Eleven variables were described: activity (motor and verbal), flight of ideas, voices/noise level, hostility/destructiveness, mood (feeling of well-being), self esteem, contacts, sleep, sexual interest and activity, work activity. Each item scores 0–4, giving a maximum score of 44. Inter-rater reliability was over 0.85. The suggested inclusion criterion for clinical trials of mania is 15 or above out of 44. Scores of 6–14 indicate partial response to treatment, scores less than 5 indicate full remission.

Additional references

Petterson V, Fyrö B, Sedvall G (1973) A new scale for longitudinal rating of manic status. *Acta Psychiatrica Scandinavica* 49: 248–56.

Mania Rating Scale

1. ACTIVITY (motor)
   0. Normal motor activity, adequate facial expressions
   1. Slightly increased motor activity, lively facial expression
   2. Somewhat excessive motor activity, lively gestures
   3. Outright excessive motor activity, on the move most of the time
      Rises one or several times during interview
   4. Constantly active, restlessly energetic, even if urged, patient cannot sit still

2. ACTIVITY (verbal)
   0. Normal, verbal activity
   1. Somewhat talkative
   2. Very talkative, no spontaneous intervals in the conversation
   3. Difficult to interrupt
   4. Impossible to interrupt, dominates completely the conversation

3. FLIGHT OF THOUGHTS
   0. Cohesive speech, no flight of thoughts
   1. Vivid associations, maintaining cohesive speech
   2. Sporadic clang associations
   3. Several clang associations
   4. Difficult to impossible to follow the patient'clang association

4. VOICE–NOISE LEVEL
   0. Natural volume of voice
   1. Speaks loudly without being noisy
   2. Voice discernible at a distance, and somewhat noisy
   3. Vociferous, voice discernible at a long distance, is noisy
   4. Shouting, screaming, singing or using other sources of noise due to hoarseness

5. HOSTILITY–DESTRUCTIVENESS
   0. No signs of impatience or hostility
   1. Touchy, but irritation easily controlled
   2. Markedly impatient, or irritable. Provocation badly tolerated
   3. Provocative, make threats, but can be calmed down
   4. Overt physical violence. Physically destructive

6. MOOD (feelings of well-being)
   0. Neutral mood
   1. Slightly elevated mood, optimistic, but still adapted to situation
   2. Moderately elevated mood, joking, laughing
   3. Markedly elevated mood, exuberant both in manner and speech
   4. Extremely elevated mood, quite irrelevant to situation

7. SELF ESTEEM
   0. Normal self esteem, slightly boasting
   1. Slightly increased self esteem, slightly boasting
   2. Moderately increased self esteem, boasting. Frequent use of superlatives
   3. Bragging, unrealistic ideas
   4. Grandiose ideas which cannot be correct

8. CONTACT
   0. Normal contact
   1. Slightly meddling, putting his oar in
   2. Moderately meddling and arguing
   3. Dominating, arranging, directing, but still in context with the setting
   4. Extremely dominating and manipulating without context with the setting

9. SLEEP (average of last 3 nights)
   0. Habitual duration of sleep
   1. Duration of sleep reduced by 25%
   2. Duration of sleep reduced by 50%
   3. Duration of sleep reduced by 75%
   4. No sleep

10. ACTIVITY (sexual)
    0. Habitual sexual interest and activity
    1. Slight increase in sexual interest and activity. Slightly flirtatious
    2. Moderate increase in sexual interest and activity
    3. Clearly flirtatious. Dress provocative
    4. Completely and inadequately occupied by sexuality

11. ACTIVITY (work and interests)
    0. Habitual work activities
    1. Work slightly up and/or quality slightly down
    2. Work somewhat up, but quality clearly down. Attention easily distracted
    3. Unable to work, tries to do several things at the same time, but nothing is brought to an end. In hospital, rate 3 if patient does not spend at least 3 hr per day in activities (hospital, job or hobbies)
    4. Unable to work, purposelessly occupied all the time. In hospital, rate 4 if patient often has to be helped with personal needs

Reprinted from *Neuropharmacology*, Vol. 17, Bech P, Rafaelsen OJ, Kramp P, Bolwig TG, The Mania Rating Scale: scale construction and inter-observer agreement, pp. 430–1, copyright © 1978, with kind permission from Elsevier Science Ltd, The Boulevard, Langford Lane, Kidlington OX5 1GB, UK.

Checklist Differentiating Pseudodementia from Dementia

Reference   Wells CE (1979) Pseudodementia. *American Journal of Psychiatry* **136**: 895–900

Time taken 15 minutes
Rating by a semi-structured interview with an experienced rater

Main indications
To differentiate pseudodementia from dementia.

Commentary
The Checklist Differentiating Pseudodementia from Dementia is a 22-item instrument focusing on clinical history, behaviour and an assessment of mental capacities. It was validated with a psychometric test battery, computerized tomography and electroencephalogram (EEG). The instrument is for clinical use only.

Checklist Differentiating Pseudodementia from Dementia

Clinical course and history	Pseudodementia	Dementia
1. Family awareness of dysfunction and its severity:		
aware	☐	
unaware		☐
2. Onset dated with:		
some precision	☐	
only within broad limits		☐
3. Duration of symptoms before medical help sought:		
short	☐	
long		☐
4. Progression of symptoms after onset:		
rapid	☐	
slow		☐
5. History of previous psychiatric dysfunction:		
present	☐	
absent		☐
Complaints and clinical behaviour		
6. Patient complains of cognitive loss:		
much	☐	
little		☐
7. Patient's complaint of cognitive dysfunction:		
detailed	☐	
vague		☐
8. Attitude towards disability:		
emphasizes disability	☐	
conceals disability		☐
9. Response to achievements:		
highlights failures	☐	
delights in accomplishments, even if trivial		☐
10. In performing even simple tasks:		
patient makes little effort	☐	
patient struggles		☐
11. In order to keep up with things:		
patient does not try	☐	
patient relies on notes, calendars etc.		☐

	Pseudodementia	Dementia
12. In emotional situations:		
patient communicates strong sense of distress _____	☐	
patient often appears unconcerned _____		☐
13. Affective change:		
pervasive_____	☐	
labile and shallow _____		☐
14. Social skills:		
prominent and early loss _____	☐	
retained_____		☐
15. Congruence between performance and apparent cognitive dysfunction:		
behavior incompatible_____	☐	
behavior compatible _____		☐
16. Nocturnal accentuation of dysfunction:		
not present_____	☐	
occurs _____		☐

Clinical assessment of mental capacities

	Pseudodementia	Dementia
17. Attention and concentration:		
well preserved _____	☐	
faulty _____		☐
18. Typical answers to questions:		
"don't know"_____	☐	
"near-miss"_____		☐
19. Answers in tests of orientation:		
"don't know"_____	☐	
inappropriate, replaces usual with "unusual", e.g. "home" when patient in hospital _____		☐
20. Memory loss for recent and remote events:		
equally severe _____	☐	
more severe for recent than for remote_____		☐
21. Memory gaps for specific periods or events:		
present _____	☐	
memory loss not patchy_____		☐
22. Performance on tasks similar in difficulty:		
marked variability_____	☐	
consistently poor _____		☐

American Journal of Psychiatry, Vol. 136, pp. 895–900, 1979. Copyright 1979, the American Psychiatric Association. Reprinted by permission.

NIMH Dementia Mood Assessment Scale (DMAS)

Reference Sunderland T, Alterman IS, Yount D, Hill JL, Tariot PN, Newhouse PA, Mueller EA, Mellow AM, Cohen RM (1988) A new scale for the assessment of depressed mood in dementia patients. *American Journal of Psychiatry* **145**: 955–9

Time taken 20–30 minutes
Rating by direct observation and a semi-structured interview of the patient by trained raters

Main indications

A measure of mood in cognitively impaired subjects.

Commentary

The NIMH Dementia Mood Assessment Scale (DMAS) was validated on 21 patients with primary degenerative dementia to the 24-item scale. It is not a diagnostic instrument for depression in dementia but a measure of mood in people with mild to moderate disease. The first 17 items of the 24-item scale assess depression, the last 7 severity of dementia. There were high inter-rater reliability and intraclass correlations, and validation was against other instruments – the Geriatric Depression Scale (GDS; page 2) and Montgomery and Åsberg Depression Rating Scale (MADRS; page 7) – to focus on observable mood and functional capacities of dementia patients. The DMAS is in part derived from the Hamilton Depression Rating Scale (page 4).

Additional reference

Sunderland T, Hill J, Lawlor B et al (1988) NIMH Dementia Mood Assessment Scale (DMAS). *Psychopharmacology Bulletin* **24**: 747–53.

Address for correspondence

Trey Sunderland
Unit of Geriatric Psychopharmacology
Laboratory of Clinical Science, NIMH
Building 10
Room 3D41
Bethesda
MD 20892
USA

NIMH Dementia Mood Assessment Scale (DMAS)

1. Self-Directed Motor Activity
0 = Remains active in day-to-day pursuits.
2 = Participates in planned activities but may need some guidance structuring free time.
4 = Needs much direction with unstructured time but still participates in planned activities.
6 = Little or no spontaneous activity initiated. Does not willingly participate in activities even with much direction.

2. Sleep (Rate A and B)
A. Insomnia
0 = No insomnia/restlessness.
2 = Restlessness at night or occasional insomnia (greater than one hour). May complain of poor sleep.
4 = Intermittent early morning awakening or frequent difficulty falling asleep (greater than one hour).
6 = Almost nightly sleep difficulties, insomnia, frequent awakening, and/or agitation, which is profoundly disturbing the patient's sleep–wake cycle.
B. Daytime Drowsiness
0 = No apparent drowsiness.
2 = May appear drowsy during the day with occasional napping.
4 = May frequently nod off during the day.
6 = Continuously attempts to sleep during the day.

3. Appetite (Rate either A or B)
A. Decreased Appetite
0 = No decreased appetite.
2 = Shows less interest in meals.
4 = Reports loss of appetite or shows greater than 1 pound/week weight loss.
6 = Requires urging or assistance in eating or shows greater than 2 pounds/week weight loss.

B. Increased Appetite
0 = No increased appetite.
2 = Shows increased interest in meals and meal planning.
4 = Snacking frequently in addition to regular meal schedule or weight gain of greater than 1 pound/week.
6 = Excessive eating through the day or weight gain of greater than 2 pounds/week.

4. Psychosomatic Complaints
0 = Not present or appropriate for physical condition.
2 = Overconcern with health issues (i.e., real or imaginery medical problems).
4 = Frequent physical complaints or repeated requests for medical attention out of proportion to existing conditions.
6 = Preoccupied with physical complains. May focus on specific complaints to the exclusion of other problems.

5. Energy
0 = Normal energy level.
2 = Slight decrease in general energy level.
4 = Appears tired often. Occasionally misses planned activities because of "fatigue."
6 = Attempts to sit alone in a chair or lie in bed much of day. Appears exhausted despite low activity level.

6. Irritability
0 = No more irritable than normal.
2 = Overly sensitive, showing low tolerance to normal frustrations; sarcastic.
4 = Impatient, demanding, frequent angry reactions.
6 = Global irritability that cannot be relieved by diversion or explanation.

7. Physical Agitation
0 = No physical restlessness or agitation noted.
2 = Fidgetiness (i.e., plays with hands or taps feet) or bodily tension.
4 = Has trouble sitting still. May move from place to place without obvious purpose.
6 = Hand wringing or frequent pacing. Unable to sit in one place for structured activity.

8. Anxiety
0 = No apparent anxiety.
2 = Apprehension or mild worry noted but able to respond to reassurance.
4 = Frequent worries about minor matters or overconcern about specific issues. Tension usually obvious in facial countenance or manner. May require frequent reassurances.
6 = Constantly worried and tense. Requires almost constant attention and reassurance to maintain control of anxiety.

9. Depressed Appearance
0 = Does not appear depressed and denies such when questioned directly.
2 = Occasionally seems sad or downcast. May admit to "spirits" being low from time to time.
4 = Frequently appears depressed, irrespective of ability to express or explain underlying thoughts.
6 = Shows mostly depressed appearance, even to casual observer. May be associated with frequent crying.

10. Awareness of Emotional State
0 = Fully acknowledges emotional condition. Expressed emotions are congruent with current situation.
2 = Occasionally denies feelings appropriate to situation.
4 = Frequently denies emotional reactions. May display some appropriate feelings with focused discussion of individual issues.
6 = Persistently denies emotional state, even with direct confrontation.

11. Emotional Responsiveness
0 = Smiles and cries in appropriate situations. Establishes eye contact regularly. Speaks and jokes spontaneously in groups.
2 = Occasionally avoids eye contact but able to respond appropriately when addressed by others. Sometimes may appear distant when sitting in social situations, as if not paying attention.
4 = Often sitting with blank stare while with others. Responses usually show limited variation of facial expression.
6 = Does not seek social interaction. Shows little emotion, even when in the presence of loved ones. Seems unable to react to emotional situations, either positively or negatively (i.e., calm or "bland").

Scale is continued overleaf

12. Sense of Enjoyment
0 = Appears to enjoy activities, friends, and family normally.
2 = Reduced animation. May display less pleasure.
4 = Infrequent display of pleasure. May show less enjoyment of family or friends.
6 = Rarely expresses pleasure or enjoyment, even when taking part in formerly consuming interests.

13. Self-Esteem
0 = No obvious loss of self-esteem or sense of inferiority.
2 = Mild decrease in self-esteem noted ocasionally. May be unable to identify strengths and accomplishments.
4 = Spontaneously self-deprecating. May display feeling of worthlessness out of proportion to objective observations.
6 = Persistent feelings of worthlessness that cannot be dispelled with reassurance.

14. Guilt Feelings
0 = Absent.
2 = Self-reproach.
4 = Spontaneously talks of being a burden to the family or caretakers. May be overly concerned with ideas of guilt or past errors but can be reassured by others.
6 = Preoccupied with guilty thoughts or feelings of shame.

15. Hopelessness/Helplessness
0 = No evidence of hopelessness or helpnessness.
2 = Questions ability to cope with life and future. May ask for assistance with simple tasks or decisions that are within his/her capacity.
4 = Pessimistic about the future but can be reassured. Frequently seeks assistance regardless of need.
6 = Feels hopeless about the future. Expresses belief of having little or no control over life.

16. Suicidal Ideation
0 = Absent. Denies any thoughts of suicide.
2 = Feels life is not worth living or states that others would be better off without him/her. Not consciously pursuing any plans for self-harm.
4 = Thoughts of possible death to self; may wish to die in his/her sleep or pray for "God to take me now."
6 = Any attempt, gesture, or specific plan of suicide.

17. Speech
0 = Normal rate and rhythm with usual tonal variability. Speech is audible, clear, and fluent.
2 = Noticeable pauses during conversation. Voice may be low, soft, or monotonous.
4 = Reduced spontaneous speech. Responses to direct questions are less fluent or mumbled. Initiates little conversation; difficult to hear.
6 = Rarely speaks spontaneously. Speech is difficult to understand.

18. Diurnal Mood Variation
A. Note whether mood appears worse in morning or evening. If no diurnal variation, mark "none."
0 = None.
1 = Worse in morning.
2 = Worse in evening.

B. When present, mark the severity of the variation. Mark "none" if no variation is present.
0 = None.
2 = Mild.
4 = Moderate.
6 = Severe.

19. Diurnal Cognitive Variation
A. Note whether general cognitive abilities appear worse in morning or evening. If no diurnal variation, mark "none."
0 = None.
1 = Worse in morning.
2 = Worse in evening.

B. When present, mark the severity of the variation. Mark "none" if no variation is present.
0 = None
2 = Mild.
4 = Moderate.
6 = Severe.

20. Paranoid Symptoms
0 = None
2 = Occasionally suspicious of harm or watching others closely. Guarded with personal questions.
4 = Shows intermittent ideas of reference or frequent suspiciousness.
6 = Paranoid delusions or overt thoughts of persecution.

21. Other Psychotic Symptoms
0 = None.
2 = Occasionally misinterprets sensory input or experiences illusions.
4 = Frequently misinterprets sensory input.
6 = Overt hallucinations or nonparanoid delusions.

22. Expressive Communication Skills
0 = Able to make self understood, even to strangers.
2 = Sometimes has difficulty communicating with others, but is able to make self understood with additional effort (e.g., visual cues).
4 = Frequently has trouble expressing ideas to others.
6 = Marked difficulty communicating ideas to others, even family members and significant others.

23. Receptive Cognitive Capacity
0 = Appears to grasp ideas normally.
2 = Experiences occasional difficulty understanding complex statements expressed by others.
4 = Frequently misunderstands or fails to comprehend issues when addressed directly, despite repeated attempts.
6 = Needs multiple modalities of communication (e.g., verbal, visual, and/or pysical prompts) to comprehend basic task.

24. Cognitive Insight
0 = Normal cognitively or shows insight into deficits.
2 = Admits to some, but not all of his/her cognitive difficulties.
4 = Intermittently denies cognitive deficits even when pointed out by others.
6 = Denies cognitive difficulties even when they are obvious to casual observers.

Scoring for DMAS 17 (1–17) = max 102
DMAS 18–24 (last 7 items) = max 42
DMAS 17 corresponds to mood scale
DMAS 18–24 – dementia severity

American Journal of Psychiatry, Vol. 145, pp. 955–959, 1988. Copyright 1988, the American Psychiatric Association. Reprinted by permission.

Emotionalism and Mood Disorders after Stroke

References House A, Dennis M, Molyneux A, Warlow C, Hawton K (1989a) Emotionalism after stroke. *British Medical Journal* 298: 991–4

House A, Dennis M, Hawton K et al (1989b) Methods of identifying mood disorders in stroke patients: experience in the Oxfordshire Community Stroke Project. *Age and Ageing* 18: 371–9

Time taken 15 minutes (reviewer's estimate)
Rating by clinician, nurse or carer

Main indications
For the assessment of emotional lability post-stroke.

Commentary
The original paper described the prevalence using the emotionalism scale in 128 patients post-stroke. Emotionalism was associated with higher measures of mood disorder and psychiatric illness, more cognitive impairment and larger lesions on CT scan, particularly in the left frontal and temporal regions. The scale asked the following questions:

(1) Have you been more tearful since the stroke than you were beforehand? Have you actually cried more in the past month (not just felt like it)?

(2) Does the weepiness come suddenly, at times when you aren't expecting it? (Suddenly means with only a few moments or no warning, not after several minutes trying to control yourself)

(3) If you feel the tears coming on, or if they have started, can you control yourself to stop them? Have you been unable to stop yourself crying in front of other people? Is that a new experience for you?

Emotionalism was present if the reply was positive to the above questions.

In a companion paper, House et al (1989b) presented a nurses' and carers' depression scale for the assessment of stroke patients, using the House Scales, the Beck Depression Inventory (BDI; page 6) and a visual analogue self-report scale. Validity measures against a standardized psychiatric interview were made. None of the measures was satisfactory – at 12 months past stroke, a cut off on the BDI of 6/7 gave a true-positive rate of 0.90 and a false-positive rate of 0.32 in the detection of depression.

Address for correspondence
Allan House
The General Infirmary at Leeds
Great George Street
Leeds LSI 3EX
UK

Carers' and Nurses' Depression Scale

In addition to the questions given in the commentary, patients were asked to complete the Beck Inventory and the MMSE. Language function was also assessed (Frenchay aphasia screening test).

Nurses' depression rating

Would you consider .... has shown evidence of the following features of depression over the past week?

Behaviour (1) Slowness of thought
(2) Social withdrawal/uncommunicativeness
(3) Self-neglect

Mood (1) Sadness or tearfulness (regardless of circumstances)
(2) Anxiety/lack of self-confidence
(3) Irritability

Thinking (1) Apathy—lack of motivation, interest or concentration
(2) Negativity—refusal to co-operate or participate
(3) Pessimism—hopelessness or suicidal ideas

Somatic (1) Disturbed sleep pattern
symptoms (2) Anorexia (with or without weight loss)
(3) Loss of libido (where appropriate)

Taking all these features into consideration, would you consider that this person is significantly depressed or otherwise emotionally disordered?

1	2	3	4
Yes definitely	Yes probably	Probably not	Definitely not

Any other comments:

Carer's depression rating

Would you say any of the following descriptions applied to .... as far as you have noticed over the past week?

(1)	Slowed up in thinking or movement	YES/NO
(2)	Wanting to keep away from other people or avoid conversation	YES/NO
(3)	Not looking after him/herself properly	YES/NO
(4)	Sad or tearful	YES/NO
(5)	Anxious or lacking in self-confidence	YES/NO
(6)	Irritable	YES/NO
(7)	Lacking in interest	YES/NO
(8)	Refusing to co-operate or join in things	YES/NO
(9)	Pessimistic or hopeless	YES/NO
(10)	Feeling suicidal	YES/NO
(11)	Sleeping poorly	YES/NO
(12)	Not eating properly	YES/NO

Do you think that he/she is depressed or suffering from any other emotional problems? YES/NO

Any other comments:

Reprinted from House A, Dennis M, Hawton K et al (1989) Methods of identifying mood disorders in stroke patients: experience in the Oxfordshire Community Stroke Project. *Age and Ageing* **18**: 371–9. By kind permission of Oxford University Press.

Chapter 2a

Neuropsychological tests

The syndrome of dementia comprises three core features: a neuropsychological deficit which is progressive over time, neuropsychiatric features (sometimes called non-cognitive features and consisting of behavioural disturbances and psychiatric symptoms) and disabilities in activities of daily living (ADL).

The quantification of neuropsychological testing began in recognizable terms, in Newcastle, in the 1950s with work by Roth and Hopkins describing questions about orientation, memory and attention/concentration. These early ideas were later incorporated into the Blessed Dementia Scale (page 40) (which comprised the Information/Memory and Concentration (IMC) test, the ADL and personality change score). It was these studies that confirmed that the dementia occurring in elderly people shared the same pathology as Alzheimer's disease (up until then considered a disease of younger people). They also related the severity of disease in life to the plaque count in the cerebral cortex, leading to the recognition that the pathology was related to the clinical signs of the disease, suggesting a connection between the two. The Mental Test Score (page 38) was developed from the Blessed IMC test, shortened to the Abbreviated Mental Test Score (AMTS; page 38) in a ten- or nine-item version (depending on whether another person was available for the purpose of recognition). A seven-item score was developed, and a six-item test (in the USA), the latter validated against neuropathological findings.

In the USA, Marshal Folstein published the Mini-Mental State Examination (MMSE; page 34), which has probably become the most widely used test, with a standardized version published recently which has gained wide acceptance. Jacobs produced another screening test around the same time, but it did not catch on. The Kew Cognitive Test (page 66) attempted to measure parietal lobe signs in addition to memory loss. Several other tests have also been published which measure cognition. These include the Face–Hand Test (FHT; page 68), the SET Test (page 58) and the Brief Cognitive Rating Scale (BCRS; page 52). Cognitive sections appear in a host of other instruments, such as the Structured Interview for the Diagnosis of the Alzheimer's Type and Multi-infarct Dementia and Dementias of other Aetiology (SIDAM; page 197) and the Geriatric Mental State Schedule (GMSS; page 200). The Alzheimer's Disease Assessment Scale (ADAS; page 42) contains cognitive and non-cognitive items, and the cognitive section has

become the gold standard of cognitive scales used in pharmaceutical trials (and is available in parallel forms). The cognitive section of the CAMDEX (page 208) (the CAMCOG) has also been widely used and validated against other measures in both clinical and community samples. The Clifton Assessment Procedures for the Elderly (CAPE; page 48) combines a cognitive and a behavioural score, the former being popular in general practice. Other cognitive tests include the Syndrom Kurztest (SKT; page 62) (which takes 15 minutes to administer) the Mattis Dementia Rating Scale (page 186) and the Severe Impairment Battery (SIB; page 67) (which can be used in the later stages of dementia to assess cognitive function). Computerized tests are also available for specialist use [the Cambridge Neuropsychological Test Automated Battery (CANTAB; page 54) and the Cognitive Drug Research Assessment System (COGDRAS; page 64)], but with the more widespread use of computers, screening tests may become available.

Time constraints for primary care mean that one of the shorter versions is best for the assessment of cognitive function. To obtain a formal score, the Mini-Mental State Examination (MMSE; page 34) (probably the standardized version) or the much shorter AMTS (page 38) is preferred, with more detailed investigation required if the patient scores below the cut off point. The ADAS and the CAMCOG are too lengthy for anything other than specialist use. The Clock Drawing Test (page 44) has become very popular because of its ease of use and non-threatening method of administration. This is an important aspect because traditional cognitive testing is often perceived as inappropriate, with questions being asked in a didactic matter and given little or no introduction. Testing cognitive function can be as skilled an interview technique as inquiring about delusions and hallucinations, and introducing the test with an explanation (and sometimes apologetically, if necessary) can usually secure co-operation. The use of autobiographical questions found in some early scales (e.g. asking the name of the person's school) has been used as a way around this, but the inability of the interviewer to verify the answers is a great drawback and the practicalities of obtaining an informant make this unworkable. The recently published 7 Minute Neurocognitive Screening Battery (page 70) promises much, but the lack of easily identifiable cut-offs means more work needs to be done before it is widely accepted.

Mini-Mental State Examination (MMSE)

Reference Folstein MF, Folstein SE, McHugh PR (1975) "Mini-Mental State": a practical method for grading the cognitive state of patients for the clinician. *Journal of Psychiatric Research* **12**: 189–98

Time taken 10 minutes
Rating by interview (some training desirable)

Main indications

Rating of cognitive function.

Commentary

The Mini-Mental State Examination (MMSE) is probably the most widely used measure of cognitive function. Much has been written about the MMSE and amendments have been suggested such as the Standardized Mini-Mental State Examination (SMMSE; page 36) (Molloy et al, 1991) and the Modified Mini-Mental State Examination (MMMSE) (Teng et al, 1987). A recent review of the MMSE detailed the particular measures of test/retest reliability, internal consistency and assessment of recognized cut-off points (Tombaugh and McIntyre, 1992). The MMSE has been suggested as being helpful in the early diagnosis of Alzheimer's disease with the addition of a verbal fluency test (Galasko et al, 1990), and the limits of the MMSE as a screening test have also been discussed (Anthony et al, 1982). Population norms have been reproduced (Crum et al, 1993). Recently, an analysis of the scale with a commentary by the original author has been published (Burns et al, 1998). The original paper showed that the MMSE was created to differentiate organic from functional organic disorders, and could be used as a quantitative measure of cognitive impairment in an attempt to measure change but was not intended to be used in any diagnostic sense. The authors noted originally that one of the uses of the MMSE was in teaching psychiatric trainees to become skilled in the evaluation of cognitive aspects of the mental state. The "Mini" qualification was added because no aspects of mood, abnormal mental experiences or disordered forms of thinking were measured. The MMSE has a maximum score of 30 points, with different domains assessed: orientation to time and place (10 points), registration of three words (3 points), attention and calculation (5 points) recall of three words (3 points), language (8 points) and visual construction (1 point). Variations have included different words, e.g. *shirt, tree, rose, elephant* and *dog*, and great debate has surrounded whether serial 7 or spelling the word *world* backwards should be used. The original validity and reliability of the MMSE were based on 206 patients with a variety of psychiatric disorders, the scale successfully separating those with dementia, depression, and those with depression and cognitive impairment. A correlation of 0.78 was found with the Weschler adult intelligence scale for verbal IQ and 0.66 for performance IQ. Test/restest reliability was 0.89 and a combination of test/restest and inter-rater reliability was 0.83. Details of extensive subsequent validity and reliabililty studies are described by Tombaugh and McIntyre (1992).

Additional references

Anthony J, LeResche L, Niaz U et al (1982) Limits of the "Mini-Mental State" as a screening test for dementia and delirium among hospital patients. *Psychological Medicine* **12**: 397–408.

Burns A, Brayne C, Folstein M (1998) Mini-Mental State: a practical method for grading the cognitive state of patients for the clinician. *International Journal of Psychiatry in Geriatric Practice* **134**: 285–94.

Crum R et al (1993) Population-based norms for the Mini-Mental State Examination by age and educational level. *Journal of the American Medical Association* **18**: 2386–91.

Galasko D, Klauber MR, Hofstetter CR et al (1990) The Mini-Mental State Examination in the early diagnosis of Alzheimer's disease. *Archives of Neurology* **47**: 49–52.

Molloy DW, Alemanelin E, Robert R (1991) Reliability of a standardized Mini-Mental State Examination compared with the traditional Mini-Mental State Examination. *American Journal of Psychiatry* **148**: 102–5.

Teng EL, Chang Chui H, Schneider LS et al (1987) Alzheimer's dementia: performance on the Mini-Mental State Examination. *Journal of Consulting and Clinical Psychology* **55**: 96–100.

Tombaugh TN, McIntyre NJ (1992) The Mini-Mental State Examination: a comprehensive review. *Journal of the American Geriatrics Society* **40**: 922–35.

Address for correspondence

Marshal Folstein
Department of Psychiatry
Tufts University School of Medicine
NEMC #1007
750 Washington Street
Boston
MA 02111
USA

Mini-Mental State Examination (MMSE)

Max score	Score	
		ORIENTATION
5	( )	What is the (year) (season) (date) (month) (day)?
5	( )	Where are we: (state) (county) (town) (hospital) (floor)?
		REGISTRATION
3	( )	Name 3 objects: (1 second to say each). Then ask the patient all three after you have said them. Give 1 point for each correct answer. Then repeat them until the patient learns all 3. Count trials and record. Number of Trials _____
		ATTENTION AND CALCULATION
5	( )	Serial 7's. 1 point for each correct. Stop after 5 answers. If the patient refuses, spell "world" backwards.
		RECALL
3	( )	Ask for 3 objects repeated above. Give 1 point for each correct.
		LANGUAGE
9	( )	Name a pencil; name a watch. (2 points) Repeat the following: "No ifs, ands or buts." (1 point) Follow a three stage command: "Take this paper in your right hand, fold it in half, and put it on the floor." (3 points) Read and obey the following: "Close your eyes." (1 point)

Write a sentence. (1 point)

Copy a design. (1 point)

Total Score_____   Assess level of consciousness along a continuum   _____

Alert   Drowsy   Stupor   Coma

Reprinted from the *Journal of Psychiatric Research*, Vol. 12, Folstein MF, Folstein SE, McHugh PR "Mini-Mental State": a practical method for grading the cognitive state of patients for the clinician. (1975), with permission from Elsevier Science.

Standardized Mini-Mental State Examination (SMMSE)

Reference   Molloy DW, Alemayehu E, Roberts R (1991) Reliability of a Standardized Mini-Mental State Examination compared with the traditional Mini-Mental State Examination. *American Journal of Psychiatry* **148**: 102–5

Time taken 5–10 minutes
Rating by interviewer, preferably with some training

Main indications

As per MMSE.

Commentary

The Standardized Mini-Mental State Examination (SMMSE) was developed in an attempt to improve the objectivity of the original MMSE (page 34), which, in the authors' experience, varied greatly. Up to six raters assessed eight elderly patients on three different occasions 1 week apart and, using a one-way analysis of variance, estimated inter-rater variance and intrarater variance. Inter- and intrarater variance was reduced by 86% and 76% respectively when the SMMSE was used and the intraclass correlation rose from 0.69 to 0.90. The SMMSE took slightly less time to administer than the SMMSE (10.5 minutes compared with 13.4 minutes; Molloy and Standish, 1997).

Essentially, the SMMSE comes with more specific instructions as to how the scale will be measured, with specific examples of the scoring of the figures and spelling

world backwards. Ball, car and man are three objects used, with alternatives provided for repeated testing.

A slightly expanded, modified Mini-Mental State (3MS) is also available (Teng and Chiu, 1987).

Additional references

Molloy DW, Standish TIM (1997) A guide to the Standardized Mini-Mental State Examination. *International Psychogeriatrics* 9 (Suppl 1): 37–43.

Teng E, Chiu C (1987) The modified mini-mental state. *Journal of Clinical Psychiatry* 48: 314–18.

Address for correspondence

DW Molloy
Geriatric Research Group
McMaster University
Hamilton Civic Hospitals
Henderson General Division
711 Concession Street
Hamilton
Ontario L8V 1C3
Canada

Standardized Mini-Mental State Examination (SMMSE)

I am going to ask you some questions and give you some problems to solve. Please try to answer as best as you can.

Max Score

1. *(Allow 10 seconds for each reply)*
a) What year is this? **1**
   (accept exact answer only)
b) What season is this? **1**
   (during last week of the old season or first week of a new season, accept either season)
c) What month of the year is this? **1**
   (on the first day of new month, or last day of the previous month, accept either)
d) What is today's date? **1**
   (accept previous or next date, e.g. on the 7th accept the 6th or 8th)
e) What day of the week is this? **1**
   (accept exact answer only)

2. *(Allow 10 seconds for each reply)*
a) What country are we in? **1**
   (accept exact answer only)
b) What province/state/county are we in? **1**
   (accept exact answer only)
c) What city/town are we in? **1**
   (accept exact answer only)
d) **(In clinic)** What is the name of this hospital/building? **1**
   (accept exact name of hospital or institution only)
   (In home) What is the street address of this house? **1**
   (accept street name and house number or equivalent in rural areas)
e) **(In clinic)** What floor of the building are we on? **1**
   (accept exact answer only)
   (In home) What room are we in? **1**
   (accept exact answer only)

3. I am going to name 3 objects. After I have said all three objects, I want you to repeat them. Remember what they are because I am going to ask you to name them again in a few minutes. **3**
   (say them slowly at approximately 1 second intervals)

Ball   Car   Man

For repeated use:

Bell	**Jar**	**Fan**
Bill	**Tar**	**Can**
Bull	**War**	**Pan**

Please repeat the 3 items for me.
(score 1 point for each correct reply on the first attempt)
Allow 20 seconds for reply, if subject did not repeat all 3, repeat until they are learned or up to a maximum of 5 times.

4. Spell the word WORLD. **5**
   (you may help subject to spell world correctly)
   *Say **now spell it backwards please**. Allow 30 seconds to spell backwards. (If the subject cannot spell world even with assistance – score 0.)*

5. Now what were the 3 objects that I asked you to remember? **3**

Ball   Car   Man

Score 1 point for each correct response regardless of order, allow 10 seconds.

6. Show wristwatch. Ask: what is this called? **1**
   Score 1 point for correct response. Accept "wristwatch" or "watch". Do not accept "clock", "time", etc. (allow 10 seconds).

7. Show pencil. Ask: what is this called? **1**
   Score 1 point for correct response, accept pencil only – score 0 for pen.

8. I'd like you to repeat a phrase after me: "no if's, and's or but's". **1**
   *(allow 10 seconds for response. Score 1 point for a correct repetition. Must be **exact**, e.g. no if's or but's – score 0)*

9. Read the words on this page and then do what it says: Hand subject the laminated sheet with CLOSE YOUR EYES on it. **1**

CLOSE YOUR EYES

*If subject just reads and does not then close eyes – you may repeat: read the words on this page and then do what it says to a maximum of 3 times. Allow 10 seconds, score 1 point **only** if subject closes eyes. Subject does not have to read aloud.*

10. Ask if the subject is right or left handed. Alternate right/left hand in statement, e.g. if the subject is right-handed say **Take this paper in your left hand**. . . Take a piece of paper – hold it up in front of subject and say the following: **3**

"Try this paper in your right/left hand, fold the paper in half once with both hands and put the paper down on the floor."

Takes paper in correct hand	1
Folds it in half	1
Puts it on the floor	1

Allow 30 seconds. Score 1 point for each instruction correctly executed.

11. Hand subject a pencil and paper. **1**
   Write any complete sentence on that piece of paper. Allow 30 seconds. Score 1 point. The sentence should make sense. Ignore spelling errors.

12. Place design, pencil, eraser and paper in front of the subject. **1**
   Say: copy this design please. Allow multiple tries until patient is finished and hands it back. Score 1 point for correctly copied diagram. The subject must have drawn a 4-sided figure between two 5-sided figures. Maximum time – 1 minute.

Total Test Score   30

Reproduced (with the permission of the Geriatric Research Group) from Molloy DW, Alemayehu E, Roberts R (1991) Reliability of a Standardized Mini-Mental State Examination compared with the traditional Mini-Mental State Examination. *American Journal of Psychiatry*, Vol. 140, pp. 102–5.

Mental Test Score (MTS)/Abbreviated Mental Test Score (AMTS)

References   Hodkinson M (1972) Evaluation of a mental test score for assessment of mental impairment in the elderly. *Age and Ageing* 1: 233–8

Qureshi K, Hodkinson M (1974) Evaluation of a 10 question mental test of the institutionalized elderly. *Age and Ageing* 3: 152–7

Time taken MTS, 10 minutes; AMTS, 3 minutes
Rating by clinician

Commentary

The Mental Test Score (MTS) was developed from the Blessed Dementia Scale (page 40), and was used in a study of over 700 patients carried out under the auspices of the Royal College of Physicians. A previous study had shown that a score of 25 and above (out of 34) was within the normal range; and the important point was made (but is often forgotten) that tests such as these do not discriminate between dementia and delirium – although longitudinal follow-up will provide quantitative changes in mental test performance. Graphic displays in the paper demonstrated questions of high and low discriminating ability. On this basis, the Abbreviated Mental Test Score (AMTS) was developed, showing that the results corresponded closely with that of the full score. The AMTS is scored out of 10 or, if there is not the facility to carry out the recognition question, out of 9. A cut-off score of 7 or 8 out of 10 (6 or 7 out of 9) is suggested to discriminate between a cognitive impairment and normality. Qureshi and Hodkinson (1974) further validated the questionnaire in patients over the age of 60 with comparisons against the Roth and Hopkins (1953) and Denham and Jeffries (1972) questionnaires.

Additional references

Roth M, Hopkins B 91953) Psychological test performance in patients over 60. Senile psychosis and affective disorders of old age. *Journal of Mental Science* **99**: 439–50.

Denham MJ, Jeffries PM (1972) Routine mental assessment in elderly patients. *Modern Geriatrics* **2**: 275–9.

Mental Test Score (MTS)/Abbreviated Mental Test Score

ORIGINAL TEST ITEMS

	Score
Name	0/1
Age	0/1
Time (to nearest hour)	0/1
Time of day	0/1
Name and address for five minutes recall; this should be repeated by the patient to ensure it has been heard correctly.	
Mr John Brown	0/1/2
42 West Street	0/1/2
Gateshead	0/1
Day of week	0/1
Date (correct day of month	0/1
Month	0/1
Year	0/1
Place: Type of place (i.e. Hospital)	0/1
Name of Hospital	0/1
Name of ward	0/1
Name of town	0/1
Recognition of two persons (doctor, nurse, etc.)	0/1/2
Date of birth (day and month sufficient)	0/1
Place of birth (town)	0/1
School attended	0/1
Former occupation	0/1
Name of wife, sib or next of kin	0/1
Date of First World War (year sufficient)	0/1
Date of Second World War (date sufficient)	0/1
Name of present Monarch	0/1
Name of present Prime Minister	0/1
Months of year backwards	0/1/2
Count 1–20	0/1/2
Count 20–1	0/1/2
Total	(34)

ABBREVIATED MENTAL TEST SCORE

1. Age
2. Time (to nearest hour)
3. Address for recall at end of test – this should be repeated by the patient to ensure it has been heard correctly: 42 West Street
4. Year
5. Name of hospital
6. Recognition of two persons (doctor, nurse, ...)
7. Date of birth
8. Year of First World War
9. Name of present Monarch
10. Count backwards 20–1

(each question scores one mark)

Source: Hodkinson M (1972) Evaluation of a mental test score for assessment of mental impairment in the elderly. *Age and Ageing* **1**: 233–8. By kind permission of Oxford University Press.

Blessed Dementia Scale [incorporating the Information–Memory–Concentration (IMC) Test and the Dementia Scale]

Reference   Blessed G, Tomlinson BE, Roth M (1968) The association between quantitative measures of dementia and of senile change in the cerebral grey matter of elderly subjects. *British Journal of Psychiatry* 114: 797–811

Time taken 30 minutes (reviewer's estimate)
Rating structured questions by observer

Main indications

Assessment of cognition and behaviour in people with dementia.

Commentary

The Blessed Dementia Scale was designed to assess quantitatively the signs of dementia to enable comparisons to be made with pathological changes. The scale is divided into two: the Information–Memory–Concentration (IMC) Test and the Dementia Scale, which incorporated changes in everyday performance habits and personality, and assessed orientation, memory and concentration, which have been shown to differentiate groups of demented and non-demented aged persons (Roth and Hopkins, 1953; Shapiro et al, 1956). Correlation of senile plaque count and the dementia score was 0.77 and against the test score 0.59, both highly significant (on 60 patients, the direction of correlation was in keeping with the hypothesis that more pathological changes were associated with worse clinical signs). The Blessed study is one of the key papers of old age psychiatry, showing for the first time that clinical functions of dementia are related to neuropathological changes.

Additional references

Roth M, Hopkins B (1953) Psychological test performance in patients over 60. 1. Senile psychosis and the affective disorders of old age. *Journal of Mental Science* 99: 439.

Shapiro MB, Post F, Löfving B et al (1956) "Memory function" in psychiatric patients over sixty; some methodological and diagnostic implications. *Journal of Mental Science* 102: 233.

Blessed Dementia Scale

Changes in performance of everyday activities

1.	Inability to perform household tasks	1	½	0
2.	Inability to cope with small sums of money	1	½	0
3.	Inability to remember short list of items, e.g. in shopping	1	½	0
4.	Inability to find way about indoors	1	½	0
5.	Inability to find way about familiar streets	1	½	0
6.	Inability to interpret surroundings (e.g. to recognize whether in hospital, or at home, to discriminate between patients, doctors and nurses, relatives and hospital staff, etc)	1	½	0
7.	Inability to recall recent events (e.g. recent outings, visits of relatives or friends to hospital, etc.)	1	½	0
8.	Tendency to dwell in the past	1	½	0

Changes in habits

9. Eating:

Cleanly with proper utensils	0
Messily with spoon only	2
Simple solids, e.g. biscuits	2
Has to be fed	3

10. Dressing:

Unaided	0
Occasionally misplaced buttons, etc.	1
Wrong sequence, commonly forgetting items	2
Unable to dress	3
11. Complete sphincter control	0
Occasional wet beds	1
Frequent wet beds	2
Doubly incontinent	3

Changes in personality, interests, drive

	No change	0
12.	Increased rigidity	1
13.	Increased egocentricity	1
14.	Impairment of regard for feelings of others	1
15.	Coarsening of affect	1
16.	Impairment of emotional control, e.g. increased petulance and irritability	1
17.	Hilarity in inappropriate situations	1
18.	Diminished emotional responsiveness	1
19.	Sexual misdemeanour (appearing de novo in old age)	1
	Interests retained	0
20.	Hobbies relinquished	1
21.	Diminished initiative or growing apathy	1
22.	Purposeless hyperactivity	1
	Total	

Information–Memory–Concentration Test
Information test

Name	1
Age	1
Time (hour)	1
Time of day	1
Day of week	1
Date	1
Month	1
Season	1
Year	1
Place—	
Name	1
Street	1
Town	1
Type of place (e.g. home, hospital, etc.)	1
Recognition of persons (cleaner, doctor, nurse, patient, relative; any two available)	2
Total	

Scores lie between 0 (complete failure) and +37 (full marks)

Memory:

(1) personal

Date of birth	1
Place of birth	1
School attended	1
Occupation	1
Name of sibs or Name of wife	1
Name of any town where patient had worked	1
Name of employers	1

(2) non-personal

*Date of World War I	1
*Date of World War II	1
Monarch	1
Prime Minister	1

(3) Name and address (5-minute recall)

Mr John Brown
  42 West Street
    Gateshead   5

Total
Concentration

Months of year backwards	2	1	0
Counting 1–20	2	1	0
Counting 20–1	2	1	0

*½ for approximation within 3 years.

Ascertain from relative/friend. Applies to last 6 months. Score lies between 0 (fully preserved capacity) and +28 (extreme incapacity)

Reproduced from the *British Journal of Psychiatry*, Blessed G, Tomlinson BE, Roth M (1968) The association between quantitative measures of dementia and of senile change in the cerebral grey matter of elderly subjects, Vol. 114, pp. 797–811. © 1968 Royal College of Psychiatrists. Reproduced with permission.

Alzheimer's Disease Assessment Scale (ADAS) – Cognitive and Non-Cognitive Sections (ADAS-Cog, ADAS-Non-Cog)

Reference Rosen WG, Mohs RC, Davis KL (1984) A new rating scale for Alzheimer's disease. *American Journal of Psychiatry* 141: 1356–64

Time taken 45 minutes
Rating by trained observer

Main indications

Standardized assessment of cognitive function and non-cognitive features. Standard measure to assess change in cognitive function in drug trials.

Commentary

The Alzheimer's Disease Assessment Scale – Cognitive and Non-Cognitive Sections (ADAS-Cog and ADAS-Non-Cog) were designed specifically to evaluate all aspects of Alzheimer's disease. The primary cognitive function included components of memory, language and praxis, while the non-cognitive features included mood state and behavioural changes. There are 11 main sections testing cognitive function and 10 assessing non-cognitive features.

Additional references

Mohs R, Knopman D, Petersen R et al (1997) Development of cognitive instruments for use in clinical trails of antidementia drugs: additions to the Alzheimer's Disease Assessment Scale that broaden its scope. *Alzheimer Disease and Associated Disorders* 11 (suppl 2): S13–S21.

Schwarb S, Koberle S, Spiegel R (1988) The Alzheimer's Disease Assessment Scale (ADAS): an instrument for early diagnosis of dementia? *International Journal of Geriatric Psychiatry* 3: 45–53.

Standish T, Molloy DW, Bédard M et al (1996) Improved reliability of the standardized Alzheimer's Disease Assessment Scale (SADAS) compared with the Alzheimer's Disease Assessment Scale (ADAS). *Journal of the American Geriatrics Society* 44: 712–16.

Zec R, Landreth E, Vicari S et al (1992) Alzheimer Disease Assessment Scale: useful for both early detection and staging of dementia of the Alzheimer type. *Alzheimer Disease and Associated Disorders* 6: 89–102.

Address for correspondence

KL Davis
Department of Psychiatry
Bronx VA Medical Center
130 West Kingsbridge Road
Bronx NY 10468
USA

Alzheimer's Disease Assessment Scale (ADAS) – Cognitive and Non-Cognitive Sections (ADAS-Cog, ADAS-Non-Cog)

Cognitive Items

1. Spoken language ability _____
2. Comprehension of spoken language _____
3. Recall of test instructions _____
4. Word-finding difficulty _____
5. Following commands _____
6. Naming: objects, fingers _____

High:	1	2	3	4	Fingers: Thumb
Medium:	1	2	3	4	Pinky Index
Low:	1	2	3	4	Middle Ring

7. Constructions: drawing _____
   Figures correct: 1   2   3   4
   Closing in: Yes _____ No _____
8. Ideational praxis _____
   Step correct:
   1 2 3 4 5
9. Orientation _____
   Day _____ Year _____ Person _____ Time of day _____
   Date _____ Month _____ Season _____ Place _____
10. Word recall: mean error score _____
11. Word recognition: mean error score _____
    Cognition total _____

Noncognitive Items (all rated by examiner)

12. Tearful _____
13. Appears/reports depressed mood _____
14. Concentration, distractibility _____
15. Uncooperative to testing _____
16. Delusions _____
17. Hallucinations _____
18. Pacing _____
19. Increased motor activity _____
20. Tremors _____
21. Increase/decrease appetite _____
    Noncognition total _____

Total Scores

Cognitive behavior _____
Noncognitive behavior _____
Word recall _____
Word recognition _____
   Total _____

Rating: x = not assessed
0 = not present
1 = very mild
2 = mild
3 = moderate
4 = moderately severe
5 = severe

Spoken language – quality of speech **not** quantity.
Comprehension – do **not** include responses to commands.
Do not include finger or object naming.
Score 0–5 steps correct
1–4 steps correct
2–3 steps correct
3–2 steps correct
4–1 steps correct
5 – cannot do one step correct

Name fingers of dominant hand and high/medium/low frequency objects.
0 = all correct; one finger incorrect and/or one object incorrect
1 = two–three fingers and/or two objects incorrect
2 = two or more fingers and three–five objects incorrect
3 = three or more fingers and six–seven objects incorrect
4 = three or more fingers and eight–nine objects incorrect

Ability to copy circle, two overlapping rectangles, rhombus and cube.

5 components in sending self a letter
1 = difficulty or failure to perform one component
2 = difficulty and/or failure to perform two components
3 = difficulty and/or failure to perform three components
4 = difficulty and/or failure to perform four components
5 = difficulty and/or failure to perform five components

Date, month, year, day of week, season, time of day, place and person.

Noncognitive behavior is evaluated over preceding week to interview.

American Journal of Psychiatry, Vol. 141, pp. 1356–64, 1984. Copyright 1984, the American Psychiatric Association. Reprinted by permission.

Clock Drawing Test

References Brodaty H, Moore CM (1997) The Clock Drawing Test for dementia of the Alzheimer's type: a comparison of three scoring methods in a memory disorders clinic. *International Journal of Geriatric Psychiatry* 12: 619–27

Shulman K, Shedletsky R, Silver I (1986) The challenge of time. Clock drawing and cognitive function in the elderly. *International Journal of Geriatric Psychiatry* 1: 135–40

Sunderland T, Hill JL, Mellow AM, Lawlor BA, Gundersheimer J, Newhouse PA, Grafman JH (1989) Clock drawing in Alzheimer's disease. *Journal of the American Geriatrics Society* 37: 725–9

Wolf-Klein GP, Silverstone FA, Levy AP, Brod MS, Breuer J (1989) Screening for Alzheimer's disease by clock drawing. *Journal of the American Geriatrics Society* 37: 730–4

Time taken 2 minutes
Rating standardized interpretation of drawing by clinican

Main indications

As a screening measure or measure of severity in dementia.

Commentary

The Clock Drawing Test reflects frontal and temporo-parietal functioning and is an easy test to carry out. A standard assessment is that the patient is asked to draw a clock face marking the hours and then draw the hands to indicate a particular time (e.g. 10 minutes to 2). The test tends to be non-threatening but there is obviously a wide variation in the way the results can be interpreted. Three methods have been described by Brodaty and Moore (1997). Shulman et al (1986) describe a six-point hierarchical error producing a global rating assessed on 75 patients, with inter-rater reliability of 0.75, a sensitivity of 86% and specificity of 72% against the Mini-Mental State Examination (MMSE; page 34). Sunderland et al (1989) described a 10-point anchored scale tested on 150 patients and controls, with inter-rater reliability of 0.86 and sensitivity of 78% with a specificity of 96% according to diagnostic criteria for Alzheimer's disease. Wolf-Klein et al (1989) described a 10-point categorical scale assessed on 312 consecutive admissions, with a sensitivity of 0.68 in the total population and a specificity of over 0.9. Brodaty and Moore (1997), on a sample of 56 patients and controls, assessed the methods of clock drawing analysis comparing them with other measures of cognitive function. The Shulman scale, when combined with the MMSE, was felt to be a valuable screening test for mild to moderate dementia of the Alzheimer's type.

Clock Drawing Test

A priori criteria for evaluating clock drawings (10 = best and 1 = worst)

10–6. Drawing of Clock Face with Circle and Numbers is Generally Intact

10. Hands are in correct position (i.e. hour hand approaching 3 o'clock)
9. Slight errors in placement of the hands
8. More noticeable errors in the placement of hour and minute hands
7. Placement of hands is significantly off course
6. Inappropriate use of clock hands (i.e. use of digital display or circling of numbers despite repeated instructions)

5–1. Drawing of Clock Face with Circle and Numbers is Not Intact

5. Crowding of numbers at one end of the clock or reversal of numbers. Hands may still be present in some fashion.
4. Further distortion of number sequence. Integrity of clock face is now gone (i.e. numbers missing or placed at outside of the boundaries of the clock face).
3. Numbers and clock face no longer obviously connected in the drawing. Hands are not present.
2. Drawing reveals some evidence of instructions being received but only a vague representation of a clock.
1. Either no attempt or an uninterpretable effort is made.

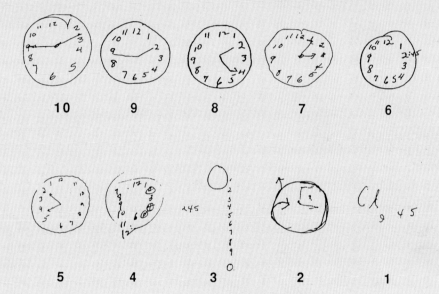

Samples of clock drawings from Alzheimer patients with evaluations of best (10) to worst (1)

Scale is continued overleaf

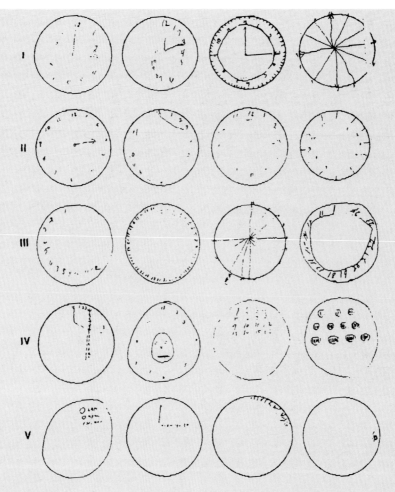

Clinical examples of clock errors

Classification of clock errors

I   Visuospatial
     (a) Mildly impaired spacing of times
     (b) Draws times outside circle
     (c) Turns page while writing numbers so that some numbers appear upside down
     (d) Draws in lines (spokes) to orient spacing

II   Errors in denoting the time as 3 o'clock
     (a) Omits minute hand
     (b) Draws a single line from 12 to 3
     (c) Writes the words '3 o'clock'
     (d) Writes the number 3 again
     (e) Circles or underlines 3
     (f) Unable to indicate 3 o'clock

III Visuospatial
     (a) Moderately impaired spacing of times (so that 3 o'clock cannot be accurately denoted)
     (b) Omits numbers
     Perseveration
     (a) Repeats the circle
     (b) Continues on past 12 to 13, 14, 15, etc.
     Right–left reversal – numbers drawn counterclockwise
     Dygraphia – unable to write numbers accurately

IV   Severely disorganized spacing
     (a) Confuses 'time' – writes in minutes, times of day, months or seasons
     (b) Draws a picture of human face on the clock
     (c) Writes the word 'clock'

V   Unable to make any reasonable attempt at a clock
     (excludes severe depression or other psychotic state)

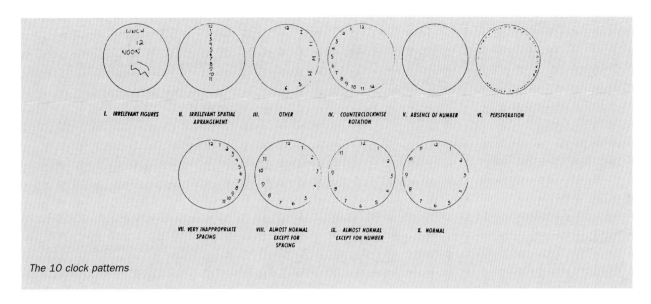

I. IRRELEVANT FIGURES   II. IRRELEVANT SPATIAL ARRANGEMENT   III. OTHER   IV. COUNTERCLOCKWISE ROTATION   V. ABSENCE OF NUMBER   VI. PERSEVERATION

VII. VERY INAPPROPRIATE SPACING   VIII. ALMOST NORMAL EXCEPT FOR SPACING   IX. ALMOST NORMAL EXCEPT FOR NUMBER   X. NORMAL

The 10 clock patterns

Sources: Sunderland T, Hill JL, Mellow AM, Lawlor BA, Gundersheimer J, Newhouse PA, Grafman JH (1989) Clock drawing in Alzheimer's disease; and Wolf-Klein GR, Silverstone FA, Levy AP, Brod MS, Breuer J (1989) Screening for Alzheimer's disease by clock drawing, *Journal of American Geriatrics Society*. Vol. 37, no. 8. pp 725–9 and 730–4, respectively; also Brodaty H, Moore CM (1997) The Clock Drawing Test for dementia of the Alzheimer's type: a comparison of three scoring methods in a memory disorders clinic; and Shulman K, Shedleksky R, Silver I (1986) The challenge of time. Clock drawing and cognitive function in the elderly, *International Journal of Geriatric Psychiatry*. Vol. 12, pp. 619–27 and Vol. 1, pp. 135–40, respectively (Copyright John Wiley & Sons Limited. Reproduced with permission).

Clifton Assessment Procedures for the Elderly (CAPE)

Reference   Pattie AH, Gilleard CJ (1979) *Manual of the Clifton Assessment Procedures for the Elderly (CAPE)*. Sevenoaks: Hodder & Stoughton Educational

Time taken 15–25 minutes (both scales)
Rating by trained interviewer

Main indications

Assessment of mental and physical functioning in elderly people.

Commentary

The Clifton Assessment Procedures for the Elderly (CAPE) consists of two related scales: the Cognitive Assessment Scale (CAS), which itself comprises the questionnaires exploring information and orientation, mental ability and a psychomotor test (the Gibson Maze; Gibson, 1977), and the Behaviour Rating Scale (BRS). The BRS grew out of the Stockton Geriatric Rating Scale (page 182). Some 18 items were derived from the original scale by dropping those with an inter-rater reliability of less than 0.4, and two items from inappropriate settings outside hospital were also dropped (Gilleard and Pattie, 1977). Measures of sensory deficits were added, but not included in the total score. Normative data on 400 subjects over the age of 60 are available (Gilleard and Pattie, 1977). Pattie and Gilleard (1975) reported the results of the Psychogeriatric Assessment Schedule and Stockton Geriatric Rating Scale in 100 consecutive admissions to a psychiatric hospital, showing that the information/orientation subtest of the CAS correctly classified 92% of patients. The scale successfully discriminated those patients who at follow-up were still in hospital and those who had been discharged (Pattie and Gilleard, 1978). A survey version of the CAPE has been described (Pattie, 1981).

The BRS has essentially the same principal areas as the Stockton Geriatric Rating Scale (physical disability, apa-thy, communication difficulties and social disturbance). Inter-rater reliability of the BRS is consistently above 0.8. The communication difficulties and social disturbance scales have slightly lower inter-rater reliabilities. Test/retest reliability on the CAS is high. Validity of the two instruments has been demonstrated in terms of correlations with other neuropsychological tests and with longitudinal studies. The scales tend to intercorrelate, but the pattern is suggestive of overlapping disabilities rather than simply reflecting one single dimension (Pattie and Gilleard, 1979).

Additional references

Gibson H (1977) *Manual of the Gibson Spiral Maze* (2nd edition). London: Hodder & Stoughton.

Gilleard C, Pattie A (1977) The Stockton Geriatric Rating Scale: a shortened version with British nominative data. *British Journal of Psychiatry* **131**: 90–4.

Pattie A (1981) A survey version of the Clifton Assessment Procedures for the Elderly. *British Journal of Clinical Psychology* **20**: 173–8.

Pattie A, Gilleard C (1975) A brief psychogeriatric assessment schedule: validation against psychiatric diagnosis and discharge from hospital. *British Journal of Psychiatry* **127**: 489–93.

Pattie A, Gilleard C (1978) The two year predictive validity of the Clifton Assessment Schedule and the Shortened Stockton Geriatric Rating Scale. *British Journal of Psychiatry* **133**: 457–60.

Clifton Assessment Procedures for the Elderly (CAPE) – Cognitive Assessment Scale (CAS)

Date of birth: **Occupation:**

Information/Orientation

Name:	*Hospital Address:*	*Colour of British Flag:*
Age:	*City:*	*Day:*
DoB:	*PM:*	*Month:*
Ward/Place:	*US President:*	*Year:*

I/O Score

Mental Ability

Count 1–20 Time:	Errors:		Alphabet: Time:	Errors:	
≤10 secs no errors		*3*	≤10 secs no errors		*3*
≤30 secs no errors		*2*	≤30 secs no errors		*2*
≤30 secs 1 error		*1*	≤30 secs 1 error		*1*
		0			*0*

Write name:		Reading: (See overleaf)	
Correct and legible	*2*	10 words or more	*3*
Can write but not correctly	*1*	6–9 words	*2*
Not able to	*0*	1–5 words	*1*
		0 words	*0*

MAb Score

Psychomotor Time	Errors	**Pm Score**
Scoring		

Score 1 point for each correct answer. The psychomotor test is the Gibson Spiral Maze.

Scale is continued overleaf

Clifton Assessment Procedures for the Elderly (CAPE) – Behaviour Rating Scale (BRS)

Please ring the appropriate number for each item

1. WHEN BATHING OR DRESSING, HE/SHE REQUIRES:
   - no assistance 0
   - some assistance 1
   - maximum assistance 2
2. WITH REGARD TO WALKING, HE/SHE:
   - shows no signs of weakness 0
   - walks slowly without aid, or uses a stick 1
   - is unable to walk, or if able to walk, needs frame, crutches or someone by his/her side 2
3. HE/SHE IS INCONTINENT OF URINE AND/OR FAECES (day or night):
   - never 0
   - sometimes (once or twice per week) 1
   - frequently (3 times per week or more) 2
4. HE/SHE IS IN BED DURING THE DAY (bed does not include couch, settee, etc.):
   - never 0
   - sometimes 1
   - almost always 2
5. HE/SHE IS CONFUSED (unable to find way around, loses possessions, etc.):
   - almost never confused 0
   - sometimes confused 1
   - almost always confused 2
6. WHEN LEFT TO HIS/HER OWN DEVICES, HIS/HER APPEARANCE (clothes and/or hair) IS:
   - almost never disorderly 0
   - sometimes disorderly 1
   - almost always disorderly 2
7. IF ALLOWED OUTSIDE, HE/SHE WOULD:
   - never need supervision 0
   - sometimes need supervision 1
   - always need supervision 2
8. HE/SHE HELPS OUT IN THE HOME/WARD:
   - often helps out 0
   - sometimes helps out 1
   - never helps out 2
9. HE/SHE KEEPS HIM/HERSELF OCCUPIED IN A CONSTRUCTIVE OR USEFUL ACTIVITY (works, reads, plays games, has hobbies, etc):
   - almost always occupied 0
   - sometimes occupied 1
   - almost never occupied 2
10. HE/SHE SOCIALISES WITH OTHERS:
    - does establish a good relationship with others 0
    - has some difficulty establishing good relationships 1
    - has a great deal of difficulty establishing good relationships 2
11. HE/SHE IS WILLING TO DO THINGS SUGGESTED OR ASKED OF HIM/HER:
    - often goes along 0
    - sometimes goes along 1
    - almost never goes along 2
12. HE/SHE UNDERSTANDS WHAT YOU COMMUNICATE TO HIM/HER (you may use speaking, writing, or gesturing):
    - understands almost everything you communicate 0
    - understands some of what you communicate 1
    - understands almost nothing of what you communicate 2
13. HE/SHE COMMUNICATES IN ANY MANNER (by speaking, writing or gesturing):
    - well enough to make him/herself easily understood at all times 0
    - can be understood sometimes or with some difficulty 1
    - can rarely or never be understood for whatever reason 2
14. HE/SHE IS OBJECTIONABLE TO OTHERS DURING THE DAY (loud or constant talking, pilfering, soiling furniture, interfering with affairs of others):
    - rarely or never 0
    - sometimes 1
    - frequently 2

15. HE/SHE IS OBJECTIONABLE TO OTHERS DURING THE NIGHT (loud or constant talking, pilfering, soiling furniture, interfering in affairs of others, wandering about, etc.):

rarely or never	0
sometimes	1
frequently	2

16. HE/SHE ACCUSES OTHERS OF DOING HIM/HER BODILY HARM OR STEALING HIS/HER PERSONAL POSSESSIONS
    – If you are sure the accusations are true, rate zero, otherwise rate one or two:

never	0
sometimes	1
frequently	2

17. HE/SHE HOARDS APPARENTLY MEANINGLESS ITEMS (wads of paper, string, scraps of food, etc.):

never	0
sometimes	1
frequently	2

18. HIS/HER SLEEP PATTERN AT NIGHT IS:

almost never awake	0
sometimes awake	1
often awake	2

EYESIGHT: (tick which applies)

can see (or can see with glasses)
partially blind
totally blind

HEARING: (tick which applies)

no hearing difficulties, without hearing aid
no hearing difficulties, though requires hearing aid
has hearing difficulties which interfere with communication
is very deaf

Brief Cognitive Rating Scale (BCRS)

Reference Reisberg B, Ferris SH (1988) Brief Cognitive Rating Scale (BCRS). *Psychopharmacology Bulletin* 24: 629–36

Time taken about 15 minutes (reviewer's estimate)
Rating by clinician

Main indications

The assessment of cognitive symptoms.

Commentary

The Brief Cognitive Rating Scale (BCRS) is part of the triad of assessments with the Global Deterioration Scale (GDS; page 166) and the Functional Assessment Staging (FAST; page 164). It is divided into five axes: concentration, recent memory, past memory, orientation and function/self-care. The scales on the five axes correlate approximately to the GDS. The validity of the scale has been assessed in a number of studies (Reisberg et al, 1983, 1985), and the validity was measured against the clinical syndrome of age-associated memory impairment and progressive degenerative dementia as well as a number of different psychometric tests. Reliability is generally about 0.9 for all the five axes in the three reliability studies published (Foster et al, 1988; Reisberg et al, 1989).

Additional references

Foster JR, Sclan S, Welkowitz J et al (1988) Psychiatric assessment in medical longterm care facilities: reliability of commonly used rating scales. *International Journal of Geriatric Psychiatry* 3: 229–35.

Reisberg B, Schneck MK, Ferris SH et al (1983) The Brief Cognitive Rating Scale (BCRS). Findings in primary degenerative dementia (PDD). *Psychopharmacology Bulletin* 19: 47–50.

Reisberg B, Ferris SH, Anand R et al (1985) Clinical assessment of cognitive decline in normal and aging and primary degenerative dementia: concordant ordinal measures. In Pinchot P et al, eds. *Psychiatry*. Vol. 5. New York: Plenum Press, 333–8.

Reisberg B, Ferris SH, Steinberg G et al (1989) Longitudinal study of dementia patients and aged controls. In Lawton MP, Herzog AR, eds. *Special research methods for gerontology*. Amityville, NY: Baywood, 195–231.

Address for correspondence

Barry Reisberg
Department of Psychiatry
Aging and Dementia Research Center
NYU Medical Center
550 First Avenue
NY 10016
USA

Brief Cognitive Rating Scale (BCRS)

Axis	Rating (Circle Highest Score)	Item
Axis I:		
Concentration	1 =	No objective or subjective evidence of deficit in concentration.
	2 =	Subjective decrement in concentration ability.
	3 =	Minor objective signs of poor concentration (e.g. on subtraction of serial 7s from 100).
	4 =	Definite concentration deficit for persons of their background (e.g. marked deficit on serial 7s; frequent deficit in subtraction of serial 4s from 40).
	5 =	Marked concentration deficit (e.g. giving months backwards or serial 2s from 20).
	6 =	Forgets the concentration task. Frequently begins to count forward when asked to count backwards from 10 by 1s.
	7 =	Marked difficulty counting forward to 10 by 1s.
Axis II:		
Recent Memory	1 =	No objective or subjective evidence of deficit in recent memory.
	2 =	Subjective impairment only (e.g. forgetting names more than formerly).
	3 =	Deficit in recall of specific events evident upon detailed questioning. No deficit in the recall of major recent events.
	4 =	Cannot recall major events of previous weekend or week. Scanty knowledge (not detailed) of current events, favorite TV shows, etc.
	5 =	Unsure of weather; may not know current President or current address.
	6 =	Occasional knowledge of some recent events. Little or no idea of current address, weather, etc.
	7 =	No knowledge of any recent events.
Axis III:		
Past Memory	1 =	No subjective or objective impairment in past memory.
	2 =	Subjective impairment only. Can recall two or more primary school teachers.
	3 =	Some gaps in past memory upon detailed questioning. Able to recall at least one childhood teacher and/or one childhood friend.
	4 =	Clear-cut deficit. The spouse recalls more of the patient's past than the patient. Cannot recall childhood friends and/or teachers but knows the names of most schools attended. Confuses chronology in reciting personal history.
	5 =	Major past events sometimes not recalled (e.g. names of schools attended).
	6 =	Some residual memory of past (e.g. may recall country of birth or former occupation).
	7 =	No memory of past.
Axis IV:		
Orientation	1 =	No deficit in memory for time, place, identity of self or others.
	2 =	Subjective impairment only. Knows time to nearest hour, location.
	3 =	Any mistake in time > 2 hrs; day of week > 1 day; date > 3 days.
	4 =	Mistakes in month > 10 days of year > 1 month.
	5 =	Unsure of month and/or year and/or season; unsure of locale.
	6 =	No idea of date. Identifies spouse but may not recall name. Knows own name.
	7 =	Cannot identify spouse. May be unsure of personal identity.
Axis V:		
Functioning and Self-Care	1 =	No difficulty, either subjectively or objectively.
	2 =	Complains of forgetting location of objects. Subjective work difficulties.
	3 =	Decreased job functioning evident to co-workers. Difficulty in traveling to new locations.
	4 =	Decreased ability to perform complex tasks (e.g. planning dinner for guests, handling finances, marketing, etc.).
	5 =	Requires assistance in choosing proper clothing.
	6 =	Requires assistance in feeding, and/or toileting, and/or bathing, and/or ambulating.
	7 =	Requires constant assistance in all activities of daily life.

Concentration: test for concentration and attentiveness directly e.g. serial 7s
Recent memory: index of cognitive deficiency
Orientation: in time, place and person

Cambridge Neuropsychological Test Automated Battery (CANTAB)

Time taken varies with each subscale. Total battery, *c.* 90 minutes

Rating by trained neuropsychologists or assistant nurse, technician or equivalent.

Main indications

A computerized battery of tests for neuropsychological evaluation.

Commentary

The Cambridge Neuropsychological Test Automated Battery (CANTAB) is a neuropsychological battery which is of proven sensitivity and specificity in differentiating patients with a number of neurological conditions from each other and from normal controls. Various sub-tests provide assessment of different cognitive functions, including learning, memory, attention (including sustained, divided and selective forms) and tests of executive function (including problem solving and planning). As a computerized battery, it can control for movement disability, it is tailored to the individual, and the tests are graded in difficulty – avoiding floor and ceiling effects. Specific batteries include separate Alzheimer and Parkinson's disease batteries, an attention battery, visual memory battery, and working memory and planning battery, also available in parallel forms. The tests are administered via a touch-screen, and are largely language- and culture-free.

Additional references

Eagger SA, Levy R, Sahakian BJ (1991) Tacrine in Alzheimer's disease. *Lancet* **337**: 989–92.

Fowler KS et al (1997) Computerized neuropsychological tests in the early detection of dementia: prospective findings. *Journal of the International Neuropsychological Society* **3**: 139–46.

Sahakian B et al (1988) A comparative study of visual/spatial memory and learning in Alzheimer type dementia and Parkinson's disease. *Brain* **111**: 695–718.

Sahakian BJ, Coull JT (1994) Nicotine and tetrahydroaminoacradine – evidence for improved attention in patients with dementia of the Alzheimer-type. *Drug Development Research* **31**: 80–8.

Sagal A et al (1991) Detection of visual memory and learning deficits in Alzheimer's disease using CANTAB. *Dementia* **2**: 150–8.

Address for correspondence

Joanna Iddon
Senior Neuropsychologist
Cenes Cognition Ltd
St John's Innovation Centre
Cowley Road
Cambridge CB4 4WS
UK

Short Portable Mental Status Questionnaire (SPMSQ)

Reference   Pfeiffer E (1975) A Short Portable Mental Status Questionnaire for the assessment of organic brain deficit in elderly patients. *Journal of the American Geriatrics Society* 23: 433–41

Time taken 2 minutes
Rating by clinical interview

Main indications

To assess organic brain function in the elderly.

Commentary

The Short Portable Mental Status Questionnaire (SPMSQ) is a short 10-question reliable instrument to detect presence of intellectual impairment and to determine the degree. It is particularly useful for clinicians whose practice includes the elderly. Validity studies were performed using a clinical diagnosis of organic brain syndrome, so it appears to be subjective. Test/retest reliability was over 0.82. The questionnaire explores short-term memory, long-term memory, orientation and the ability to conduct serial operations.

Address for correspondence

E Pfeiffer, MD
USF Suncoast Gerontology Center
12901 Bruce B Downs Boulevard
MDC 50
Tampa, FL 33612
USA

Short Portable Mental Status Questionnaire (SPMSQ)

Instructions: Ask questions 1–10 in this list and record all answers. Ask question 4a only if patient does not have a telephone. Record total number of errors based on ten questions.

Allow one more if subject has had only a grade school education.
Allow one less error if subject has had education beyond high school.
Allow one more error for black subjects, using identical educational criteria.

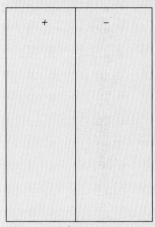

1. What is the date today?_____
                       Month   Day   Year
2. What day of the week is it?_____
3. What is the name of this place? _____
4. What is your telephone number? _____
4a. What is your street address? _____
    (Ask only if patient does not have a telephone)
5. How old are you?_____
6. When were you born?_____
7. Who is the President of the U.S. now? _____
8. What was President just before him? _____
9. What was your mother's maiden name?_____
10. Subtract 3 from 20 and keep subtracting 3 from each new number, all the way down.

TOTAL NUMBER OF ERRORS

        0–2   Errors   Intact Intellectual Functioning
        3–4   Errors   Mild Intellectual Impairment
        5–7   Errors   Moderate Intellectual Impairment
        8–10 Errors   Severe Intellectual Impairment

To be completed by interviewer

Patient's Name: _____   Date:_____

              Sex: 1. Male   Race: 1. White
                      2. Female   2. Black
                                               3. Other

Years of education: _____   1. Grade School
                                           2. High School
                                         3. Beyond High School

Interviewer's name:_____

Reproduced from Pfeiffer E (1975) Short Portable Mental Status Questionnaire for the assessment of organic brain deficit in elderly patients. *Journal of the American Geriatrics Society,* Vol. 23, no. 10, pp. 433–41.

SET Test

Reference   Isaacs B, Akhtar AJ (1972) The SET Test: a rapid test of mental function in old people. *Age and Ageing* **1**: 222–6

Time taken 5 minutes, often 2
Rating by interviewer

Main indications

Assessment of mental function in older people.

Commentary

The object of the SET Test was to provide a brief test of mental function in older people which was not perceived as a threat. The test is essentially a variant of verbal fluency. The original paper described the results of the test in 64 elderly people over the age of 65 who were seen in their own homes by a doctor who also carried out the Mill Hill Vocabulary Test, Raven's Progressive Colour Matrices and a modified version of the Crichton Royal Behavioural Rating Scale (page 171). There were highly significant correlations between the SET Test and the scores on these scales.

The SET Test

The test is introduced to the subject as a challenge rather than a threat, the appropriate words being "let's see how good your memory is", or some variant of this. The subject is then asked "I want you to tell me all the colours you can think of". The examiner may repeat the instructions as often as required, but should offer no other help. There is no time limit, this part of the test being complete when the subject has offered ten different colours, in which case he is awarded a score of ten; or when he cannot think of any more, or begins to repeat himself, in which case his score is the number of different colours he has given. The end-point is usually clear, the subject coming to an abrupt stop with an admission of failure such as "That's all I can think of", or a defensive rationalization like "There are lots more".

The test is then repeated three times more by asking in turn for animals, fruits and towns. A maximum of 10 points is awarded for each of the four sets and a maximum of 40 for the total.

Source: Isaacs B, Akhtar AJ (1972) The SET Test: a rapid test of mental function in old people. *Age and Ageing* **1**: 222–6. By kind permission of Oxford University Press.

Short Mental Status Questionnaire

Reference   Robertson D, Rockwood K, Stolee P (1982) A Short Mental Status Questionnaire. *Canadian Journal on Aging* **1**: 16–20

Time taken about 5 minutes
Rating by interviewer

Main indications

Assessment of mental status in elderly people.

Commentary

The justification for the development of another scale measuring cognitive function was on the need to develop a short questionnaire for use in the Saskatchewan Health Survey where questions such as "Who is the President of the United States?" were felt to be less relevant to elderly Canadians compared with Americans, and the validity of asking the patient to recall his or her mother's maiden name was of doubtful significance in view of the inability to verify that information. The questions about monarchs and presidents were replaced by asking the name of the Prime Minister of Canada and recalling three words instead of a fictitious name and address, and, as calculations appear to have a high error rate, counting from 20 down to 1 was suggested. Fifty elderly subjectes were examined with a test/retest correlation of 0.89. While the questioner identified moderate and severe cognitive impairment satisfactorily it was difficult, on the basis of the test alone, to differentiate those with mild impairment from normal controls.

Short Mental Status Questionnaire

1. What is your full name? — Correct forename and surname
2. What is your address? — Correct street address and municipality
3. What year is this? — Correct year
4. What month is this? — Correct month
5. What day of the week is this? — Correct day of week (not date)
6. How old are you? — Correct age, verified by another person, or from date of birth
7. What is the name of the Prime Minister of Canada? — Correct answer to include surname of current Prime Minister
8. When did the First World War start? — Year 1914
9. Remember these three items. I will ask you to recall them in a few minutes . . . **bed, chair, window**. Have subject repeat items correctly before proceeding.
10. Count backwards from 20 to 1 — No error. Any uncorrected error = 0
    (If necessary like this, 20, 19 and so on)
11. Repeat the three items I asked you to remember — All items correct = 1
    Any uncorrected error = 0

Short Orientation–Memory–Concentration Test

Reference Katzman R, Bown T, Fuld P, Peck A, Schechter R, Schimmel H (1983) Validation of a Short Orientation–Memory–Concentration Test of cognitive impairment. *American Journal of Psychiatry* **140**: 734–9

Time taken less than 5 minutes (reviewer's estimate)
Rating by clinician

Main indications

A brief six-item cognitive test developed from the longer Blessed Information and Concentration test.

Commentary

The Short Orientation–Memory–Concentration Test is a six-item test that was developed out of the larger 26-item Mental Status Questionnaire, which was carried out on a group of people in a nursing facility (322 subjects in total). When post-mortems were carried out on 38 sub-jects, the 26 questions were subject to multivariant analyses and the six items most correlated with senile plaque counts in the cerebral cortex were described – year, time of day, counting backwards from 20 to 1, months backwards, the memory phase (name and address) and month. The scale, once developed, was tested on three additional populations: 170 subjects admitted to the same nursing facility on whom the original study was performed, 42 subjects in a dementia ward and 52 subjects at a senior citizens day centre. The shorter scale stood up statistically very well in comparison with the longer scale. The correlation between the scores and plaque counts at post-mortem was highly significant (0.52) and very similar to the correlation of the 26-item test.

Short Orientation–Memory–Concentration Test

Items	Maximum error	Score		Weight		
1　What year is it now?	1	___	×	4	=	___
2　What month is it now?	1	___	×	3	=	___
Memory phrase	Repeat this phrase after me: John Brown, 42 Market Street, Chicago					
3　About what time is it? (within 1 hour)	1	___	×	3	=	___
4　Count backwards 20 to 1	2	___	×	2	=	___
5　Say the months in reverse order	2	___	×	2	=	___
6　Repeat the memory phrase	5	___	×	2	=	___

Score of 1 for each incorrect response; maximum weighted error score = 24

American Journal of Psychiatry, Vol. 140, pp. 734–739, 1983. Copyright 1983, the American Psychiatric Association. Reprinted by permission.

Syndrom Kurztest (SKT)

Reference   Erzigkeit H (1989) The SKT: a short cognitive performance test as an instrument for the assessment of clinical efficacy of cognition enhancers. In Bergener M, Reisberg B, eds. *Diagnosis and treatment of senile dementia.* Berlin: Springer-Verlag, 164–74

Lehfeld H, Erzigkeit H (1997) The SKT – a short cognitive performance test for assessing deficits of memory and attention. *International Psychogeriatrics* **9** (suppl 1): 115–21

Time taken 10–15 minutes
Rating by anyone trained in the use of the test

Main indications

The Syndrom Kurztest (SKT) is a short cognitive performance test to assess memory and attention. The SKT was specially designed to be a brief and practicable measure of cognitive function.

Commentary

The test is available in five parallel forms to allow repeated administration. There are nine subtests: object naming, object recall, learning, reading numbers from blocks, arranging the blocks, replacing them in their original position, simple recognition and interference task, and two memory performance tasks. Reliability of the test is between 0.6 and 0.8, face validity has been shown and significant correlations occur between the SKT results and other psychometric tests as well as neuroimaging parameters – CT and EEG. The SKT has also been shown to be sensitive to the effects of drugs.

Additional references

Erzigkeit H (1991) The development of the SKT project. In Hindmarch I, Hippius H, Wilcox J, eds. *Dementia: molecules, methods and measures.* Chichester: Wiley, 101–8.

Overall J, Schaltenbrand R (1992) The SKT neuropsychological test battery. *Journal of Geriatric Psychiatry and Neurology* 5: 220–7.

Address for correspondence

H Lehfeld
Psychiatrische Universitätsklinik Erlangen
Schwabachanlage 6
91054 Erlangen
Germany

Cognitive Abilities Screening Instrument (CASI)

Reference Teng EL, Hasegawa K, Homma A, Imai Y, Larson E, Graves A, Sugimoto K, Yamaguchi T, Sasaki H, Chiu D, White LR (1994) The Cognitive Abilities Screening Instrument (CASI): a practical test for cross-cultural epidemiological studies of dementia. *International Psychogeriatrics* 6: 45–58

Time taken 15–20 minutes
Rating by trained interviewer

Main indications

A cognitive test providing a quantitative assessment (from 0 to 100) for a wide range of cognitive skills.

Commentary

The Cognitive Abilities Screening Instrument (CASI) consists of items similar to those used in a number of existing scales such as the Hasegawa Dementia Screening Scale (Hasegawa, 1983), and the Mini-Mental State Examination (MMSE; page 34), according to DSM-III-R criteria, is included. A number of different versions of the CASI are available, in English and in Japanese, and the study has been described in the USA and in Japan (Teng et al, 1994). Training is required (provided by the authors).

Additional references

Hasegawa K (1983) The clinical assessment of dementia in the aged: a dementia screening scale for psychogeriatric patients. In Bergener M, Lehr U, Lang E et al, eds. *Ageing in the eighties and beyond*. New York: Springer, 207–18.

Teng EL, Chui HC (1987) The Modified Mini-Mental State Examination. *Journal of Clinical Psychiatry* 48: 314–18.

Teng EL, Haegama K, Homma A, Imai V, Larson E, Graves A, Sugimoto K, Yamaguchi T, Sasaki H, Chin D, White L (1994) *International Psychogeriatrics* 6(1): 45–58.

Address for correspondence

EL Teng, c/o L White
EDB Program, National Institute on Ageing
Gateway Building, Room 3C309
National Institute of Health
Bethesda
MD 20892
USA

Main items of the Cognitive Abilities Screening Instrument (CASI)

Where were you born?
When were you born?
How old are you?
How many minutes are there in an hour?
In what direction does the sun set?
Registration and recall of 3 words
Repeating words backwards
Serial 3's
Today's date
Day of the week
Season
Orientation to place
Number of animals with 4 legs

A comparison of objects, e.g. an orange and a banana are both fruit
What action would you take if you saw you neighbour's house catching fire?
Repeat "he would like to go home?"
Obey command "raise your hand"
Write "he would like to go home"
Copy 2 interlocking pentagons
Three-stage command
Recognition of body parts
Recognition of objects
Recall of objects

Cognitive Drug Research Assessment System (COGDRAS)

Reference   Simpson PM, Surmon DJ, Wesnes KA, Wilcock GK (1991) The Cognitive Drug Research computerized Assessment System for demented patients: a validation study. *International Journal of Geriatric Psychiatry* 6: 95–102

Time taken approximately 30 minutes
Rating by trained personnel

Main indications

A computerized battery to assess the effects of drugs on cognitive functions in dementia.

Commentary

The Cognitive Drug Research Assessment System (COGDRAS) was developed to assess the effects of drugs on cognitive function. The version presented is validated for use in patients suffering from dementia. Refinements of the system included: avoidance of negative feedback; larger presentation of words and digits; the presence of trained technical support; and the ability to modify the programme if the patient is distracted. The following tests were used in the study: immediate verbal recognition; picture presentation; number vigilance task; choice reaction time; memory scanning task; delayed word recognition and picture recognition. The COGDRAS-D was administered to 51 patients attending a memory clinic and validated by other neuropsychological tests such as the Mini-Mental State Examination (MMSE; page 34) and the Kew Cognitive Test (page 66). Patients with dementia showed impairments in speed of choice reaction and in all the memory tests. Test/retest reliability was good, and the results showed that the system had comparable properties to the previous versions.

Additional reference

Simpson PM, Wesnes KA, Christmas L (1989) A computerised system for the assessment of drug-induced performance changes in young, elderly and demented populations. *British Journal of Clinical Pharmacology* 27: 711–12P.

Address for correspondence

KA Wesnes
Cognitive Drug Research
13 The Grove
Reading RG1 4RB
UK

Cognitive Drug Research Assessment System (COGDRAS)

Immediate verbal recognition

A series of 12 words is presented visually at the rate of one every three seconds. Immediately after, the 12 words are presented in random order with 12 different words and the patient required to press a button each time to signal whether or not the word was from the originally presented list.

Picture presentation

A series of 14 pictures is presented on the monitor at the rate of one every three seconds.

Number vigilance task

A number is constantly displayed just to the right of the centre of the screen. A series of 90 digits is presented in the centre at the rate of 80 per minute. The patient has to press the YES button every time the digit in the centre matches the one constantly displayed.

Choice reaction time

Either the word YES or the word NO is presented in the centre of the monitor. The patient is instructed to press the YES or NO button as appropriate as quickly as possible. There are 20 trials and the intertrial interval varies randomly between one and 2.5 seconds.

Memory scanning task

Three digits are presented singly at the rate of one every 1.2 seconds for the patient to remember. A series of 18 digits is then presented and for each one the patient must press the YES button if he/she believes it was one of three presented or NO if not.

Delayed word recognition

The 12 words originally presented are presented again with 12 new distractors. Again the patient must decide whether or not each word was from the original list, pressing the YES or NO button accordingly.

Picture recognition

The 14 pictures presented earlier are presented again with 14 new ones in a randomized order. The patient signals recognition by pressing the YES or NO button as appropriate.

Reproduced from Simpson PM, Surmon DJ, Wesnes KA, Wilcock GK (1991) The Cognitive Drug Research computerized Assessment System for demented patients: a validation study. *International Journal of Geriatric Psychiatry* **6**: 95–102. Copyright John Wiley & Sons Limited. Reproduced with permission.

Kew Cognitive Test

Reference   Hare M (1978) Clinical checklist for diagnosis of dementia. *British Medical Journal* 2: 266–7

Time taken 5–10 minutes (reviewer's estimate)
Rating by clinical interview

Main indications

Assessment of memory, speech and parietal function in dementia.

Commentary

The Kew Cognitive Test assesses cognitive function in the three areas of memory, aphasia and parietal signs using a simple 15-item questionnaire, five in each category. Two studies have used a modified version of the test, the study by Hare (1978) and McDonald (1969). Hare (1978) examined 200 people admitted to a psychogeriatric assess-ment unit, repeated 4 or 6 weeks later. Patients with deficits in language ability or praxis had a significantly poorer outcome than those with memory deficits alone. McDonald used the test (among others) to divided patients into two groups showing that heterogeneity exist-ed in terms of age and mortality with an older group who did not have parietal lobe signs and a better prognosis compared with a younger group with parietal dysfunction and higher mortality.

Additional reference

McDonald C (1969) Clinical heterogeneity in senile dementia. *British Journal of Psychiatry* **115**: 267–71.

Kew Cognitive Test

Memory
What year are we in?
What month is it?
Can you tell me two countries we fought in the Second World War?
What year were you born?
What is the capital city of England?

Aphasia
What do you call this (a watch)?
What do you call this (a wrist strap or band)?
What do you call this (a buckle or clasp)?

What is a refrigerator for?
What is a thermometer for?
What is a barometer for?

Parietal signs
Show me your left hand
Touch your left ear with your right hand
Name the coin in hand named (as 10p or two shillings)
No tactile inattention present
Normal two point discrimination
Draw a square

This table was first published in the *BMJ* [Hare M, Clinical checklist for diagnosis of dementia, 1978, Vol. 2, pp. 266–7] and is reproduced by permission of the *BMJ*.

Severe Impairment Battery (SIB)

Reference   Saxton J, McGonigle-Gibson K, Swihart A, Miller M, Boller F (1990) Assessment of severely impaired patients: description and validation of a new neuropsychological test battery. *Psychological Assessment* 2: 298–303

Time taken 30–40 minutes (reviewer's estimate)
Rating by trained interviewer

Main indications

Assessment of cognitive function, particularly in severe dementia.

Commentary

The Severe Impairment Battery (SIB) has the strength of assessing cognitive function in patients with moderate to severe dementia. Items are single words or one-step commands combined with gestures. Nine areas are assessed (see below), and the score is between 0 and 100. It appears sensitive to change. Panisset et al (1994) examined 69 patients with severe dementia using the SIB and found it to be a helpful neuropsychological measure in people with severe dementia.

Additional references

Albert M, Cohen C (1992) The Test for Severe Impairment, an instrument for the assessment of patients with severe cognitive dysfunction. *Journal of American Geriatric Society* 40: 449–53.

Panisset M, Roudier M, Saxton J et al (1994) Severe Impairment Battery: a neuropsychological battery for severely impaired patients. *Archives of Neurology* 51: 41–5.

Severe Impairment Battery Domains

Domain	Questions
Orientation	Name
	Place (town)
	Time (month and time of day)
Attention	Digit span
	Counting to visual and auditory stimuli
Language	Auditory and reading comprehension
	Verbal fluency (food and months of the year)
	Naming from description, pictures of objects, objects, colors and forms
	Repetition
	Reading
	Writing
	Copying of written material
Praxis	How to use a cup, a spoon
Visuospatial	Discrimination of colors and forms
Construction	Spontaneous drawing, copying and tracing a figure
Memory	Immediate short- and long-term recall for examiner's name, objects, colors, forms and a short sentence
Orientation to name	When the patient's name is called from behind
Social interaction	Shaking hands, following general direction

Source: Panisset M, Roudier M, Saxton J et al (1994) Severe Impairment Battery: a neuropsychological battery for severely impaired patients. *Archives of Neurology* **51**: 41–5.

Mental Status Questionnaire (MSQ)/Face–Hand Test (FHT)

Reference   Kahn RL, Goldfarb AI, Pollack M, Peck A (1960) Brief objective measures for the determination of mental status in the aged. *American Journal of Psychiatry* 117: 326–8

Time taken MSQ – 5 minutes, FHT – 5 minutes
(reviewer's estimate)
Rating by trained interviewer

Main indications

Assessment of cognitive function.

Commentary

These tests reflect an early attempt to describe a quantative measure of cognitive function. The Mental Status Questionnaire (MSQ) consists of ten questions, the point being made that the questions themselves are well known but the difference is that they are administered in a standardized way and the method of marking the number of errors gives a quantitative measure of mental functioning. The Face–Hand Test (FHT) was based on a test described by Fink et al (1952) and used because it is culture-free and can be used with patients who have impaired communication. As the response to the FHT is the same in 90% of cases whether the eyes are open or not, it was given with eyes open. It is said to be sensitive to brain damage. The paper reported the results on 1077 residents of nursing homes and mental hospitals. Diagnostic categories were assigned by psychiatric interview within a month of the assessment. Some 94% of patients scoring full marks on the MSQ and 70% scoring as negative on the FHT were rated as having none or mild chronic brain syndrome (CBS). The results were similar for patients with CBS and psychosis and those rated as having management problems.

Additional reference

Fink M, Green MA, Bender MB (1952) *Neurology* 2: 48.

Mental Status Questionnaire (MSQ)/Face–Hand Test (FHT)

1. What is the name of this place?
2. Where is it located (address)?
3. What is today's date?
4. What is the month now?
5. What is the year?
6. How old are you?
7. When were you born (month)?
8. When were you born (year)?
9. Who is the president of the United States?
10. Who was the president before him?

The Face–Hand Test: This test was first described by Fink et al (1952) as a diagnostic procedure for brain damage. The test consists of touching the patient simultaneously on the cheek and on the dorsum of the hand, and asking him to indicate where he was touched. Ten trials are given: 8 face–hand combinations divided between 4 contralateral (e.g. right cheek and left hand) and 4 ipsilateral (e.g. right cheek and right hand) stimuli, and 2 interspersed symmetric combinations of face–face and hand–hand. After the second trial, if the patient only reports one stimulus, he is asked, "Were you touched any place else?" in order to give him the concept of twoness. If the patient fails consistently to locate both stimuli correctly within the 10 trials, he is classed as positive. The main types of errors are extinction, in which only 1 stimulus is indicated (almost always the face), and displacement, in which 2 stimuli are indicated but 1 of them, generally the hand stimulus, is displaced to another part of the body (e.g. if the person indicates both cheeks when the face and hand were actually touched). A patient is rated negative if he is consistently correct within the 10 trials. Frequently he makes an error on the first 4 trials, but is consistently correct after perceiving the 2 symmetric stimuli.

Cognitive Capacity Screening Examination

Reference Jacobs JW, Bernhard MR, Delgado A, Strain JJ (1977) Screening for organic mental syndromes in the medically ill. *Annals of Internal Medicine* 86: 40–6

Time taken 5 minutes
Rating by clinician

Main indications
Assessment of mental status in medically ill patients.

Commentary
The Cognitive Capacity Screening Examination was produced with the express intention of overcoming the difficulties in assessing mental function in medical patients. Standard examinations were considered inadequate because of the time taken for their administration, their lack of sensitivity and the need to give the whole test – taking into consideration the patients' education and cultural background and the variability of symptoms. The Mini-Mental State Examination (MMSE; page 34) was felt to have the shortcoming of having the specific purpose of screening psychiatric patients. The 30-item questionnaire was administered to different groups of patients to assess validity and reliability: 24 medical patients, 29 psychiatric patients, a further 69 medical patients and 25 normal controls. These groups revealed that a score of 20 or above was unlikely in the presence of an organic brain syndrome. The majority of psychiatric patients scored above that score, one third of medical admissions scored below 20 and only one of the normal controls scored below that score. Inter-rater reliability was 100%.

Cognitive Capacity Screening Examination

1. What day of the week is this? ___
2. What month? ___
3. What day of month? ___
4. What year? ___
5. What place is this? ___
6. Repeat the numbers 8 7 2. ___
7. Say them backwards. ___
8. Repeat these numbers 6 3 7 1. ___
9. Listen to these numbers 6 9 4. Count 1 through 10 out loud, then repeat 6 9 4. (Help if needed. Then use numbers 5 7 3.) ___
10. Listen to these numbers 8 1 4 3. Count 1 through 10 out loud, then repeat 8 1 4 3. ___
11. Beginning with Sunday, say the days of the week backwards. ___
12. 9 + 3 is ___
13. Add 6 (to the previous answer or "to 12"). ___
14. Take away 5 ("from 18"). ___
    Repeat these words after me and remember them, I will ask for them later: HAT, CAR, TREE, TWENTY-SIX.
15. The opposite of fast is slow. The opposite of up is ___

16. The opposite of large is ___
17. The opposite of hard is ___
18. An orange and a banana are both fruits. Red and blue are both ___
19. A penny and a dime are both ___
20. What were those words I asked you to remember? (HAT) ___
21. (CAR) ___
22. (TREE) ___
23. (TWENTY-SIX) ___
24. Take away 7 from 100, then take away 7 from what is left and keep going: 100 − 7 is ___
25. Minus 7 ___
26. Minus 7 (write down answers; check correct subtraction of 7) ___
27. Minus 7 ___
28. Minus 7 ___
29. Minus 7 ___
30. Minus 7 ___

Total correct (maximum score = 30) ___

7 Minute Neurocognitive Screening Battery

Reference Solomon PR, Hirschoff A, Kelly B et al (1998) A 7 minute neurocognitive screening battery highly sensitive to Alzheimer's disease. *Archives of Neurology* 55: 349–55

Time taken Mean 7 minutes 42 seconds (range 6–11 minutes)
Rating by trained interviewer

Main indications

A screening test for cognitive impairment to distinguish patients with dementia and normal controls.

Commentary

The 7 Minute Neurocognitive Screening Battery consists of four tests representing four cognitive areas affected in Alzheimer's disease. These are: memory, verbal fluency, visuospatial and visioconstruction and orientation for time. The screening instrument was designed so that it could be rapidly administered by a technician, requiring no clinical judgement or training in its use. It was capable of distinguishing patients with Alzheimer's disease from those with normal ageing, and it was based on recent understanding of the fundamental differences between Alzheimer's disease and normal ageing. 60 patients with Alzheimer's disease and 30 controls were examined. Test/retest reliability was evaluated in 25 of each, with overall test/retest reliability of the scale being between 0.83 and 0.92. Inter-rater reliability was 0.93 using logistic regression. Each of the four tests was able to detect patients with Alzheimer's disease in 92% of cases and to detect 96% of healthy subjects, as high sensitivity was apparent with patients with very mild, mild and moderate disease. Age, sex and education do not appear to affect the results. The results are presented in a way which does not make it easy to extract exact cut-off points on the various tests. The entire battery seems better predicted than any individual scale.

7 Minute Neurocognitive Screening Battery

The four tests used were:

Enhances Cued Recall

Category Fluency
Benton Orientation Test
Clock Drawing

Revised Hasegawa's Dementia Scale (HDS-R)

Reference   Imai Y and Hasegawa K (1994) The revised Hasegawa's dementia scale (HDS-R) – evaluation of its usefulness as a screening test for dementia. *Journal of Hong Kong College of Psychiatry* 4: 20–24

Time taken 5 minutes (reviewer's estimate)
Rating by interview

Main indications

Assessment of cognitive function as a means for screening for dementia.

Commentary

The Revised Hasegawa's Dementia Scale was developed from the original Hasegawa scale, published in 1983, which comprised 11 questions. 5 questions were deleted (place of the subject's birth, the last year of World War 2, the number of days in a year, the prime minister of Japan, and the length of time the individual has been at the place of interview). Immediate and delayed recall of 3 words and list generating fluency were added. The revised version consists of 9 questions with a maximum score of 30. Imai and Hasegawa (1994) reported on the results of

157 subjects, 95 of whom had dementia. Cronbach's alpha was 0.90. Using a cut-off point of 20/21, a sensitivity of 0.90 and a specificity of 0.82 were achieved in discriminating people with dementia from controls. A correlation with the Mini-Mental State Examination (MMSE; page 34) was 0.94. The scale was able to distinguish between stages of dementia rated on the Global Deterioration Scale (GDS; page 166).

Address for correspondence

Yukimichi Imai
Department of Psychiatry
St Marianna University
School of Medicine
2-16-1 Sugao Miyamae-Ku
Kawasaki 216
Japan

Revised Hasegawa's Dementia Scale (HDS-R)

1.	How old are you? (+/– 2 yrs.)		0	1	
2.	Year, month, date, day?	Year	0	1	
	1 point each.	Month	0	1	
		Date	0	1	
		Day	0	1	
3.	What Is this place?				
	Correct answer In 5 sec: 2 points.		0	2	
	Correct choice between "hospital? office?"		0	1	
4.	Repeating 3 words. 1 point each. (To use only one version per test.)	a)	0	1	
	Version A: "a) cherry blossom b) cat c) tram".	a)	0	1	
	Version B: "a) plum blossom b) dog c) car".	b)	0	1	
5.	100-7=? If correct, 1 point.	93	0	1	
	If not: skip to item #6.				
	-7 again=? If correct, 1 point.	86	0	1	
6.	Repeat 6-8-2 backwards.		0	1	
	If not: skip to Item #7.				
	Repeat 3-5-2-9 backwards.		0	1	
7.	Recall 3 words. For each word	a)	0	1	2
	2 points for spontaneous recall.	b)	0	1	2
	1 point for correct recall after category cue.	c)	0	1	2
8.	Show live unrelated common object, then take them back and ask for recall.		0	1	2
	1 point each.		3	4	5
9.	Name all vegetables that come to mind.				
	No time limit. May remind once.		0	1	2
	Terminate when there is no further answer after a 10 sec Interval. For each vegetable		3	4	5
	name after the 5th one: 1 point.				
	1. ___ 2. ___ 3. ___ 4. ___ 5. ___				
	6. ___ 7. ___ 8. ___ 9. ___ 10. ___				
	Total score				/30

Reproduced, with permission, from Imai Y and Hasegawa K (1994) The revised Hasegawa's dementia scale (HDS-R) – evaluation of its usefulness as a screening test for dementia. *Journal of Hong Kong College of Psychiatry* **4**: 20–24.

Neuropsychiatric assessments

These are traditionally considered to consist of psychiatric symptoms and behavioural disturbances (also known as non-cognitive features to distinguish them from cognitive deficits such as amnesia, aphasia, apraxia and agnosia). Compared with the assessment of cognitive impairment, these non-cognitive features have only relatively recently been subject to quantitative assessment. There are a large number of scales which purport to assess a wide range of features, including many neuropsychiatric problems found in the more severe stages of the illness. Often, the scales measure symptoms and signs which have more in common with lay descriptions of behaviour such as agitation, unco-operativeness and obstreporousness. They are often assessed in common with deficits in Activities of Daily Living, because of the high association between the two. Many of the scales represent a laudable attempt to assess the degree of disturbance present and use this as a measure for the amount of time carers need to spend with an individual. A significant advance has been the development of scales to measure more specific symptom profiles in patients. Measures of aggression have been devised, as have scales dealing specifically with agitation. A number of instruments have recently been published that provide a global measure of psychiatric symptoms, and as such are akin to the quantified assessments of cognitive function produced twenty years ago.

The BEHAVE-AD (behavioral symptoms in Alzheimer's disease: phenomenology and treatment) scale (page 75) was one of the first to be published, and has the advantage of being sensitive to change, making it suitable to measure the effects of drugs. A cluster of other scales include the Manchester and Oxford Universities Scale for the Psychopathological Assessment of Dementia (MOUSEPAD; page 82) derived from the Present Behavioural Examination (PBE; page 86), the Neuropsychiatric Inventory (NPI; page 78), the Columbia University Scale for Psychopathology in Alzheimer's Disease (CUSPAD; page 79) and the Consortium to Establish a Registry for Alzheimer's Disease (CERAD) Behavioral Rating Scale (page 88). These have relatively little to chose between them, and each has its own proponents and detractors. Reliability and validity data are

available for them all, and all have been published in peer-reviewed journals. The NPI is an efficient scale and has been used by pharmaceutical companies assessing the effects drugs have on these features. Many include questions of depression, and so overlap with those scales described in Chapter 1 is to be found.

Specific measures of aggression can be found [e.g. the Rating Scale for Aggressive Behaviour in the Elderly (RAGE; page 92), an observational scale for the assessment of inpatients, the Overt Aggression Scale (OAS; page 94), which measures the severity and frequency of all types of aggression, and the Ryden Aggression Scale (page 104), which is all-encompassing]. Agitation is best assessed by the Cohen-Mansfield Agitation Inventory (CMAI; page 110) which has a short and a long form plus a direct observational scale, something also found in the Pittsburgh Agitation Scale (PAS; page 112). A much shorter version of the scale exists [Brief Agitation Rating Scale (BARS; page 108)]. Measures for irritability and apathy also exist. This leaves a host of other tools which assess a wide range of behavioural disturbances in patients and which the reader has to familiarize him or herself with to decide which is the most appropriate for use. These include: the BEAM-D (page 120), the Comprehensive Psychopathological Rating Scale (CPRS; page 190), the Dysfunctional Behaviour Rating Instrument (DBRI; page 114) (validated on community patients), the Dementia Behavior Disturbance Scale (page 111), the Nurses' Observation Scale for Geriatric Patients (NOSGER; page 210) and the Neurobehavioral Rating Scale (NRS; page 96) (which includes cognitive tests). The Clinical Rating Scale for Symptoms of Psychosis in Alzheimer's Disease (SPAD; page 122) measures specifically psychotic features.

The choice of scale depends on the question to be answered. If a rating of a specific behaviour is required (e.g. to measure the effects of an intervention such as a behaviour programme or drug), then one of the specific scales should be chosen. If the rater wishes to have a more general measure of the dependency of a ward or section of a nursing home to compare them with another group, then a more global measure is appropriate which may also include an assessment of cognition and activities of daily living.

BEHAVE-AD

Reference   Reisberg B, Borenstein J, Salob SP, Ferris SH, Franssen E, Georgotas A (1987) Behavioral symptoms in Alzheimer's disease: phenomenology and treatment. *Journal of Clinical Psychiatry* **48** (suppl 5): 9–15

Time taken 20 minutes
Rating by clinician

Main indications

The BEHAVE-AD was designed particularly to be useful in prospective studies of behavioural symptoms and in pharmacological trials to look at behavioural symptoms in patients with Alzheimer's disease.

Commentary

The BEHAVE-AD is the original behaviour rating scale in Alzheimer's disease, the items having been lifted originally from a chart review of 57 outpatients with Alzheimer's disease. The areas covered were the main domains of symptomatology: paranoid and delusional ideation, hallucinations, activity disturbances, aggressiveness, diurnal rhythm disturbances, affective disturbances, and anxieties/phobias. A global rating of the trouble the various behaviours are to the caregiver is also noted. Reference is to the 2 weeks prior to the interview, which is directed to an informed carer.

Sclan et al (1996) determined inter-rater reliability of the scale transculturally, including patients from France. Inter-rater reliability was excellent, with agreement coefficients ranging from 0.65 to 0.91. Similar consistency was found in the French version. Measures were carried out on 140 patients with probable Alzheimer's disease, with the finding that the BEHAVE-AD scores were most severe in the moderate and moderately severe stages of the illness. Patterson et al (1990) reported similar very good reliability ratings (kappa value 0.62–1.00 on 20 of the 25 items with percentage agreement of between 82 and 100%). Reisberg et al (1989) demonstrated the variability of the different symptoms at the different stages of the disease [measured with the Global Deterioration Scale (GDS; page 166)].

Additional references

Patterson M, Schnell A, Martin R et al (1990) Assessment of behavioral and affective symptoms in Alzheimer's disease. *Journal of Geriatric Psychiatry and Neurology* **3**: 21–30.

Reisberg B, Franssen E, Sclan S et al (1989) Stage specific incidence of potentially remediable behavioral symptoms in aging and Alzheimer's disease; a study of 120 patients using the BEHAVE-AD. *Bulletin of Clinical Neuroscience* **54**: 95–112.

Sclan S, Saillon A, Franssen E et al (1996) The behavior pathology in Alzheimer's disease rating scale (BEHAVE-AD): reliability and analysis of symptom category scores. *International Journal of Geriatric Psychiatry* **11**: 819–30.

Address for correspondence

Barry Reisberg
Aging and Dementia Research Program
Department of Psychiatry
NYU Medical Center
550 First Avenue
NY 10016
USA

Scale is continued overleaf

Part 1: Symptomatology
Assessment Interval: Specify: ——— wks.
Total Score: ———

a. Paranoid and Delusional Ideation

1. "People are Stealing Things" Delusion
0 = Not present.
1 = Delusion that people are hiding objects.
2 = Delusion that people are coming into the home and hiding objects or stealing objects.
3 = Talking and listening to people coming into the home.

2. "One's House is Not One's Home" Delusion
0 = Not present.
1 = Conviction that the place in which one is residing is not one's home (e.g. packing to go home; complaints, while at home, of "take me home").
2 = Attempt to leave domiciliary to go home.
3 = Violence in response to attempts to forcibly restrict exit.

3. "Spouse (or Other Caregiver) is an Imposter" Delusion
0 = Not present.
1 = Conviction that spouse (or other caregiver) is an imposter.
2 = Anger toward spouse (or other caregiver) for being an imposter.
3 = Violence towards spouse (or other caregiver) for being an imposter.

4. "Delusion of Abandonment" (e.g. to an Institution).
0 = Not present.
1 = Suspicion of caregiver plotting abandonment or institutionalization (e.g. on telephone).
2 = Accusation of a conspiracy to abandon or institutionalize.
3 = Accusation of impending or immediate desertion or institutionalization.

5. "Delusion of Infidelity"
0 = Not present.
1 = Conviction that spouse and/or children and/or other caregivers are unfaithful.
2 = Anger toward spouse, relative, or other caregiver for infidelity.
3 = Violence toward spouse, relative, or other caregiver for supposed infidelity.

6. "Suspiciousness/Paranoia" (other than above)
0 = Not present.
1 = Suspicious (e.g. hiding objects that he/she later may be unable to locate).
2 = Paranoid (i.e. fixed conviction with respect to suspicions and/or anger as a result of suspicions).
3 = Violence as a result of suspicions.
Unspecified?
Describe

7. Delusions (other than above)
0 = Not present.
1 = Delusional
2 = Verbal or emotional manifestations as a result of delusions.
3 = Physical actions or violence as a result of delusions.
Unspecified?
Describe

b. Hallucinations

8. Visual Hallucinations
0 = Not present.
1 = Vague: not clearly defined.
2 = Clearly defined hallucinations of objects or persons (e.g. sees other people at the table).
3 = Verbal or physical actions or emotional responses to the hallucinations.

9. Auditory Hallucinations
0 = Not present.
1 = Vague: not clearly defined.
2 = Clearly defined hallucinations of words or phrases.
3 = Verbal or physical actions or emotional response to the hallucinations.

10. Olfactory Hallucinations
0 = Not present.
1 = Vague: not clearly defined.
2 = Clearly defined
3 = Verbal or physical actions or emotional responses to the hallucinations.

11. Haptic Hallucinations
0 = Not present.
1 = Vague: not clearly defined.
2 = Clearly defined.
3 = Verbal or physical actions or emotional responses to the hallucinations.

12. Other Hallucinations
0 = Not present.
1 = Vague: not clearly defined.
2 = Clearly defined
3 = Verbal or physical actions or emotional responses to the hallucinations.
Unspecified?
Describe

c. Activity Disturbances

13. Wandering: Away From Home or Caregiver
0 = Not present.
1 = Somewhat, but not sufficient to necessitate restraint.
2 = Sufficient to require restraint.
3 = Verbal or physical actions or emotional responses to attempts to prevent wandering.

14. Purposeless Activity (Cognitive Abulia)
0 = Not present.
1 = Repetitive, purposeless activity (e.g. opening and closing pocketbook, packing and unpacking clothing, repeatedly putting on and removing clothing, opening and closing drawers, insistent repeating of demands or questions).
2 = Pacing or other purposeless activity sufficient to require restraint.
3 = Abrasions or physical harm resulting from purposeless activity.

15. Inappropriate Activity
0 = Not present.
1 = Inappropriate activities (e.g. storing and hiding objects in

inappropriate places, such as throwing clothing in wastebasket or putting empty plates in the oven; inappropriate sexual behavior, such as inappropriate exposure).
2 = Present and sufficient to require restraint.
3 = Present, sufficient to require restraint, and accompanied by anger or violence when restraint is used.

d.   Aggressiveness
16. Verbal Outbursts
0 = Not present.
1 = Present (including unaccustomed use of foul or abusive language).
2 = Present and accompanied by anger.
3 = Present, accompanied by anger, and clearly directed at other persons.

17. Physical Threats and/or Violence
0 = Not present.
1 = Threatening behavior.
2 = Physical violence.
3 = Physical violence accompanied by vehemence.

18. Agitation (other than above)
0 = Not present.
1 = Present.
2 = Present with emotional component.
3 = Present with emotional and physical component.
Unspecified?
Describe

e.   Diurnal Rhythm Disturbances
19. Day/Night Disturbance
0 = Not present.
1 = Repetitive wakenings during night.
2 = 50% to 75% of former sleep cycle at night.
3 = Complete disturbance of diurnal rhythm (i.e. less than 50% of former sleep cycle at night).

f.   Affective Disturbance
20. Tearfulness
0 = Not present.
1 = Present.
2 = Present and accompanied by clear affective component.
3 = Present and accompanied by affective and physical component (e.g. "wrings hands" or other gestures).

21. Depressed Mood: Other
0 = Not present.
1 = Present (e.g. occasional statement "I wish I were dead," without clear affective concomitants).

2 = Present with clear concomitants (e.g. thoughts of death).
3 = Present with emotional and physical component (e.g. suicide gestures).
Unspecified?
Describe

g.   Anxieties and Phobias
22. Anxiety Regarding Upcoming Events (Godot Syndrome)
0 = Not present.
1 = Present: Repeated queries and/or other activities regarding upcoming appointments and/or events.
2 = Present and disturbing to caregivers.
3 = Present and intolerable to caregivers.

23. Other Anxieties
0 = Not present.
1 = Present.
2 = Present and disturbing to caregivers.
3 = Present and intolerable to caregivers.
Unspecified?
Describe

24. Fear of being Left Alone
0 = Not present.
1 = Present: Vocalized fear of being alone.
2 = Vocalized and sufficient to require specific action on part of caregiver.
3 = Volcalized and sufficient to require patient to be accompanied at all times.

25. Other Phobias
0 = Not present.
1 = Present.
2 = Present and of sufficient magnitude to require specific action on part of caregiver.
3 = Present and sufficient to prevent patient activities.
Unspecified?
Describe

Part 2: Global Rating
With respect to the above symptoms, they are of sufficient magnitude as to be:
0 = Not at all troubling to the caregiver or dangerous to the patient.
1 = Mildly troubling to the caregiver or dangerous to the patient.
2 = Moderately troubling to the caregiver or dangerous to the patient.
3 = Severely troubling or intolerable to the caregiver or dangerous to the patient.

Source: Reisberg B, Borenstein J, Salob SP, Ferris SH, Franssen E, Georgotas A, Behavioral symptoms in Alzheimer's disease: phenomenology and treatment, *Journal of Clinical Psychiatry*, Vol. 48 (Suppl 5), pp. 9–15, 1987. Copyright © 1986 Barry Reisberg. Reprinted by permission.

Neuropsychiatric Inventory (NPI)

Reference   Cummings JL, Mega M, Gray K, Rosenberg-Thompson S, Carusi DA, Gornbein J (1994) The Neuropsychiatric Inventory: comprehensive assessment of psychopathology in dementia. *Neurology* **44**: 2308–14

Time taken 10 minutes

Rating by clinician in interview with a carer

Main indications

The Neuropsychiatric Inventory (NPI) evaluates a wider range of psychopathology than comparable instruments, and may help distinguish between different causes of dementia; it also records severity and frequency separately.

Commentary

The NPI is a relatively brief interview assessing 10 behavioural disturbances: delusions; hallucinations; dysphoria; anxiety; agitation/aggression; euphoria; disinhibition; irritability/lability; apathy; and aberrant motor behaviour. It uses a screening strategy to cut down the length of time the instrument takes to administer, but it obviously takes longer if replies are positive. It is scored from 1 to 144. Severity and frequency are independently assessed. The authors reported on 40 caregivers, and content and concurrent validity and inter-rater and test/retest reliability were assessed. Some 45 assessments were used for the inter-rater reliability and 20 for test/retest reliability. Concurrent validity was found to be satisfactory using a panel of appropriated experts; concurrent reliability was determined by comparing the NPI subscale with subscales of the BEHAVE-AD (page 75) and the Hamilton Depression Rating Scale (page 4). Highly significant correlations were found. A high level of internal consistency (0.88) was found using a Cronbach's coefficient. Inter-rater reliability revealed agreement in over 90 ratings, and test/retest reliability (a second interview within 3 weeks) was very highly significant. A training pack and further information is available from the author.

Address for correspondence

JL Cummings
Neurobehavior Unit
Psychiatry Service (116F)
West Los Angeles, VAMC
11301 Wilshire Blvd
Los Angeles
CA 90073
USA

Neuropsychiatric Inventory (NPI)

Description of the NPI

The NPI consists of 12 behavioral areas

Delusions	Apathy
Hallucinations	Disinhibition
Agitation	Irritability
Depression	Aberrant motor behaviour
Anxiety	Night-time behaviors
Euphoria	Appetite and eating disorders

Frequency is rated as
1. Occasionally – less than once per week
2. Often – about once per week
3. Frequently – several times a week but less than every day
4. Very frequently – daily or essentially continuously present

Severity is rated as
1. Mild – produce little distress in the patient
2. Moderate – more disturbing to the patient but can be redirected by the caregiver
3. Severe – very disturbing to the patient and difficult to redirect

Distress is scored as
0 – no distress
1 – minimal
2 – mild
3 – moderate
4 – moderately severe
5 – very severe or extreme

For each domain there are 4 scores. Frequency, severity, total (frequency × severity) and caregiver distress. The total possible score is 144 (ie. A maximum of 4 in the frequency rating × 3 in the severity rating × 12 remaining domains) This relates to changes, usually over the 4 weeks prior to completion.

Source: Cummings JL, Mega M, Gray K, Rosenberg-Thompson S, Carusi DA, Gornbein J (1994) The Neuropsychiatric Inventory: comprehensive assessment of psychopathology in dementia. *Neurology* **44**: 2308–14.

Columbia University Scale for Psychopathology in Alzheimer's Disease (CUSPAD)

Reference   Devanand DP, Miller L, Richards M, Marder K, Bell K, Mayeux R, Stern Y (1992) Columbia University Scale for Psychopathology in Alzheimer's Disease. *Archives of Neurology* **49**: 371–6

Time taken 10–15 minutes

Rating most items on a categorical measure of presence or absence in the last month. Interview carried out with carer

Main indications

As a screening instrument for psychopathology in Alzheimer's disease.

Commentary

The Columbia University Scale for Psychopathology in Alzheimer's Disease (CUSPAD) uses operational definitions based on existing definitions of symptomatology. An important development is the differentiation of the delusion as being either fixed (i.e. not amenable to correction) or otherwise. A measure of whether the feature is persistent (more than three times a week) or transient is also made. If the symptom is present, depression items are scored on a five-point scale. The study consisted of reliability on 20 patients between a psychiatrist and lay inter-viewer. Further interviews were carried out with 91 patients with Alzheimer's disease to form the basis of a follow-up study. Inter-rater reliability was high, varying from 0.80 to 1.0 in the conjoint interviews and 0.30 to 0.73 in the independent interviews. The distinction between paranoid ideation and paranoid delusions was underscored by the striking difference in prevalence between a broad and narrow definition of the symptom (narrow corresponding to a true delusion, broad to the wider concept). The strength of the scale is its proven reliability by lay interviewers and its further definition of psychotic symptoms.

Address for correspondence

DP Devanand
New York State Psychiatric Institute
722 West 168 Street
New York
NY 10032
USA

Scale is continued overleaf

Columbia University Scale for Psychopathology in Alzheimer's Disease (CUSPAD)

1. DELUSIONS (past month)

For all **delusions** ask:
(a) Was this the case some of the time or most of the time?

Score –		
	Persistent	0
	Transient	1
	N/A	2

(b) Will the patient accept the truth if corrected?

Score –	No	0
	Yes	1
	N/A	2

General

In the past month, has the patient talked about any strange ideas or unusual beliefs?

	No	0
	Yes	1

If "Yes", can you describe them for me? _____
_____
_____

Paranoid Delusions (past month)

(a) Has the patient felt that others are stealing things from him/her?

	No	0
	Yes	1

(b) Has the patient suspected that his/her wife/husband is unfaithful? (circle N/A if patient is single or widowed)

	No	0
	Yes	1
	N/A	2

(c) Has the patient had any other unfounded suspicions?

	No	0
	Yes	1

If "Yes", can you describe them? _____
_____
_____

Delusions of Abandonment (past month)

Has the patient suspected or accused the caregiver of plotting to leave him/her?

	No	0
	Yes	1

Somatic Delusions (past month)

Has the patient has any false beliefs that he/she has cancer or another physical illness?

	No	0
	Yes	1

Misidentification syndromes (past month)

(a) Has the patient stated that people are in the house/home when nobody is there?

	No	0
	Yes	1

(b) Has the patient looked into the mirror and said it is someone else?

	No	0
	Yes	1

(c) Has the patient misidentified people, for example, said that the spouse/caregiver is an impostor?

	No	0
	Yes	1

(d) Has the patient said that his/her house or home is not his/her home?

	No	0
	Yes	1

(e) Has the patient believed that the characters on television are real or in the room? (Circle N/A if the patient has no access to a television)

	No	0
	Yes	1
	N/A	2

Other Delusions (past month)

Has the patient had any other false beliefs or other strange ideas that I have not asked you about?

	No	0
	Yes	1

If "Yes", can you describe them? _____
_____
_____

2. HALLUCINATIONS (past month)

(a) Has the patient heard voices or sounds when no one is there? (Auditory)

	No	0
	Yes: Vague	1
	Clear	2

(b) Has the patient seen visions? (Visual)

	No	0
	Yes: Vague	1
	Clear	2

(c) Has the patient reported unusual smells like burning rubber, gas or rotten eggs? (Olfactory)

	No	0
	Yes: Vague	1
	Clear	2

(d) Has the patient felt that things are crawling under his/her skin?

No 0
Yes: Vague 1
Clear 2

(e) Has the patient reported any other hallucinations?

No 0
Yes: Vague 1
Clear 2

3. ILLUSIONS (past month)

Has the patient reported that one thing is something else, for example, saying that a pillow looks like a person or a light bulb looks like a fire starting?

No 0
Yes: Vague 1
Clear 2

If "Yes", can you describe them? _____
_____
_____

4. BEHAVIORAL DISTURBANCES (past month)

(a) Has the patient wandered away from home or from the caregiver?

No 0
Yes 1

(b) Has the patient made verbal outburts?

No 0
Yes 1

(c) Has the patient used physical threats and/or violence?

No 0
Threatening behavior 1
Physical violence 2

(d) Has the patient shown agitation or restlessness?

No 0
Yes 1

(e) Has the patient been more confused at night or during evening, compared to the day?

No 0
Yes 1

5. DEPRESSION (past month)

If the answer to items (a) to (c) below is "Yes", circle the appropriate level of severity. If the answer is "No", circle "N/A".

(a) Has the patient been sad, depressed, blue or down in the dumps?

No 0
Yes 1

If "Yes", how do you know they are sad, e.g. do they cry or complain they feel sad?

Write down details: _____
_____
_____

Was he/she depressed?:   N/A   0
  occasionally   1
  some of the time   2
  most of the time   3
  all of the time   4

(b) Has the patient had difficulty sleeping?   No   0
  Yes   1

If "Yes", is there: N/A   0
  slight difficulty   1
  at least 2 hours sleep at night   2
  less than 2 hours sleep at night   3
  excessive sleep/sleepiness   4

(c) Has the patient's appetite changed?   No   0
  Yes   1

If "Yes", circle one: N/A   0
  slightly decreased   1
  no appetite – food is tasteless   2
  need persuasion to eat at all   3
  excessive appetite   4

Symptomatology is absolute not relative.

Reproduced (with permission from the American Medical Association) from Devanand DP, Miller L, Richards M, Marder K, Bell K, Mayeux R, Stern Y (1992) Columbia University Scale for Psychopathology in Alzheimer's Disease. *Archives of Neurology* **49**: 371–6. Copyright 1992. American Medical Association.

Manchester and Oxford Universities Scale for the Psychopathological Assessment of Dementia (MOUSEPAD)

Reference Allen NHP, Gordon S, Hope T, Burns A (1996) Manchester and Oxford Universities Scale for Psychopathological Assessment of Dementia (MOUSEPAD). *British Journal of Psychiatry* **169**: 293–307

Time taken 15–30 minutes
Rating by experienced clinician, most items on a 3-point severity scale. Interview with carers

Main indications

The measurement of psychiatric symptoms and behavioural changes in patients with dementia.

Commentary

There have been a number of different scales assessing non-cognitive features of dementia, and this is one of them. The Manchester and Oxford Universities Scale for the Psychopathological Assessment of Dementia (MOUSEPAD) is based on the longer Present Behavioural Examination (PBE; Hope and Fairburn, 1992), but was developed as being a shorter instrument and one with an equal emphasis on psychiatric symptomatology as much as behavioural changes. The 59-item instrument was developed from questions in the PBE as well as questions derived from empirical studies of the phenomenology of Alzheimer's disease (Burns et al, 1990). The paper presents reliability, sensitivity and validity. Thirty patients were interviewed four times over 6 weeks. The MOUSEPAD has the ability to measure the presence of phenomena in the last month as well as since the onset of dementia defined as the presence of the first change, whether this be memory loss, personality change or otherwise. Test/retest reliability in the main symptoms areas was generally above 0.6. Inter-rater reliability was of a similar magnitude. The range of kappa values for test/retest reliability was 0.4–0.93, 0.56–1.0 for inter-rater reliability and 0.43–0.67 for validity. It

should be noted that the scale contains no items for depression, and the Cornell Scale for Depression in Dementia (page 8), is suggested as the additional instrument (Alexopoulos et al, 1988). Validity was compared with the PBE itself and, while ratings varied, generally there was excellent agreement. A global rating of change suggested that the MOUSEPAD is sensitive to change but that the degree of change observed was slight. Separate ratings of severity and frequency are made.

Additional references

Alexopoulos G, Abrahams R, Young R et al (1988) Cornell Scale for Depression in Dementia. *Biological Psychiatry* **23**: 271–84.

Burns A, Jacoby R, Levy R (1990) Psychiatric phenomena in Alzheimer's disease. I. Disorders of thought content. *British Journal of Psychiatry* **157**: 72–6.

Hope RA, FairburnCG (1992) The Present Behavioural Examination (BPE): the development of an interview to measure current behavioural abnormalities. *Psychological Medicine* **22**: 223–30.

Address for correspondence

Harry Allen
Consultant Psychiatrist
York House
Manchester Royal Infirmary
Oxford Road
Manchester 13
UK

Manchester and Oxford Universities Scale for the Psychopathological Assessment of Dementia (MOUSEPAD)

Descriptive psychopathology of dementia

Name _____

Date

No.

Informant

First, establish the duration of the dementia syndrome in months: How long ago was the first symptom you noticed?
(Cases referred to are 'she'/'her' purely for convenience)

Delusions
(These beliefs should be held firmly, be false, **last for more than seven days** and occur in the absence of acute physical illness.)

	Yes/no	Severity	Months from onset	Duration in months	In last month? Y/N	Convince otherwise
Has she ever said:						
she is being watched or spied upon?	–	–	–	–	–	–
her food or drink is being poisoned?	–	–	–	–	–	–
she is being followed?	–	–	–	–	–	–
her possessions are being hidden?	–	–	–	–	–	–
her possessions are being stolen?	–	–	–	–	–	–
her house is not her own home?	–	–	–	–	–	–
her spouse is having an affair?	–	–	–	–	–	–
she is involved in an amorous affair?	–	–	–	–	–	–
she is about to be abandoned by her family?	–	–	–	–	–	–
someone else is in the house?	–	–	–	–	–	–

Hallucinations
(These experiences can be considered present if the patient has spontaneously complained of the phenomenon or if there is evidence that she has been seen interacting with an apparently false perception. They must have occurred in the absence of acute illness and have lasted for **more than seven days**. NB. Do not rate here patients talking to mirror image, to photographs or to television – these should be rated under misidentifications.)

Has she heard voices or other sounds where there have been none apparent?

	Yes/no	Severity	Months from onset	Duration in months	In last month? Y/N
If so, have they been:					
voices?					
from known persons	–	–	–	–	–
from unknown persons	–	–	–	–	–
does she appear to understand the voices? Yes/No	–	–	–	–	–
music	–	–	–	–	–
animals	–	–	–	–	–
other noises	–	–	–	–	–

Has she seen things where there have been none apparent?

	Yes/no	Severity	Months from onset	Duration in months	In last month? Y/N
If so, have they been:					
people					
known persons	–	–	–	–	–
unknown persons	–	–	–	–	–
dwarf-like figures	–	–	–	–	–
children	–	–	–	–	–
animals	–	–	–	–	–
other					
Has the patient reported strange smells when none have been apparent?	–	–	–	–	–
Has the patient reported strange sensations in her body?	–	–	–	–	–
Has the patient reported an unusual taste in her food or drink	–	–	–	–	–

Scale is continued overleaf

Misidentifications
*(These experiences must have **lasted for at least seven days** and have occurred in the absence of acute physical illness.)*

Has she acted unusually when seeing herself in the mirror?

	Yes/no	Severity	Months from onset	Duration in months	In last month? Y/N
If so, has she:					
claimed that her image is not her own self?	–	–	–	–	–
spent time conversing with her own image?	–	–	–	–	–
Has she ever apparently believed:					
that a close relative or carer is not who they claim to be?	–	–	–	–	–
that they have been replaced by an imposter?	–	–	–	–	–
that TV images or photographs are real events?	–	–	–	–	–
that she is infested with small animals?	–	–	–	–	–

Reduplications
*(These experiences must have **lasted for at least seven days** and have occurred in the absence of acute physical illness.)*

Has she ever said that things have been reduplicated?:
(e.g. that there are two of anyone or anything in existence)

If so what?					
Spouses or carers	–	–	–	–	–
Houses or other inanimate objects	–	–	–	–	–
Animate objects (pets etc.)	–	–	–	–	–

Behavioural changes in dementia
Note any physical problems which might significantly alter ratings (e.g. arthritis might affect her walking around). If physical problem makes rating inappropriate rate 8 and explain.

	Yes/no	Severity	Months from onset	Duration in months	In last month? Y/N
Walking					
Does she walk around more often than she used to just before the memory problems started?					
If yes then rate:					
1: mild: sits most days for more than 15 minutes at a time, awake					
2: severe: will not sit, most days, for as long as 15 minutes at a time, awake	–	–	–	–	–
Does she follow you (or anyone else) around?					
0: follows others around less than 30 minutes each day					
1: follows others around, most days, for more than 30 minutes but less than 2 hours					
2: follows others around for more than 2 hours, most days	–	–	–	–	–
Does she wander out of the house or home (beyond the garden)?					
0: absent or occasional only (less than 1 hour on a typical day)					
1: for less than 3 hours most days					
2: for more than 3 hours most days	–	–	–	–	–

Eating

Has her weight changed since onset of problems?   No/clearly gained/clearly lost

	Yes/no	Severity	Months from onset	Duration in months	In last month? Y/N
Does she eat more than just before the onset of problems than she used to?					
1: eats a little more					
2: eats half as much again, or more	–	–	–	–	–
Does she eat more quickly than just before the onset of problems than she used to?					
1: eats a little more quickly					
2: eats much more quickly	–	–	–	–	–
Have you ever had to limit how much she eats because otherwise she would try to eat too much?					
1: on a few occasions only					
2: need to control intake much of the time	–	–	–	–	–
Does she eat more sweet things than she used to? (More of a sweet tooth)	Yes/No				

	Yes/no	Severity	Months from onset	Duration in months	In last month? Y/N
Sleep					
Is she restless/wakeful during the night?	–	–	–	–	–
Does she confuse night and day?	–	–	–	–	–
Does she "doze" during the day, more than she did before the onset of her problems?	–	–	–	–	–
Sexual behaviour					
Does she talk inappropriately about sex?	–	–	–	–	–
Does she act in a sexually disinhibited manner?	–	–	–	–	–
Aggression					
Has she been physically or verbally aggressive since onset of memory problems (**more** aggressive than before onset of dementia)?			Yes/No		
If yes, under what circumstances?					
While she was being cared for (e.g. washing, dressing)?			Yes/No		
Unprovoked or impatient?			Yes/No		
In response to hallucinations or mistaken ideas you were going to harm her?			Yes/No		
Is the aggression:					
physical – against other people	–	–	–	–	–
– against objects	–	–	–	–	–
verbal	–	–	–	–	–
Does she have outbursts of					
laughing	–	–	–	–	–
crying	–	–	–	–	–
Other types of behaviour in the last month			Yes/No		
Does she move objects and hide them, or put them in strange places?			–		
Does she mislay things?			–		

Rate symptoms, hallucinations, misidentifications and behavioural changes as follows (can be current or occurred in the past):
0 = Absent
1 = Mild (< 1 × week)
2 = Moderate (1 day/week or more but < 4/7 days)
3 = Severe – present at least 4 × week
8 = Not applicable/not asked
9 = Interviewee does not know
Must explain why 8 or 9 given in any question.

Reproduced from the *British Journal of Psychiatry*, Allen NHP, Gordon S, Hope T, Burns A (1996) Manchester and Oxford Universities Scale for Psychopathological Assessment of Dementia (MOUSEPAD). Vol. 169, pp. 293–307. © 1996 Royal College of Psychiatrists. Reproduced with permission.

Present Behavioural Examination (PBE)

Reference   Hope T, Fairburn CG (1992) The present behavioural examination (PBE): the development of an interview to measure current behaviour abnormalities. *Psychological Medicine* 22: 223–30

Time taken   up to 1 hour
Rating   by trained observer

Main indications

Assessment of current behaviour of people with dementia.

Commentary

This is an extremely detailed assessment of the behaviour of people with dementia, equating to the Present State Examination for psychiatric patients and representing the gold standard in such scales. It is a lengthy interview assessing a number of different domains (number of questions in brackets): mental health (15); walking (28); eating (30); diurnal rhythm (19); aggressive behaviour (44); sexual behaviour (5); continence (26); individual behavioural abnormality (20). There are 121 main questions in total, with a further 66 subsidiary questions if a corresponding main question is answered positively. Some 115 of 121 main questions are on a discontinuous scale (i.e. between a 2- and 7-point severity rating scale), with the remaining six on an unlimited ordinal scale. Inter-rater and test/retest reliability is presented, inter-rater reliability ranging from between 0.65 and 1.0 and between 0.16 and 0.74 for test/retest reliability. Some 96% of items were rated the same by each rater in the inter-rater reliability study and 83% in the test/retest reliability study.

Address for correspondence

Tony Hope
Reader in Medicine
Warneford Hospital
Oxford OX3 7JX
UK

CERAD Behavioral Rating Scale

Reference   Tariot PN, Mack JL, Patterson MB, Edland SD, Weiner MF, Fillenbaum G, Blazina L, Teri L, Rubin E, Mortimer JA, Stern Y and the Behavioral Pathology Committee of the Consortium to Establish a Registry for Alzheimer's Disease (1995) The behavioral rating scale for dementia of the Consortium to Establish a Registry for Alzheimer's Disease. *American Journal of Psychiatry* **152**: 1349–57

Time taken 20–30 minutes (reviewer's estimate)
Rating by a trained examiner who meets a predetermined certification standard

Main indications

Rating of psychopathology in patients with probable Alzheimer's disease.

Commentary

This rating scale comes out of the large CERAD (Consortium to Establish a Registry for Alzheimer's Disease) initiative. The scale has 46 questions, most rated on a five-point severity scale but some with a categoric yes/no response. The items were gleaned from existing scales and designed to be administered to a knowledgeable informant. Items were rated by frequency in view of the difficulty of making judgements of severity. Rating is limited to the previous month, although notes can be made of signs and symptoms occurring before that. The original sample consisted of 303 subjects attending 16 Alzheimer centres within the USA. Eight factors were revealed: depressive features; psychotic features; defective self-regulation; irritability/agitation; vegetative features; apathy; aggression; and affective lability. Inter-rater reliability ranges between 91 and 100% with a kappa value ranging from 0.77 to 1.0, the vast majority being over 0.9. A further study (Patterson et al, 1997) followed 64 health controls and 261 patients with Alzheimer's disease over 12 months to assess changes in behaviour over time. Test/retest reliability over 1 month was good, with correlation coefficients between 0.7 and 0.89 for patients with Alzheimer's disease [categorized in terms of scores on the Mini-Mental State Examination (MMSE; page 34)]. There was relatively little change in total behaviour rating scores over 12 months, although there was a decrease in the total score in the normal control group and an increase in patients with Alzheimer's disease whose MMSE score was between 16 and 20. It was suggested that additive scores of correlated items would be a better measure of change in behaviour over time rather than a simple summation of total scores in view of the variability of behaviour over time.

Additional references

Patterson MB, Mack JL (1997) CERAD Behavior Rating Scale for Dementia (BRSD). *Alzheimer Disease and Associated Disorders* **11** (suppl 2): S90–1.

Patterson MB, Mack JL, Mackell JA et al (1997) A longitudinal study of behavioral pathology across five levels of dementia severity in Alzheimer's disease: the CERAD behavior rating scale for dementia. *Alzheimer Disease and Associated Disorders* **11** (Suppl 2): S40–4.

Address for correspondence

Pierre N Tariot
Psychiatry Unit
Monroe Community Hospital
435 East Henrietta Road
Rochester
NY 14620

CERAD Behavioral Rating Scale

1. Has {S} **said** that {S} feels anxious, worried, tense, or fearful? (For example, has {S} expressed worry or fear about being left alone? Has {S} said {S} is anxious or afraid or certain situations?) If so, describe.   A

2. Has {S} shown **physical signs** of anxiety, worry, tension, or fear? (For example, is {S} easily startled? Does {S} appear nervous? Does {S} have a tense or worried facial expression?) If so, describe.   A

3. Has {S} appeared sad or blue or depressed?   A

4. Has {S} expressed feelings of hopelessness or pessimism?   A

5. Has {S} cried within the past month?   A

6. Has {S} said that {S} feels guilty? (For example, has {S} blamed {S's} self for things {S} did in the past?) If yes, describe nature and extent of guilt.   A

7. Has {S} expressed feelings of poor self-esteem? For example, has {S} said that {S} feels like a failure or that {S} feels worthless? This item is intended to reflect global loss of self-esteem rather than simply a concern over loss of, for example, a particular ability.   A

8. Has {S} said {S} feels life is not worth living? Or has {S} expressed a wish to die or done something that suggested {S} was considering suicide? If yes, specify what subject said or did.   A

   If yes or a rating of 8, ask: Has {S} ever made a suicide attempt?
   Include any suicidal gestures in rating this probe.

   0 No
   1 Yes
   9 NA

9. Have there been times when {S} doesn't enjoy the things {S} does as much as {S} used to before {S's} dementia began? This item refers to any specific loss of enjoyment so long as {S} actually engages in the activity in question. {S} need not be an active participant in this activity; {S} need only be present.   B

10. Do you find {S} sometimes can't seem to **get started** on things {S} used to do before {S's} dementia began, even though {S} is **capable** of doing them? (For example, do you find {S} won't start a task or pastime on {S's} own, but with a little encouragement {S} goes ahead and carries it out?) This item refers to any failure to initiate activities, so long as the activities are those which S is still capable of carrying out when given the opportunity.   B

11. Has {S} seemed tired or lacking in energy?   A

12. Was {S's} sleeping pattern in the past month different from the way it was before {S's} dementia began? (For example, does {S} sleep more or less than {S} used to? Does {S} sleep at a different time of day than {S} used to?) If yes, describe change.   B

13. Has {S} had difficulty falling asleep or remaining asleep? If yes, describe.   A

14. Has {S's} appetite during the past month changed from the way it was before {S's} dementia began? (For example, at meal times does {S's} desire to eat seem different?) "Appetite" refers to S's response to food when it is presented in the usual manner.   B
   If yes, circle either increased or decreased appetite, according to informant's judgment.

   1 Increased
   2 Decreased

15. In the past month, has {S} gained or lost weight without intending to?   B
   If yes, circle amount gained or lost.
   Gained:

   1 Up to 5 lbs.
   2 More than 5 lbs.

   Lost:

   1 Up to 5 lbs.
   2 More than 5 lbs.

16. Has {S} had physical complaints that seemed out of proportion to {S's} actual physical problems?   A

17. In the past month, has {S's} sexual interest been different from the way it was before {S's} dementia began? If yes, describe.   B

18. Has {S} shown sudden changes in {S's} emotions? (For example, does {S} go from laughter to tears quickly?)   A

19. Have there been times when {S} was agitated or upset? This item refers to **observable** signs of emotional distress, such as verbal comments, facial expressions, or gestures. It is the **emotional components that distinguishes this item from item 24.**   A

20. Have there been times when {S} was easily irritated or annoyed?   A

21. Has {S} been uncooperative? (For example, does {S} refuse to accept appropriate help? Does {S} insist on doing things {S's} own way?)   A

22. Has {S} been threatening or verbally abusive toward others?   A

23. Has {S} been physically aggressive toward people or things? (For example, has {S} shoved or physically attacked people or thrown or broken objects?)   A

Scale is continued overleaf

24. Has {S} seemed restless or overactive? (For example, does {S} fidget or pace? Does {S} finger things or seem unable to sit still?) When the overactive behavior is associated with emotional agitation that is rated in item 19, it should **not** be rated here also. A

25. Has {S} done things that seem to have no clear purpose or a confused purpose? (For example, does {S} open and close drawers? Does {S} put things in inappropriate places? Does {S} hoard things or rummage through things?) If S's behavior shows a high level of motor activity rather than confusion or lack of purpose, it should be rated under item 24. A

26. Has there been a particular time of day during which {S} seemed more confused than at other times? B

    1 Daytime

If yes, circle time of day   2 Evening (6:00 pm to bedtime)

    3 Night

27. Has {S} wandered or tried to wander for no apparent reason? "Wandering" includes wandering away from one's residence or caregiver, as well as within the residence. If yes, describe incidents. A

28. Has tried to leave home or get away from whoever was taking care of {S} **with** an apparent purpose or destination in mind? If yes, describe incidents. A

29. Has {S} done socially inappropriate things? (For example, does {S} make vulgar remarks? Does {S} talk excessively to strangers? Has {S} sexually exposed {S's} self or done other things such as making gestures of touching people inappropriately? This item is intended to reflect a loss of propriety, not simply confusion. If inappropriate behavior can be rated under a more specific item, such as abusive behavior (item 22) or aggressive behavior (item 23), it should not be rated here. A

30. Does {S} tend to say the same things repeatedly? This item refers to repetitive statements, including questions, phrases, demands, etc. A

31. Does {S} withdraw from social situations? (For example, does {S} avoid groups of people or prefer to be alone? Does {S} avoid participating in activities with others?) A

32. Does {S} seek out more visual or physical contact with {S's} caregivers than before {S's} dementia began? (For example, has {S} seemed "clingy"? Does {S} follow you about and seem to want to be in the same room with you?) B

33. Has {S} misidentified people? (For example, has {S} confused one familiar person with another, or has {S} thought that a familiar person was a stranger?) "Misidentification" means an actual belief that one person was another, not simply a misnaming or failure to remember who someone is, and it refers to someone actually seen by {S}. A

34. Has {S} looked at {S's} -self in a mirror and not recognized {S's} -self? A

35. Has {S} misidentified things? Has {S} thought common things were someting else? (For example, has {S} said that a pillow was a person or that a light bulb was a fire?) If yes, describe. A

36. Has {S} done or said anything that suggests {S} believes people are harming, threatening, or taking advantage of {S} in some way? (For example, with no good reason has {S} thought things have been given away or stolen; has {S} thought {S} was mischarged or over charged for purchase; has {S} seemed suspicious or wary?) A

    0 Yes

If yes, ask: If you try to correct {S}, will {S} accept the truth?   1 No

    9 N/A

37. Has {S} done or said anything that suggests {S} thinks {S's} spouse is unfaithful? A

    0 Yes

If yes, ask: If you try to correct {S}, will {S} accept the truth?   1 No

    9 N/A

38. Has {S} done or said anything that suggests {S} thinks {S's} spouse or caregiver is plotting to abandon {S}? A

    0 Yes

If yes, ask: If you try to correct {S}, will {S} accept the truth?   1 No

    9 N/A

39. Has {S} done or said anything that suggests {S} thinks {S's} spouse or caregiver is an imposter? A

    0 Yes

If yes, ask: If you try to correct {S}, will {S} accept the truth?   1 No

    9 N/A

40. Has {S} done or said anything that suggests {S} thinks that characters on television are real? (For example, has {S} talked to them, acted as if they could hear or see {S}, or said that they were friends or neighbors?) A

    0 Yes

If yes, ask: If you try to correct {S}, will {S} accept the truth?   1 No

    9 N/A

41. Has {S} done or said anything that suggests {S} believes that there are people in or around the house beyond those who are actually there? A

    0 Yes

If yes, ask: If you try to correct {S}, will {S} accept the truth?   1 No

    9 N/A

42. Has {S} done or said anything that suggests {S} believes that a dead person is still alive, even though {S} used to know they were dead? Do not rate memory problems. If {S} simply cannot remember whether a particular person has died, it should not be rated as a mistaken belief. A

		0 Yes
	If yes, ask: If you try to correct {S}, will {S} accept the truth?	1 No
		9 N/A
43.	Has {S} done or said anything that suggests {S} thinks where {S} lives is not really {S's} home, even though {S} used to consider it home?	A
		0 Yes
	If yes, ask: If you try to correct {S}, will {S} accept the truth?	1 No
		9 N/A
44.	Has {S} heard voices or sounds when there was no sound? If yes, describe.	A
	If yes, rate for clarity.	Vague 0 Clear 1
45.	Has {S} seen things or people that were not there? If yes, describe.	A
	If yes, rate for clarity.	Vague 0 Clear 1
46.	Before we stop, I want to be sure we've covered all of {S's} problems, except, of course, for those related to memory loss. Has {S} done anything else in the past month that seemed strange or created difficulties? Has {S} said anything that suggests {S} has some unusual ideas or beliefs that I haven't asked you about? If response concerns purely cognitive symptoms, do not rate. If response contains behaviors that can be rated under other items, do so. Any behavior that is rated here should be described. Indicate the most frequently occurring problem and rate it.	A

S = subject.

Code A:
0 = Not occurred since illness began
1 = 1–2 days in past month
2 = 3–8 days in past month (up to 2 × week)
3 = 9–15 days in past month
4 = 16 days or more in past month
8 = Occurred since illness began, but not in past month
9 = Unable to rate

Code B:
0 = Not occurred since illness began
1 = Yes, has occurred in past month
8 = Occurred since illness began, but not in past month
9 = Unable to rate

American Journal of Psychiatry, Vol. 152, pp. 1349–1357, 1995. Copyright 1995, the American Psychiatric Association. Reprinted by permission.

Rating Scale for Aggressive Behaviour in the Elderly (RAGE)

Reference   Patel V, Hope RA (1992) A rating scale for aggressive behaviour in the elderly – the RAGE. *Psychological Medicine* **22**: 211–21

Time taken less than 5 minutes
Rating by trained interviewer

Main indications

Designed to be of value in studies involving the treatment and correlates of aggressive behaviour in psychogeriatric inpatients.

Commentary

The authors of the Rating Scale for Aggressive Behaviour in the Elderly (RAGE) note the wide availability of global rating scales, but while *useful* they are not reliable in assessing specific problems such as aggressive behaviour. The RAGE scale was specifically designed to be filled in by ward-based nursing staff. Aggression was defined as "... an overt act involving the delivery of noxious stimuli to (but not necessarily aimed at) another organism, object or self which is clearly not accidental". The original set of items was generated following interviews with carers of 40 patients with dementia and the observation period was defined as the past few days (chosen to balance the risk of missing the behaviour if the period is too short and decreased sensitivity if the period is too long). On the basis of feedback from professionals, the scale was revised and underwent inter-rater reliability, test/retest reliability and validation using direct observation. Inter-rater reliability was 0.94 with 86% agreement. Test/retest reliability over 6 hours, 7 and 14 days was excellent. Sensitivity was evaluated by validating the scale scores against descriptions by the nursing staff for changes in behaviour. Other analyses incude intraclass correlation, split half reliability, correlation of individual items and principal components analysis.

Address for correspondence

Tony Hope
Reader in Medicine
Warneford Hospital
Oxford OX3 7JX
UK

Rating Scale for Aggressive Behaviour in the Elderly (RAGE)

Has the patient in the past 3 days . . .

1.	Been demanding or argumentative?	0	1	2	3
2.	Shouted, yelled, or screamed?	0	1	2	3
3.	Sworn or used abusive language?	0	1	2	3
4.	Disobeyed ward rules, e.g. deliberately passed urine outside the commode?	0	1	2	3
5.	Been uncooperative or resisted help, e.g. whilst being given a bath or medication?	0	1	2	3
6.	Been generally in a bad mood, irritable or quick to fly off the handle?	0	1	2	3
7.	Been critical, sarcastic or derogatory, e.g. saying someone is stupid or incompetent?	0	1	2	3
8.	Been inpatient or got angry if something does not suit him/her?	0	1	2	3
9.	Threatened to harm or made statements to scare others?	0	1	2	3
10.	Indulged in antisocial acts, e.g. deliberately stealing food or tripping someone?	0	1	2	3
11.	Pushed or shoved others?	0	1	2	3
12.	Destroyed property or thrown things around angrily, e.g. towels, medicines?	0	1	2	3
13.	Been angry with him/herself?	0	1	2	3
14.	Attempted to kick anyone?	0	1	2	3
15.	Attempted to hit others?	0	1	2	3
16.	Attempted to bite, scratch, spit at, or pinch others?	0	1	2	3
17.	Used an object (such as a towel or a walking stick) to lash out or hurt someone?	0	1	2	3

In the past 3 days, has the patient inflicted any injury . . .

18.	On him/herself?	0	1	2	3
19.	On others?	0	1	2	3

    0   no
    1   mild e.g. a scratch
    2   moderate e.g. a bruise
    3   severe e.g. a fracture

20. Has the patient in the past 3 days been required to be placed under sedation or in isolation or in physical restraints, in order to control his/her aggressiveness?
    0 no; 1 yes

21. Taking all factors into consideration, do you consider the patient's behaviour in the last 3 days to have been aggressive?
    0 not at all
    1 mildly
    2 moderately
    3 severely

Total score:
Any additional comments:

Rating on frequency basis over last 3 days

0 = Never
1 = At least once in past 3 days
2 = At least once every day in past 3 days
3 = More than once every day in past 3 days

Source: Patel V, Hope RA (1992) A rating scale for aggressive behaviour in the elderly – the RAGE. *Psychological Medicine* **22**: 211–21. Reprinted by kind permission of Cambridge University Press.

Overt Aggression Scale (OAS)

Reference Yudofsky SC, Silver JM, Jackson W, Endicott J, Williams D (1986) The Overt Aggression Scale for the objective rating of verbal and physical aggression. *American Journal of Psychiatry* **143**: 35–9

Time taken 5 minutes (reviewer's estimate)

Rating by nurses and nursing aides

Main indications

The scale is designed as an objective rating of verbal and physical aggression specifically to quantify the severity of the aggression and to distinguish those with chronic hostility from those with episodic outbursts.

Commentary

The Overt Aggression Scale (OAS) is divided into four categories: verbal aggression; physical aggression against objects; physical aggression against self; and physical aggression against other people. It is primarily designed to be used in psychiatric settings, and records the severity of the aggression, the timing and duration of the incident and the intervention. Correlation coefficients were greater than 0.5 in 95% of ratings and greater than 0.75 in 52%. The total aggression score had a correlation coefficient of 0.87. Buss and Durkee (1959) describe a hostility scale which forms the basis for many aggression ratings.

Additional reference

Buss A, Durkee A (1957) An inventory for assessing different kinds of hostility. *Journal of Consulting Psychology* **21**: 343–9.

Address for correspondence

SC Yudofsky
Allegheny General Hospital
320 East North Avenue
Pittsburgh
PA 15212
USA

Overt Aggression Scale (OAS)

AGGRESSIVE BEHAVIOR (check all that apply)

Verbal Aggression

__ Makes loud noise, shouts angrily.
__ Yells mild personal insults, e.g. "You're stupid!"
__ Curses viciously, uses foul language in anger, makes moderate threats to others or self.
__ Makes clear threats of violence toward others or self ("I'm going to kill you") or requests to help control self.

Physical Aggression Against Self

__ Picks or scratches skin, hits self, pulls hair (with no or minor injury only).
__ Bangs head, hits fist into objects, throws self onto floor or into objects (hurst self without serious injury).
__ Small cuts or bruises, minor burns.
__ Mutilates self, causes deep cuts, bites that bleed, internal injury, fracture, loss of consciousness, loss of teeth.

Physical Aggression Against Objects

__ Slams door, scatters clothing, makes a mess.
__ Throws objects down, kicks furniture without breaking it, marks the wall.
__ Breaks objects, smashes windows.
__ Sets fires, throws objects dangerously.

Physical Aggression Against Other People

__ Makes threatening gesture, swings at people, grabs at clothes.
__ Strikes, kicks, pushes, pulls hair (without injury to them).
__ Attacks others, causing mild-moderate physical injury (bruises, sprain, welts).
__ Attacks others, causing severe physical injury (broken bones, deep lacerations, internal injury).

Time incident began: __ __:__ __ a.m. / p.m.　　　　Duration of incident: __ __:__ __ (hours:minutes)

INTERVENTION (check all that apply)

__ None.　　　　__ Immediate medication given by mouth.　　__ Use of restraints.

__ Talking to patient.　　__ Immediate medication given by injection.　__ Injury requires immediate medical treatment for patient.

__ Closer observation.　　__ Isolation without seclusion (time out).　　__ Injury requires immediate treatment for other person.

__ Holding patient.　　__ Seclusion.

COMMENTS

American Journal of Psychiatry, Vol. 143, pp. 35–39, 1986. Copyright © 1986, the American Psychiatric Association. Reprinted with permission.

Neurobehavioral Rating Scale (NRS)

Reference   Sultzer DL, Levin HS, Mahler ME, High WM, Cummings JL (1992) Assessment of cognitive, psychiatric, and behavioral disturbances in patients with dementia: the Neurobehavioral Rating Scale. *Journal of the American Geriatrics Society* 40: 549–55

Time taken 30–40 minutes
Rating by observer

Main indications

Characterizes the cognitive, psychiatric and behavioural disturbance in patients with dementia.

Commentary

The Neurobehavioural Rating Scale (NRS) is a comprehensive instrument assessing a very wide range of changes, containing most of the items of the Brief Psychiatric Rating Scale (BPRS; page 194). The original validation study was performed on 83 patients with dementia (61 with Alzheimer's Disease and 22 with multi-infarct dementia). High correlations were found between the scale and depressive symptoms on the Hamilton Depression Rating Scale (page 4). Inter-rater reliability had been previously reported in patients with head injury. Principal components analysis revealed six factors: cognition/insight, agitation/disinhibition, behavioural retardation, anxiety/depression, verbal output disturbance and psychosis.

Additional references

Corrigan JD, Dickerson J, Fisher E et al (1990) The Neurobehavioral Rating Scale: replication in an acute inpatient rehabilitation setting. *Brain Injury* 4: 215–22.

Hilton G, Sisson R, Freeman E (1990) The Neurobehavioral Rating Scale: an inter-rater reliability study in the HIV seropositive population. *Journal of Neuroscience Nursing* 22: 36–42.

Levin HS, High WM, Goethe KE et al (1987) The Neurobehavioral Rating Scale: assessment of the behavioral sequelae of head injury by the clinician. *Journal of Neurology, Neurosurgery and Psychiatry* 50: 183–93.

Address for correspondence

DL Sultzer
Behavioral Neurosciences Section
B-111
West LA VA Medical Center
11301 Wilshire Blvd
Los Angeles
CA 90073
USA

Neurobehavioral Rating Scale (NRS)

___ 1.   Inattention/Reduced Alertness
         Decreased alertness; unable to sustain attention; easily distracted.
___ 2.   Somatic Concern
         Volunteers complaints or elaborates excessively about somatic symptoms.
___ 3.   Disorientation
         Confusion for person, place, or time.
___ 4.   Anxiety
         Worry, apprehension, or overconcern.
___ 5.   Expressive Deficit
         Aphasia, with nonfluent features.
___ 6.   Emotional Withdrawal
         Lack of spontaneous interaction; poor relatedness during interview.
___ 7.   Conceptual Disorganization
         Thought process is loose, disorganized, or tangential.
___ 8.   Disinhibition
         Socially inappropriate comments or actions.
___ 9.   Guilt Feelings
         Self-blame or remose for past behavior.
___ 10. Memory Deficit
         Difficulty learning new information.
___ 11. Agitation
         Excessive motor activity (e.g. restlessness, kicking, arm flailing, roaming).
___ 12. Inaccurate Insight
         Poor insight; exaggerated self-opinion; overrates level of ability.
___ 13. Depressed Mood
         Sadness, hopelessness, despondency, or pessimism.
___ 14. Hostility/Uncooperativeness
         Animosity, belligerence, or oppositional behavior.
___ 15. Decreased Initiative/Motivation
         Fails to initiate or persist in tasks; reluctant to accept new challenges.
___ 16. Suspiciousness
         Mistrust.
___ 17. Fatigability
         Rapidly tires on tasks or complex activities; lethargic.
___ 18. Hallucinations
         Sensory perceptions without corresponding external stimuli.
___ 19. Motor Retardation
         Slowed movements or speech; not primary weakness.
___ 20. Unusual Thought Content
         Odd, strange, or bizarre thoughts; delusions.
___ 21. Blunted Affect
         Reduced emotional tone; reduced range or intensity of affect.
___ 22. Excitement
         Increased emotional tone; elevated mood; euphoria.
___ 23. Poor Planning
         Unrealistic goals; poorly formulated plans for the future.
___ 24. Mood Lability
         Rapid changes in mood that are disproportionate to the situation.
___ 25. Tension
         Postural and facial expression of anxiety; autonomic hyperactivity.
___ 26. Comprehension Deficit
         Difficulty understanding verbal or written instructions.
___ 27. Speech Articulation Defect
         Misarticulation or slurring of words that affects intelligibility.
___ 28. Fluent Aphasia
         Aphasia, with fluent features.

Reproduced from Sultzer DL, Levin HS, Mahler ME, High WM, Cummings JL (1992) Assessment of cognitive, psychiatric, and behavioral disturbances in patients with dementia: the Neurobehavioral Rating Scale. *Journal of the American Geriatrics Society,* Vol. 40, no. 6, pp. 549–55.

Caretaker Obstreperous-Behavior Rating Assessment (COBRA) Scale

Reference Drachman DA, Swearer JA, O'Donnell BF, Mitchell AL, Maloon A (1992) The Caretaker Obstreperous-Behavior Rating Assessment (COBRA) Scale. *Journal of the American Geriatrics Society* 40: 463–70

Time taken 20 minutes (author's estimate)
Rating by observer

Main indications

For the assessment of "obstreperous" behaviours in dementia (defined as difficult and troublesome behaviours).

Commentary

The Caretaker Obstreperous-Behavior Rating Assessment (COBRA) Scale is divided into four main areas: aggressive/assaultive, disordered ideas/personality, mechanical/motor and vegetative, with a total of 30 items. It measures both frequency and severity. A summary score is produced. The scale was validated on 67 patients with dementia. Inter-rater reliability (on seven patients) was between 0.73 and 0.99 for eight of the twelve summary measures and between 0.30 and 0.63 for four. Test/retest reliability correlaton coefficients were significant at $p < 0.01$. Validity was assessed with comparison to cognitive measures and global ratings of dementia.

Address for correspondence

DA Drachman
Department of Neurology
University of Massachusetts Medical Center
55 Lake Avenue North
Worcester
MA 01655
USA

Caretaker Obstreperous-Behavior Rating Assessment (COBRA) Scale

Illustrative examples of the operational definitions used in the COBRA Scale for each of the behavioral categories

Behavioral category	Target behavior	Operational definition
Aggressive/assaultive	Physical attack	Effort or actual physical injury to other, e.g. hit, kick, bite, scratch, etc. If the attack did not end in contact, it was because the patient was physically restrained.
Ideas/personality	Bradyphrenia	Responds slowly to questions and only after a long delay.
Mechanical/motor	Wandering	Aimlessly walks without guidance, frequently away from where he/she should be.
Vegetative	Change in sexuality	
	Hypersexuality	Increased and aggressive interest in sexual activities;
	Hyposexuality	Loss of interest in all sexual activities.

These are **Target Behaviors**
8 OBs = Aggressive/Assaultive
9 OBs = Disordered ideas/Personality
7 OBs = Mechanical/Motor
6 OBs plus subdivisions = vegetative

Videos provided for each OB to facilitate recognition/description by caretaker.

Frequency and severity scales – an intensity assessment for each target OB.

Frequency
0 = Behavior **not** occurred within past 3 months.
1 = |
2 = |
3 = ↓
4 = Behavior occurred daily or more often.

Severity – rate disruptiveness of behavior
0 = No appreciable disruptive effect.
1 = |
2 = |
3 = ↓
4 = Significant danger.
Ceiling scores to differentiate maximum possible effects.

COBRA Scale summary scores

I. Total number of OBs in each category

Behavior	Number present
1. Aggressive/Assaultive	____
2. Ideas/Personality	____
3. Mechanical/Motor	____
4. Vegetative	____

II. Highest severity score in each category

Behavior	Highest Severity Score
5. Aggressive/Assaultive	____
6. Ideas/Personality	____
7. Mechanical/Motor	____
8. Vegetative	____

III. Most severe OBs—all categories
    9. Highest severity score for any OB ____
    10. How many OBs had scores >3? ____

IV. Most frequent OBs—all categories
    11. Highest frequency score for any OB ____
    12. How many OBs had scores >3? ____

Determines behavioral categories, number of different OBs, severity of disruption of OBs and frequency of OB occurrence

Reproduced from Drachman DA, Swearer JA, O'Donnell BF, Mitchell AL, Maloon A (1992) The Caretaker Obstreperous-Behavior Rating Assessment (COBRA) Scale. *Journal of the American Geriatrics Society,* Vol. 40, no. 5, pp. 463–70.

Nurses' Observation Scale for Inpatient Evaluation (NOSIE)

Reference   Honigfeld G, Klett CJ (1965) Nurses' Observation Scale for Inpatient Evaluation: a new scale for measuring improvement in chronic schizophrenia. *Journal of Clinical Psychology* 21: 65–71

Time taken 20 minutes
Rating by nursing staff

Main indications

To assess change in psychopathology in patients with schizophrenia.

Commentary

The Nurses' Observation Scale for Inpatient Evaluation (NOSIE) was designed as a sufficiently sensitive scale to measure change resulting from therapy in older people with schizophrenia but could also be applied in clinical research to any elderly patient or for use in drug trials. The 100 initial items had been drawn from existing scales, and two scales were described: a rating scale of 80 items and a directly derived 30-item scale using only the items derived from a factor analysis which were most sensitive to therapeutic effects. The NOSIE-80 was derived from the initial 100 items by dropping 20 with insufficient inter-rater reliability.

Scoring is based on a three-day observation of the patient on a five-scale frequency score. Seven factors are identified in the NOSIE-80: social competence, social interests, personal neatness, co-operation, irritability, manifest psychosis and psychotic depression. The NOSIE-30 has six factors – co-operation and psychotic depression are absent, with the addition of retardation. Inter-rater reliability was found to be satisfactory.

Additional reference

Honigfeld G, Gillis RD, Klett CJ (1966) NOSIE-30: a treatment-sensitive ward behavior scale. *Psychological Reports* 19: 180–2.

Nurses' Observation Scale for Inpatient Evaluation (NOSIE)

Instructions: For each of the 30 items below you are to rate this patient's behavior during the last **three days only**. Indicate your choice by placing a circle around the correct number before each item.

0 Never
1 Sometimes
2 Often
3 Usually
4 Always

1.	Is sloppy	0	1	2	3	4
2.	Is impatient	0	1	2	3	4
3.	Cries	0	1	2	3	4
4.	Shows interest in activities around him	0	1	2	3	4
5.	Sits, unless directed into activity	0	1	2	3	4
6.	Gets angry or annoyed easily	0	1	2	3	4
7.	Hears things that are not there	0	1	2	3	4
8.	Keeps his clothes neat	0	1	2	3	4
9.	Tries to be friendly with others	0	1	2	3	4
10.	Becomes easily upset if something doesn't suit him	0	1	2	3	4
11.	Refuses to do the ordinary things expected of him	0	1	2	3	4
12.	Is irritable and grouchy	0	1	2	3	4
13.	Has trouble remembering	0	1	2	3	4
14.	Refuses to speak	0	1	2	3	4
15.	Laughs or smiles at funny comments or events	0	1	2	3	4
16.	Is messy in his eating habits	0	1	2	3	4
17.	Starts up a conversation with others	0	1	2	3	4
18.	Says he feels blue or depressed	0	1	2	3	4
19.	Talks about his interests	0	1	2	3	4
20.	Sees things that are not there	0	1	2	3	4
21.	Has to be reminded what to do	0	1	2	3	4
22.	Sleeps, unless directed into activity	0	1	2	3	4
23.	Says that he is not good	0	1	2	3	4
24.	Has to be told to follow hospital routine	0	1	2	3	4
25.	Has difficulty completing even simple tasks on his own	0	1	2	3	4
26.	Talks, mutters, or mumbles to himself	0	1	2	3	4
27.	Is slow moving and sluggish	0	1	2	3	4
28.	Giggles or smiles to himself without any apparent reason	0	1	2	3	4
29.	Quick to fly off the handle	0	1	2	3	4
30.	Keeps himself clean	0	1	2	3	4

Source: Guy (W), Ed.: ECDEU Assessment Manual for Psychopharmacology. Ed. revised. Rockville, Maryland, U.S. Department of Health, Education and Welfare, 1976.

Reproduced from Honigfeld G, Klett C (1965) Nurses' Observational Scale for Inpatient Evaluation (NOSIE): a new scale for measuring improvement in chronic schizophrenia. *Journal of Clinical Psychology* **21**: 65–71. Copyright © 1965, John Wiley & Sons, Inc. Reprinted with permission.

Disruptive Behavior Rating Scales (DBRS)

Reference   Mungas D, Weiler P, Franzi C, Henry R (1989) Assessment of disruptive behavior associated with dementia: the Disruptive Behavior Rating Scales. *Journal of Geriatric Psychiatry and Neurology* **2**: 196–202

Time taken 10 minutes (reviewer's estimate)

Rating by nurses or carers looking after a patient

Main indications

Assessment of disruptive behaviour in patients with dementia.

Commentary

The Disruptive Behavior Rating Scales (DBRS) rate the severity of four categories of disruptive behaviour: physical aggression, verbal aggression, agitation and wandering. The behaviours were defined to minimize clinical judgement in making the ratings, which are made on a five-point severity scale. The scale was designed to assess a narrower range of behaviour than similar scales but to do so in a more detailed manner. A checklist is completed daily and the DBRS ratings made on a weekly basis. Inter-rater reliability gave values of greater than 0.83. Validity was measured against nursing assessment, and principal components analysis was used to measure convergent and discriminant validity showing four main factors: wandering, agitation and aggression.

Address for correspondence

D Mungas

Alzheimer's Disease and Diagnostic Treatment Center

UC Davis Medical Center

2000 Stockton Blvd

Sacramento

CA 95817

USA

Disruptive Behavior Rating Scales (DBRS)

Definition of behaviors

Physical aggression

Overt behavior with clear aggressive intent that is directed at either persons or objects.
Accidental behavior that otherwise fits this definition should not be rated as physical aggression.

Verbal aggression

Verbral behavior with clear aggressive intent directed at persons or objects.

Agitation

Overt behavior that indicates restlessness, hyperactivity, or subjective distress.
Verbal or physical aggressive behavior not directed at a specific target should be rated as agitation.

Wandering

Leaving authorized premises in a manner that clearly indicates that the individual does not have a rational plan for or awareness of where he/she is going.
Total disruptive behaviour: an average of measures one through four.

Name: _____

Week beginning:_____

					Day			
Behavior		1	2	3	4	5	6	7
1.	Hitting							
2.	Kicking							
3.	Biting							
4.	Spitting							
5.	Throwing things							
6.	Using weapons							
7.	Other physical aggression							
8.	Yelling/screaming							
9.	Swearing							
10.	Threatening physical harm							
11.	Critizing							
12.	Scolding							
13.	Other verbal aggression							
14.	Pacing							
15.	Hand wringing							
16.	Unable to sit/lie still							
17.	Rapid speech							
18.	Increased psychomotor activity							
19.	Repeated expressions of distress							
20.	Other signs of agitation							
21.	Wandering							

Rating:

0 = insufficient data
1 = does not occur
2 = occurs but no intervention results
3 = occurs and intervention required
4 = occurs and has major effect, e.g. injury or results in major intervention
5 = occurs and has severe effect or extreme intervention

Reprinted with kind permission of the *Journal of Geriatric Psychiatry and Neurology*, **2**: 196–202, Mungas D, Weiler P, Franzi C, Henry R (1989) Assessment of disruptive behavior associated with dementia: the Disruptive Behavior Rating Scales.

Ryden Aggression Scale

Reference   Ryden MB (1988) Aggressive behavior in persons with dementia who live in the community. *Alzheimer Disease and Associated Disorders* **2**: 342–55

Time taken 20 minutes
Rating by informant

Main indications

To measure aggressive behaviour in community-based persons with dementia.

Commentary

The Ryden Aggression Scale is based on Lanza's model of aggression, and looks at three subscales to measure physical, verbal and sexually aggressive behaviour. The inventory consists of 25 items, each of which is a specific observable aggressive behaviour. It was initially used in a pilot study on 183 community living patients with dementia. Overall inter-rater consistency was 0.88 with test/retest reliability of 0.86.

Additional reference

Lanza M (1983) Origins of aggression. *Journal of Psychosocial Nursing and Mental Health Services* 12: 11–16.

Address for correspondence

Muriel B Ryden
Associate Professor
School of Nursing
University of Minnesota
6-101 Unit F
308 Harvard Street SE
Minneapolis
MN 55455
USA

Ryden Aggression Scale

DIRECTIONS: This rating scale is to be completed by the persons who are most knowledgeable about the individual's behavior.

Below is a list of specific behaviors. To the right of each behavior is a statement about frequency. For each behavior, _circle_ the statement that best describes how often the person demonstrates this behavior.

Ratings are to be based on information you have as to how the person has acted in the past, but you need not have actually observed each of the behaviors reported.

EXAMPLE: If the person doubled up his/her fist without hitting once or twice every week, you would complete the item as shown below.

| MAKING THREATENING GESTURES | Never | Less than once a year | 1–11 times a year | 1–3 times a month | (1–6 times a week) | 1 or more times daily |

EXAMPLE: If the person has never bit anyone, you would complete the item as shown below.

| BITING | (Never) | Less than once a year | 1–11 times a year | 1–3 times a month | 1–6 times a week | 1 or more times daily |

Be sure to respond to _every_ item by circling the response that best describes how often the person demonstrates that particular behavior. Do not leave any items unanswered.

PHYSICALLY AGGRESSIVE BEHAVIOR

	(0)	(1)	(2)	(3)	(4)	(5)
1. PUSHING/SHOVING	Never	Less than once a year	1–11 times a year	1–3 times a month	1–6 times a week	1 or more times daily
2. SLAPPING	Never	Less than once a year	1–11 times a year	1–3 times a month	1–6 times a week	1 or more times daily
3. HITTING/PUNCHING	Never	Less than once a year	1–11 times a year	1–3 times a month	1–6 times a week	1 or more times daily
4. PINCHING/ SQUEEZING	Never	Less than once a year	1–11 times a year	1–3 times a month	1–6 times a week	1 or more times daily
5. PULLING HAIR	Never	Less than once a year	1–11 times a year	1–3 times a month	1–6 times a week	1 or more times daily
6. SCRATCHING	Never	Less than once a year	1–11 times a year	1–3 times a month	1–6 times a week	1 or more times daily
7. BITING	Never	Less than once a year	1–11 times a year	1–3 times a month	1–6 times a week	1 or more times daily
8. SPITTING	Never	Less than once a year	1–11 times a year	1–3 times a month	1–6 times a week	1 or more times daily
9. ELBOWING	Never	Less than once a year	1–11 times a year	1–3 times a month	1–6 times a week	1 or more times daily
10. KICKING	Never	Less than once a year	1–11 times a year	1–3 times a month	1–6 times a week	1 or more times daily
11. TACKLING	Never	Less than once a year	1–11 times a year	1–3 times a month	1–6 times a week	1 or more times daily
12. MAKING THREATENING GESTURES	Never	Less than once a year	1–11 times a year	1–3 times a month	1–6 times a week	1 or more times daily
13. THROWING AN OBJECT	Never	Less than once a year	1–11 times a year	1–3 times a month	1–6 times a week	1 or more times daily
14. STRIKING A PERSON WITH AN OBJECT	Never	Less than once a year	1–11 times a year	1–3 times a month	1–6 times a week	1 or more times daily
15. BRANDISHING A WEAPON	Never	Less than once a year	1–11 times a year	1–3 times a month	1–6 times a week	1 or more times daily
17. DAMAGING PROPERTY	Never	Less than once a year	1–11 times a year	1–3 times a month	1–6 times a week	1 or more times daily

If the person has shown other physically aggressive behavior that was not listed above, please describe the behavior.

| HOW OFTEN DOES IT OCCUR? | Never | Less than once a year | 1–11 times a year | 1–3 times a month | 1–6 times a week | 1 or more times daily |

Scale is continued overleaf

Ryden Aggression Scale

VERBALLY AGGRESSIVE BEHAVIOR	(0)	(1)	(2)	(3)	(4)	(5)
18. NAME CALLING	Never	Less than once a year	1–11 times a year	1–3 times a month	1–6 times a week	1 or more times daily
19. MAKING VERBAL THREATS	Never	Less than once a year	1–11 times a year	1–3 times a month	1–6 times a week	1 or more times daily
20. CURSING, DIRECTED AT A PERSON	Never	Less than once a year	1–11 times a year	1–3 times a month	1–6 times a week	1 or more times daily
21. HOSTILE, ACCUSATORY LANGUAGE DIRECTED AT A PERSON	Never	Less than once a year	1–11 times a year	1–3 times a month	1–6 times a week	1 or more times daily

If the person has shown other verbally aggressive behavior that was not listed above, please describe the behavior.

HOW OFTEN DOES IT OCCUR?	Never	Less than once a year	1–11 times a year	1–3 times a month	1–6 times a week	1 or more times daily

SEXUALLY AGGRESSIVE BEHAVIOR

Many of the following behaviors are ways in which we customarily show love and affection for each other. Such behaviors are considered to be sexually aggressive ONLY IF THEY ARE AGAINST THE EXPRESSED WILL AND/OR DESPITE THE RESISTANCE OF THE OTHER PERSON.

If the person has not acted sexually toward anyone against their will and/or despite their resistance, then circle "Never" opposite each behavior. If the person has ever done any of the listed behaviors in a sexually aggressive way, then circle the item opposite each behavior that indicates how often this happened.

	(0)	(1)	(2)	(3)	(4)	(5)
22. KISSING	Never	Less than once a year	1–11 times a year	1–3 times a month	1–6 times a week	1 or more times daily
23. HUGGING	Never	Less than once a year	1–11 times a year	1–3 times a month	1–6 times a week	1 or more times daily
24. TOUCHING BODY PARTS	Never	Less than once a year	1–11 times a year	1–3 times a month	1–6 times a week	1 or more times daily
25. INTERCOURSE	Never	Less than once a year	1–11 times a year	1–3 times a month	1–6 times a week	1 or more times daily
26. MAKING OBSCENE GESTURES	Never	Less than once a year	1–11 times a year	1–3 times a month	1–6 times a week	1 or more times daily

If the person has shown other sexually aggressive behavior that was not listed above, please describe the behavior.

HOW OFTEN DOES IT OCCUR	Never	Less than once a year	1–11 times a year	1–3 times a month	1–6 times a week	1 or more times daily

Source: Ryden MB (1988) Aggressive behavior in persons with dementia who live in the community. Alzheimer Disease and Associated Disorders 2: 342–55. Reproduced with permission from Lippincott-Raven Publishers.

Agitated Behavior Mapping Instrument (ABMI)

References Cohen-Mansfield J, Watson V, Meade W, Gordon M, Leatherman J, Emor C (1989) Does sundowning occur in residents of an Alzheimer unit? *International Journal of Geriatric Psychiatry* **4**: 294–8

Cohen-Mansfield J, Marx MS, Rosenthal AS (1989) A description of agitation in a nursing home. *Journal of Gerontology* **44**: M77–M84

Time taken see below

Rating by trained observers (rating from the manual and appropriate training are essential – contact Jiska Cohen-Mansfield at address below for further details)

Main indications

For the observation of behavioural disturbance in residents of nursing facilities.

Commentary

The Agitated Behavior Mapping Instrument (ABMI) is a way of quantifying agitated behaviour by direct observation. It is based on the Cohen-Mansfield Agitation Inventory (CMAI, Cohen-Mansfield, 1986). Twenty-five specific agitated behaviours are assessed encompassing the following categories: verbal non-aggressive, physical non-aggressive, verbal aggressive and physical aggressive behaviours. A training programme familiarizes observers with behaviour mapping techniques in general and continues throughout the course of any study. Observers are instructed to remain at an unobtrusive distance from the resident and, in this study, observe residents for 3 minutes during each hour of a 24-hour day stratified randomly over a period of 2 months.

Eight residents were observed over a 1-hour period and a rating made if a particular behaviour remained constant during the 3-minute observation periods. Numerical values were assigned in accordance with this.

Additional references

Cohen-Mansfield J (1986) Agitated behaviors in the elderly. II. Preliminary results in the cognitively deteriorated. *Journal of the American Geriatrics Society* **34**: 722–7.

Cohen-Mansfield J, Billig N (1986) Agitated behaviors in the elderly. I. A conceptual review. *Journal of the American Geriatrics Society* **34**: 711–21.

Address for correspondence

Jiska Cohen-Mansfield
Director of Research
Hebrew Home
Greater Washington
6121 Montrose Road
Rockville
MD 20852
USA

The Cohen-Mansfield Agitation Inventory (CMAI) – Short Form

1. Cursing or verbal aggression
2. Hitting (including self), Kicking, Pushing, Biting, Scratching, Aggressive spitting (include at meals)
3. Grabbing onto people, Throwing things, Tearing things or destroying property
4. Other aggressive behaviors or self-abuse including: Intentional falling, Making verbal or physical sexual advances, Eating/drinking/chewing inappropriate substances, Hurt self or other
5. Pace, aimless wandering, Trying to get to a different place (e.g., out of the room, building)
6. General restlessness, Performing repetitious mannerisms, tapping, strange movements
7. Inappropriate dress or disrobing
8. Handling things inappropriately
9. Constant request for attention or help
10. Repetitive sentences, calls, questions or words
11. Complaining, Negativism, Refusal to follow directions
12. Strange noises (weird laughter or crying)
13. Hiding things, Hoarding things
14. Screaming

Rating:
1 = Never; 2 = < 1 × per week; 3 = Once or several times/week; 4 = Once or several times a day
5 = A few times an hour or continuous for ½ hour or more
If more than one occurred per group then summate occurrences.

NB This is the short form CMAI. Other forms exist, e.g. Community Form CMAI, Disruptiveness Relatives CMAI

Brief Agitation Rating Scale (BARS)

Reference   Finkel SI, Lyons JS, Anderson RL (1993) A Brief Agitation Rating Scale (BARS) for nursing home elderly. *Journal of the American Geriatrics Society* 41: 50–2

Time taken 5 minutes (reviewer's estimate)
Rating by caregiver

Main indications

A brief scale to assess agitation in nursing home residents based on the Cohen-Mansfield Agitation Inventory (CMAI; page 110).

Commentary

The Brief Agitation Rating Scale (BARS) was developed after the CMAI was administered to 232 nursing home residents by inteviewers trained by a psychiatrist. The BARS was developed following a three-stage process. First, correlations of individual items against total score were rated, with those having a high correlation selected for possible inclusion. Secondly, inter-rater reliability was assessed. Thirdly, items were selected to be representative of the original CMAI scale. Cronbach's alpha showed reliability of 0.74–0.82, depending on the time of day when the scale was completed. Inter-rater reliability as assessed by intraclass correlation was 0.73. Validity was assessed using the BEHAVE-AD (page 75) and the Behavioural Syndrome Scale for Dementia (quoted in the paper). Correlations were generally high, although greater on those taken throughout the day than those in the evening or at night.

The following ten behaviours were rated in the BARS: hitting, grabbing, pushing, pacing or aimless wandering, performing repetitive mannerisms, restlessness, screaming, repetitive sentences or questions, strange noises and complaining.

Additional reference

Devanand DP, Brown RP, Sackeim HA et al (1990) Behavioural syndromes in Alzheimer's disease. *International Psychogeriatrics* 2.

Address for correspondence

SI Finkel
Department of Psychiatry and Behavioral Sciences
446 E Ontario #830
Chicago
IL 60611

Cohen-Mansfield Agitation Inventory (CMAI) – Long Form

References   Cohen-Mansfield J (1986) Agitated behaviors in the elderly. II. Preliminary results in the cognitively deteriorated. *Journal of the American Geriatrics Society* **34**: 722–7

Cohen-Mansfield J, Marx MS, Rosenthal AS (1989) A description of agitation in a nursing home. *Journal of Gerontology* **44**: M77–M84

Time taken 10–15 minutes
Rating by carers (rating from the manual and appropriate training are essential – contact Jiska Cohen-Mansfield at address below for further details)

Main indications

To look at agitated behaviour in patients with cognitive impairment.

Commentary

A seven-point rating scale assessing the frequency with which patients manifest up to 29 agitated behaviours.

Address for correspondence

Jiska Cohen-Mansfield
Director of Research
Hebrew Home
Greater Washington
6121 Montrose Road
Rockville
MD 20852
USA

Cohen-Mansfield Agitation Inventory (CMAI) – Long Form

1. Pace, aimless wandering
2. Inappropriate dress or disrobing
3. Spitting (include at meals)
4. Cursing or verbal aggression
5. Constant unwarranted request for attention or help
6. Repetitive sentence or questions
7. Hitting (including self)
8. Kicking
9. Grabbing onto people
10. Pushing
11. Throwing things
12. Strange noises (weird laughter or crying)
13. Screaming
14. Biting
15. Scratching
16. Trying to get to a different place (e.g., out of the room, building)
17. Intentional falling
18. Complaining
19. Negativism
20. Eating/drinking inappropriate substances
21. Hurt self or other (cigarette, hot water, etc.)
22. Handling things inappropriately
23. Hiding things
24. Hoarding things
25. Tearing things or destroying property
26. Performing repetitive mannerisms
27. Making verbal sexual advances
28. Making physical sexual advances
29. General restlessness

As manifest during last fornight
Rating:
1 = Never
2 = < 1 × week
3 = 1–2 × per week
4 = Several times a week
5 = Once or twice per day
6 = Several times per day
7 = Several times an hour

Dementia Behavior Disturbance Scale

Reference   Baumgarten M, Becker R, Gauthier S (1990) Validity and reliability of the Dementia Behavior Disturbance Scale. *Journal of the American Geriatrics Society* **38**: 221–6

Time taken 10–15 minutes (reviewer's estimate)
Rating in an interview with the patient's primary caregiver, or as a self-administered scale by the carer

Main indications
Measurement of behavioural disturbances in dementia.

Commentary
The Dementia Behavior Disturbance Scale is a 28-item scale developed to avoid some of the problems with earlier scales, for example the confusion of collecting information about cognitive and non-cognitive features in the same instrument. A need for assessment outside the clinical setting was also considered. Two samples were assessed: community-residing patients assessed at a geriatric assessment unit and patients taking part in a drug trial. Test/retest reliability (2 weeks later) was 0.71, internal consistency was 0.84 and construct validity was described in terms of positive correlations with the Behavioural and Mood Disturbance Scale (BMDS; page 253).

Address for correspondence
M Baumgarten
Community Health Department
St Justine Hospital
3175 Cote St Catherine
Montreal
Quebec H3T 1C5
Canada

Dementia Behavior Disturbance Scale

Asks same question repeatedly
Loses, misplaces, or hides things
Lack of interest in daily activities
Wakes up at night for no obvious reason
Makes unwarranted accusations
Sleeps excessively during the day
Paces up and down
Repeats the same action over and over
Is verbally abusive, curses
Dresses inappropriately
Cries or laughs inappropriately
Refuses to be helped with personal care
Hoards things for no obvious reason
Moves arms or legs in a restless or agitated way

Empties drawers or closets
Wanders in the house at night
Gets lost outside
Refuses to eat
Overeats
Is incontinent of urine
Wanders aimlessly outside or in the house during the day
Makes physical attacks (hits, bites, scratches, kicks, spits)
Screams for no reason
Makes inappropriate sexual advances
Exposes private body parts
Destroys property or clothing
Is incontinent of stool
Throws food

Patient's primary caregiver is respondent. There are five possible responses corresponding to behaviour frequency in preceding week:

0 = Never
4 = All the time

Thus, higher scores indicate more disturbance.

Pittsburgh Agitation Scale (PAS)

Reference Rosen J, Burgio L, Kollar M, Cain M, Allison M, Fogleman M, Michael M, Zubenko GS (1994) The Pittsburg Agitation Scale: a user-friendly instrument for rating agitation in dementia patients. *American Journal of Geriatric Psychiatry* **2**: 52–9

Time taken less than 1 minute
Rating by direct observation for between 1 and 8 hours by clinical staff

Main indications

To assess agitation in patients with dementia.

Commentary

The Pittsburgh Agitation Scale (PAS) provides a quantification of the severity of disruptive behaviour within four general behaviour groups: aberrant vocalizations; motor agitation; aggressiveness; resisting care on a scale ranging from 0 to 4. The score reflects the most disruptive or severe behaviour within each behaviour group, and thus an improvement in the PAS score may reflect a decline in a severely disruptive behaviour but other symptoms of agitation may exist. The score is useful when taken in the context that levels of agitation can vary within environments, and should the patient change environments the scores may alter. Inter-rater reliability exceeded 0.80 – validity was assessed by the number of interventions needed.

Address for correspondence

Jules Rosen
Western Psychiatric Institute and Clinic
3811 O'Hara Street
Pittsburgh
PA 15213
USA

Pittsburgh Agitation Scale (PAS)

Hours of sleep this rating period

Circle only the highest intensity score for each behavior group that you observed during this rating period. Use the anchor points as a guide to choose a suitable level of severity. (Not all anchor points need be present. Choose the more severe level when in doubt.)

Behavior groups

Aberrant vocalization

(repetitive requests or complaints, nonverbal vocalizations, e.g., moaning, screaming)

Intensity during rating period

0. Not present
1. Low volume, not disruptive in milieu, including crying
2. Louder than conversational, mildly disruptive, redirectable
3. Loud, disruptive, difficult to redirect
4. Extremely loud screaming or yelling, highly disruptive, unable to redirect

Motor agitation

(pacing, wandering, moving in chair, picking at objects, disrobing, banging on chair, taking others' possessions. Rate "intrusiveness" by normal social standards, not by effect on other patients in milieu. If "intrusive" or "disruptive" due to noise, rate under "Vocalization.")

0. Not present
1. Pacing or moving about in chair at normal rate (appears to be seeking comfort, looking for spouse, purposeless movements)
2. Increased rate of movements, mildly intrusive, easily redirectable
3. Rapid movements, moderately intrusive or disruptive, difficult to redirect
4. Intense movements, extremely intrusive or disruptive, not redirectable verbally

Aggressiveness

(score "0" if aggressive only when resisting care)

0. Not present
1. Verbal threats
2. Threatening gestures; no attempt to strike
3. Physical toward property
4. Physical toward self or others

Resisting care

(circle associated activity)
Washing
Dressing
Eating
Meds
Other

0. Not present
1. Procrastination or avoidance
2. Verbal/gesture of refusal
3. Pushing away to avoid task
4. Striking out at caregiver

Were any of the following used during this rating period because of behavior problems? (Circle interventions used.)

Seclusion
PRN Meds (specify)
Restraint
Other interventions

Reproduced from Rosen J, Burgio L, Kollar M, Cain M, Allison M, Fogleman M, Michael M, Zubenko GS (1994) The Pittsburg Agitation Scale: a user-friendly instrument for rating agitation in dementia patients. *American Journal of Geriatric Psychiatry* **2**: 52–9, with permission.

Dysfunctional Behaviour Rating Instrument (DBRI)

Reference   Molloy DW, McIlroy WE, Guyatt GH, Lever JA (1991) Validity and reliability of the Dysfunctional Behaviour Rating Instrument. *Acta Psychiatrica Scandinavica* **84**: 103–6

Time taken 10–15 minutes (reviewer's estimate)
Rating by nurse observer

Main indications

Rating of behaviour in community-living elderly people.

Commentary

The Dysfunctional Behaviour Rating Instrument (DBRI) was developed as a short, simple, comprehensive instrument to be completed by the caregiver which measures the frequency of, and caregiver's responses to, a range of behaviours found in elderly people with cognitive impairment. The specific goal was to assess the effect of behavioural disturbances on carers of patients suffering from dementia. Some 240 consecutive referrals were assessed in addition to the DBRI, the Mini-Mental State Examination (MMSE; page 34) and the Lawton and Brody Instrumental Activities of Daily Living Scale (IADL; page 128). The scale consists of 25 questions rated on a six-point scale. Inter-rater reliability was assessed using a subgroup of 35 subjects and caregivers who were assessed three times at three week intervals.

Construct validity of the DBRI was assessed by comparing it with the BPC, the Standardized MMSE (page 36) and the IADL Scale. The intraclass correlation coefficient for intra-observer reliability of DBRI was 0.75. Validity was shown by early significant correlation between the DBRI items and the BPC items. Significant negative correlations were found between the MMSE and the DBRI.

Additional reference

Molloy DW, Bédard M, Guyatt GH, Lever J (1996) Dysfunctional Behavior Rating Instrument. *International Psychogeriatrics* **8** (suppl 3): 333–41.

Address for correspondence

DW Molloy
Henderson General Hospital
711 Concession Street
Hamilton
Ontario L8V 1C3
Canada

Dysfunctional Behaviour Rating Instrument (DBRI)

1. Ask same questions over and over
2. Repeats stories over and over
3. Refused to cooperate
4. Became angry
5. Was withdrawn (did not speak or do anything unless he/she was asked)
6. Was demanding
7. Was afraid to be left alone
8. Was aggressive
9. Was hiding things
10. Was suspicious
11. Had temper outbusts
12. Had delusions, i.e. thought that:
    Spouse was "not my wife/husband"
    Home was "not my home"
    There were "people in the house"
    That "people were stealing things"
    Other:
13. Hallucinations:
    Saw things that were not there
    Heard things or people that were not there
    Other:
14. Was agitated, e.g. pacing
15. Was crying
16. Was frustrated
17. Wandered, got lost in house, property or elsewhere
18. Was up at night
19. Wanted to leave
20. Kept changing mind
21. Embarrassing behaviour in public
22. Are there any other behaviours not mentioned above that [patient's name] had?

If yes, how often does this occur?
Rating:

0 = never
1 = about every 2 weeks
2 = about 1 × week
3 = > 1 × week
4 = at least 1 × day
5 = > 5 × a day

Then – how much of a problem is this?
Rating:

0 = No problem
1 = Very little problem
2 = Little problem
3 = Somewhat of a problem
4 = Moderate problem
5 = Great deal of a problem

Reproduced (with permission from the Geriatric Research Group) from Molloy DW, McIlroy WE, Guyatt GH, Lever JA (1991) Validity and reliability of the Dysfunctional Behaviour Rating Instrument. *Acta Psychiatrica Scandinavica* **84**: 103–6.

Irritability, Aggression and Apathy

Reference Burns A, Folstein S, Brandt J, Folstein M (1990) Clinical assessment of irritability, aggression and apathy in Huntington and Alzheimer's Disease. *Journal of Nervous and Mental Disease* 178: 20–6

Time taken 10 minutes
Rating by semi-structured interview with informant

Main indications
The scale is designed to measure non-cognitive features of irritability and apathy in dementia.

Commentary
The Irritability, Aggression and Apathy scale incorporated the Yudofsky Aggression Scale in conjunction with questions relating to irritability and pathy. It was validated on 31 patients with Alzheimer's disease and 26 with Huntington's disease. Inter-rater reliability was over 0.85, scores correlated with those on the Psychogeriatric Dependency Rating Scales (PGDRS; page 174) and were significantly greater than controls.

Additional references
Yudofsky SC, Silver JM, Jackson W et al (1986) The Overt Aggression Scale for the objective rating of verbal and physical aggression. *Am J of Psychiatry* **143** 35–39.

Address for correspondence
Alistair Burns
Dept of Psychiatry
Withington Hospital
Manchester M20 8LR
UK

Irritability, Aggression and Apathy

Please answer the following questions about your ____ according to how he/she is not, compared with how he/she was before his/her health problems began. (It may be necessary to emphasize that the questionnaire relates to behaviour since the nset of illness and not in the very recent past. An open-ended question such as "what effect has your ____ illness had on him/her" may be used.)

Irritability

1. How irritable would you say he/she was?   Score

   1   2   3   4   5

     not at all   extremely   ____

     irritable   irritable

		Never (score = 1)	Sometimes (score = 2)	Always (score = 3)
2.	Does he/she sulk after he/she is angry?	____	____	____
3.	Does he/she "pout" if he/she does not get his/her own way?	____	____	____
4.	Does he/she get into arguments?	____	____	____
5.	Does he/she raise his/her voice in anger?	____	____	____
			Total score	____
				(maximum = 17)

Apathy

1. Has his/her interest in everyday events changed?   Score

   1   2   3   4   5

   much more   just the   much less

   interested   same   interested   ____

2. How long does he/she stay lying in bed or sitting in a chair doing nothing during the day?

   1   2   3   4   5

   no more than   all the

   anyone else   time   ____

3. How active is he/she in day to day activities?

   1   2   3   4   5

   very active   normal   very inactive   ____

4.   How busy does he/she keep him/herself?

1	2	3	4	5
same hobbies as usual	less so but still has hobbies	prefers doing nothing but does with prompting	prefers watching TV or watches others doing things	if left alone does nothing

____

5.   Does the patient seem withdrawn from things?

1	2	3	4	5
not at all	a little more than usual	more than usual	much more than usual	yes, definitely

____

Total score ____
(maximum = 25)

Reproduced from Burns A, Folstein S, Brandt J, Folstein M (1990) Clinical assessment of irritability, aggression and apathy in Huntington and Alzheimer's Disease. *Journal of Nervous and Mental Disease*, Vol. 178, no. 1, pp. 20–6.

Reliability, Validity and Clinical Correlates of Apathy in Parkinson's Disease

Reference   Starkstein SE, Mayberg HS, Preziosi TJ, Andrezejewski P, Leiguarda R, Robinson RG (1992)
Reliability, validity and clinical correlates of apathy in Parkinson's disease. *Journal of Neuropsychiatry and Neurosciences* **4**: 134–9

Time taken 5–10 minutes (reviewer's estimate)
Rating by clinician during interview with patient

Main indications

Assessment of apathy in patients with Parkinson's disease.

Commentary

This scale is an abridged version of a larger scale (Marin, 1990). The scale consists of 14 items rated on a three-point scale. The total score possible is 42; the higher the score the greater the apathy. Inter-rater and test/retest reliability (Spearman correlation) was above 0.80 and internal consistency, as demonstrated by Cronbach's alpha, was 0.76. Validity was assessed by asking a clinician to rate apathy independently, and whilst there did not seem to be an association between apathy and depression, apathy was associated with deficits of verbal memory and time-dependent tasks. A number of neuropsychological tests confirmed the validity of the scale and there seems no reason why the scale (properly validated) could not be used to assess apathy in other conditions.

Additional reference

Marin R (1990) Differential diagnosis and classification of apathy. *American Journal of Psychiatry* 147: 22–30.

Address for correspondence

Sergio E Starkstein
Institute of Neurological Investigation
Ayacucho 2166/68
1112 Buenos Aires
Argentina

Reliability, Validity and Clinical Correlates of Apathy in Parkinson's Disease

1. Are you interested in learning new things?
2. Does anything interest you?
3. Are you concerned about your condition?
4. Do you put much effort into things?
5. Are you always looking for something to do?
6. Do you have plans and goals for the future?
7. Do you have motivation?
8. Do you have the energy for daily activities?
9. Does someone have to tell you what to do each day?
10. Are you indifferent to things?
11. Are you unconcerned with many things?
12. Do you need a push to get started on things?
13. Are you neither happy nor sad, just in between?
14. Would you consider yourself apathetic?

Scoring:

Questions 1–8:   3 points = not at all
                 2 points = slightly
                 1 point = some
                 0 point = a lot

Questions 9–14: 3 points = a lot
                 2 points = some
                 1 point = slightly
                 0 point = not at all

Scores range from 0 to 42
Higher scores indicate more severe apathy

Reproduced from Starkstein SE, Mayberg HS, Preziosi TJ, Andrezejewski P, Leiguarda R, Robinson RG (1992) Reliability, validity and clinical correlates of apathy in Parkinson's disease. *Journal of Neuropsychiatry and Neurosciences* **4**: 134–9, with permission.

BEAM-D

Reference   Sinha D, Zemlan FP, Nelson S, Bienenfeld D, Thienhaus O, Ramaswamy G, Hamilton S (1992) A new scale for assessing behavioral agitation in dementia. *Psychiatry Research* **41**: 73–88

Time taken 20 minutes (reviewer's estimate)
Rating by trained raters

Main indications

To assess the effects of treatment on behavioural problems of inpatients with dementia.

Commentary

Some 45 patients with a diagnosis of primary degenerative dementia were assessed. The BEAM-D scale consists of 16 items – target behaviour and inferred states. Inter-rater reliabilities ranged from 0.70 to 1.0, with individual kappa statistics varying from 0.56 to 1.0. Concurrent validity was assessed using the Brief Psychiatric Rating Scale (BPRS; page 194) and the Sandoz Clinical Assessment – Geriatric (SCAG; page 188).

Address for correspondence

FP Zemlan
Alzheimer's Research Center
University of Cincinnati
College of Medicine
Cincinnati
OH 45267–0559
USA

BEAM-D

Target behaviors

1. Hostility/aggression
Verbal and nonverbal expressions of anger and resentment
0 = No information; not assessed; unable to assess.
1 = Patient has neither expressed nor manifested any
hostile/aggressive behavior.
2 = Patient has openly expressed verbally aggressive/hostile
behavior – at least one ot two separate instances.
3 = Patient has been overtly aggressive at least one to two
separate instances; physically assaultive behavior may
be manifested.
4 = Patient has been overtly aggressive – at least three or
more separate instances; physically assaultive behavior
may be manifested.

2. Destruction of property (belonging to self or others)
Extent to which the patient willfully damages, or causes
destruction of property.
0 = No information; not assessed; unable to assess.
1 = Patient has not damaged personal or others' property.
2 = At least one or two separate instances.
3 = At least three or four separate instances.
4 = Continuously engaged in destructive activities.

3. Disruption of others' activities
Extent to which the patient disrupts the activities of others.
0 = No information; not assessed; unable to assess.
1 = Patient has not interrupted the activities of others at any
time.
2 = 3 or fewer instances.
3 = 4 or more instances.
4 = Continuously disruptive to others.

4. Uncooperativeness
Extent to which the patient is responsive and receptive to
the feelings and needs of others.
0 = No information; not assessed; unable to assess.
1 = Rarely exhibits inconsiderate, discourteous behavior.
2 = Generally unconcerned about the needs and feelings of
others.
3 = Inconsiderate of and unconcerned about the needs and
feelings of others; neither cooperativeness nor courtesy;
patient's presence is still tolerated by others.
4 = Consistently inconsiderate of and unconcerned about
the needs and feelings of others; patient's presence is
infrequently tolerated by others.

5. Noncompliance
0 = No information; not assessed; unable to assess.
1 = Patient has been responsive to requests made of
him/her.
2 = Several occasions been noncompliant.
3 = Frequently noncompliant with requests.
4 = Consistently noncompliant with requests.

6. Attention-seeking behavior
0 = No information; not assessed; unable to assess.
1 = Patient has not exhibited attention-seeking behavior.
2 = Occasionally exhibited attention-seeking behavior.
3 = Frequently exhibited attention-seeking behavior.
4 = Continuously exhibited attention-seeking behavior. This
occurs several times per day.

7. Sexually inappropriate behavior
0 = No information; not assessed; unable to assess.
1 = No sexually inappropriate behavior observed.
2 = Patient observed to touch, kiss, hug others in socially
inappropriate settings.
3 = Patient occasionally exposes himself/herself.
4 = Patient frequently (tries to) expose(s) self and
masturbate(s).

8. Wandering
0 = No information; not assessed; unable to assess.
1 = Patient has not wandered from designated area.
2 = Patient has on at least 1 to 2 instances wandered from
designated area.
3 = Patient has on at least 3 to 4 instances wandered from
designated area.
4 = Patient has wandered on several (numerous) occasions.
Patient may be restrained for this behavior.

9. Hoarding behavior
0 = No information; not assessed; unable to assess.
1 = Patient has not shown any hoarding behavior.
2 = Patient has occasionally collected/hidden objects.
3 = Patient has regularly collected/hidden objects.
4 = Patient has constantly engaged in hoarding behavior.

Inferred states
1. Depression
2. Delusions
3. Hallucinations
4. Anxiety
5. Appropriateness/stability of affect
6. Increased/decreased appetite
7. Sleep

Insomnia–Early
0 = No information; not assessed; unable to assess.
1 = No difficulty falling asleep.
2 = Complains of occasional difficulty falling asleep–i.e.,
more than ½ hour.
3 = Complains of nightly difficulty falling asleep.

Insomnia–Middle
0 = No information; not assessed; unable to assess.
1 = No difficulty.
2 = Patient complains of being restless and disturbed during
the night.
3 = Waking during the night–any getting out of bed rated 2
(except for purposes of voiding).

Insomnia–Late
0 = No information; not assessed; unable to assess.
1 = No difficulty.
2 = Waking in early hours of the morning but goes back to
sleep.
3 = Unable to fall asleep again if he gets out of bed.

Rating:
Score: 1–6 as:
0 = No information, not able/not assessed; 1 = None; 2 = Mild; 3 = Moderate; 4 = Severe

Reprinted from *Psychiatry Research*, 41, Sinha D et al, A new scale for assessing behavioural agitation in dementia, 73–88,
© 1992, with permission from Elsevier Science.

Clinical Rating Scale for Symptoms of Psychosis in Alzheimer's Disease (SPAD)

Reference Reisberg B, Ferris SH (1985) A clinical rating scale for symptoms of psychosis in Alzheimer's disease. *Psychopharmacology Bulletin* **21:** 101–4

Time taken 10 minutes (reviewer's estimate)
Rating by clinician on the basis of a caregiver report

Main indications

Assessment of psychotic features in patients with Alzheimer's disease.

Commentary

The Clinical Rating Scale for Symptoms of Psychosis in Alzheimer's Disease (SPAD) represents the precursor of the BEHAVE-AD (page 75). It consists of nine questions regarding psychiatric symptoms and rated on a three-point scale of frequency. The stimulus for development appears to have been the lack of measures to assess changes in behavioural disturbances in dementia, only one example of which had been found in the literature (Barnes et al, 1982).

Additional reference

Barnes R, Veith R, Okimoto J et al (1982) Efficacy of antipsychotic medications in behaviorally disturbed dementia patients. *American Journal of Psychiatry* **139:** 1170–4.

Address for correspondence

Barry Reisberg
Clinical Director
Millhauser Laboratories
New York University Medical Center
550 First Avenue
New York
NY 10016
USA

Clinical Rating Scale for Symptoms of Psychosis in Alzheimer's Disease (SPAD)

Score* Symptomatology	Not present 0	Mild 1	Moderate 2	Severe 3
I. "People are stealing things"	Not present	Delusion that people are hiding objects	Delusion that people are coming into the home and hiding or stealing objects	Talking and listening to people coming into the home
II. "One's house is not one's home"	Not present	Conviction that the place in which one is residing is not one's home (e.g. packing to go home)	Attempt to leave domiciliary to go home	Violence in response to attempts to forcibly restrict exit
III. "Spouse (or other caregiver) is an imposter"	Not present	Conviction that spouse (or other caregiver) is an imposter	Anger toward spouse (or other caregiver) for being an imposter	Violence toward spouse (or other caregiver) for being an imposter
IV. "Delusion of abandonment" (e.g. to an institution)	Not present	Suspicion of caregiver plotting abandonment or institutionalization (e.g. on telephone)	Accusation of a conspiracy to abandon or institutionalize	Accusation of impending or immediate desertion or institutionalization
V. Cognitive Abulia (purposeless activity)	Not present	Repetitive purposeless activity (e.g. packing and unpacking clothing; repeatedly putting on and removing clothing; insistent repeating of demands or questions)	Pacing	Abrading
VI. Day/night disturbance	Not present	Repetitive wakenings during night	50 to 75% of former sleep cycle at night	Complete disturbance of diurnal rhythm (i.e. less than 50% of former sleep cycle at night)
VII. Visual hallucinatory experiences	Not present	Occasional (less than 5 in preceding 6-month period) episodes noted	Frequent (more than 5 in preceding 6-month period), definite (clearly defined hallucinations of objects or persons noted) episodes	Daily (or more frequent) hallucinatory experiences (minimum of 3 consecutive days)
VIII. Auditory hallucinatory experiences	Not present	Occasional (less than 5 in preceding 6-month period) episodes noted	Frequent (more than 5 in preceding 6-month period), definite (clearly defined hallucinations of words or phrases noted) episodes	Daily (or more frequent) hallucinatory experiences (minimum of 3 consecutive days)
IX. Other behavioral symptoms which may respond to neuroleptics (specify all that apply and total severity rating)	☐	☐	☐	☐

*General criteria for scoring:
(a)   To be scored by clinician on the basis of primary caregivers' experiences;
(b)   Information may be obtained from more than one primary caregiver with respect to the presence of each symptom;
(c)   Score "0" if a symptom is not present;
      Score "1" if symptom is present and judged to be mild by the primary caregiver;
      Score "2" if symptom is present and judged to be of moderate severity by the primary caregiver;
      Score "3" if symptom is present and judged to be severe by the primary caregiver.

Georagsobber Vatieschaal voor de Intramurale Psychogeriatrie (GIP)

Reference   Verstraten PFJ (1988) The GIP: an observational ward behavior scale. *Psychopharmacology Bulletin* 24: 717–19

Time taken 10 minutes (reviewer's estimate)

Rating by ward staff

Main indications

Assessment of behaviour in psychogeriatric inpatients.

Commentary

The Georagsobber Vatieschaal voor de Intramurale Psychogeriatrie (GIP) reports four separate behaviour subtypes: social; cognitive; psychomotor; and affective. This has been expanded to a total of 14 selected scales, and in total the GIP contains 82 items with an average of about six items in each scale. Patients are rated on each item by underlying one of four possible items indicating the frequency of the behaviour stated in that item during the last two weeks. The scale was validated on 567 patients from psychogeriatric hospital wards, nursing home residents and day care visitors. Inter-rater reliability (correlation coefficiency) ranged from 0.53 to 0.90. Interval consistency was greater than 0.75.

Address for correspondence

Peter FJ Verstraten
Stationsstraat 36
5451 AN Mill
The Netherlands

Georagsobber Vatieschaal voor de Intramurale Psychogeriatrie (GIP)

- social behavior types:
  1. nonsocial behavior;
  2. apathetic behavior;
  3. distorted consciousness;
  4. loss of decorum; and
  5. rebellious behavior
- cognitive behavior types:
  6. incoherent behavior
  7. distorted memory; and
  8. disoriented behavior;
- psychomotor behavior types:
  9. senseless repetitive behavior; and
  10. restless behavior;
- emotional or affective behavior types:
  11. suspicious behavior;
  12. melancholic or sorrowful behavior;
  13. dependent behavior; and
  14. anxious behavior.

Rated on a 4-point scale: never – always/often/continuously

Reproduced from Verstraten PFJ (1988) The GIP: an observational ward behavior scale. *Psychopharmacology Bulletin* **24**: 717–19.

Nursing Home Behavior Problem Scale (NHBPS)

Reference Ray WA, Taylor JOA, Lichtenstein MJ and Meador KG (1992) The Nursing Home Behavior Problem Scale. *Journal of Gerontology* 47: M9–16.

Time taken 3–5 minutes

Rating by nurse or nursing assistant who knows the patient

Main indications

The measurement of specific behaviour problems in the nursing home setting which are so disruptive as to lead to the use of medications or physical restraint.

Commentary

The Nursing Home Behavior Problem Scale (NHBPS) is a 29 item scale based on existing scales, omitting some passive behaviours and including others which specifically call for the prescription of medication. The study reported on 500 residents in 2 nursing home populations. Six sub-scales were described — uncooperative/aggressive, irra-tional/restless, sleep problems, annoying behaviour, inappropriate behaviour and dangerous behaviour. Validation was with the Nurses' Observation Scale for Inpatient Evaluation (NOSIE; page 100) and the Cohen-Mansfield Agitation Inventory (CMAI; page 110). Correlations with these scales were –0.747 and +0.911 respectively. Inter-rater reliability for the subscales ranged from 0.467 for dangerous behaviour to 0.768 for sleep problems.

Address for correspondence

Wayne A Ray
Department of Preventive Medicine and
Department of Psychiatry
Vanderbilt University School of Medicine
Nashville, TN
USA

Nursing Home Behavior Problem Scale (NHBPS)

DIRECTIONS
Please rate this resident's behavior during the last 3 days only. Indicate your choice by circling a number for each item, using this key:

0 = Never 1 = Sometimes 2 = Often 3 = Usually 4 = Always

Resists care
Becomes upset or loses temper easily
Enters others rooms inappropriately
Awakens during the night
Talks. mutters, or mumbles to herself
Tries to hurt herself
Refuses care
Fights or is physically aggressive: hits, slaps, kicks, bites, spits, pushes, pulls
Fidgets. Is unable to sit still, restless
Has difficulty falling asleep
Goes to the bathroom in inappropriate places (not incontinence)
Says things that do not make sense

Damages or destroys things on purpose
Screams, yells, or moans loudly
Argues, threatens, or curses
Tries to get in or out of wheelchair, bed, or chair unsafely
Asks or complains about her health, even though it is unjustified
Has inappropriate sexual behavior
Sees or hears things that are not there
Disturbs others during the night
Wanders, tries to escape or go to off-limits places
Accuses others of things that are not true
Asks for attention or help, even though it is not needed
Is uncooperative
Paces: walks or moves in wheelchair aimlessly back and forth
Tries to escape physical restraints
Complains or whines
Does something over and over, even though it doesn't make sense
Tries to do things that are dangerous

Chapter 2c

Activities of daily living

The main use of activities of daily living (ADL) scales is in people with dementia whose functioning is impaired secondarily to cognitive decline. Their use in other conditions is analogous to that in any cognitively impaired older person, with the exception that an individual who is severely depressed or psychotic may not function because of apathy or withdrawal. Activities of daily living can be categorized into two types: basic physical activities such as eating, toileting, washing, walking and dressing (sometimes referred to as physical self maintenance) and instrumental activities, which are more complex tasks including shopping, using the telephone, cooking, housekeeping, self medicating and use of transport. Measurement of function is an essential part of clinical practice and is one of the major outcomes used in the assessment of interventions in dementia. It is also one of the main determinants of people being admitted to long-term care. The development of these types of scales is underscored by the distinction between impairments, functional limitations and disability. Functional disability refers to dependence in basic daily activities taken in the context of a physical and social environment as opposed to problems with work or social interactions. It is the lack of ability to cope within a set environment which renders the person disabled rather than simply impaired.

Scales can be divided into those which are generic or disease-specific and those which are self report, informant or performance (i.e. observer) scales. Generic scales include the Barthel Index, which was originally in the rehabilitation field and measures functional abilities in older people but has been adapted for and validated for use in use in people with dementia. It taps more functional items than other scales in that it includes items such as the ability to walk up and down stairs. Criticism of the use of these scales in specific conditions such as dementia revolves round their presumed insensitivity to functional loss resulting from physical impairments, rather than that resulting from and secondary to cognitive deficits. Measures on ADL scores vary between the sexes and between cultures, and so variation in a demented group would not be surprising. However, generic scales tend to have been tested on larger numbers of patients, often in a variety of settings, and reliability and validity are well documented.

Specific instruments used in dementia are mainly observer and performance tests, the latter being particularly labour-inten-

sive, especially if carried out by a trained observer. Depending on the severity of dementia and the setting, it may be important to know which functions are intact in terms of basic daily living tasks or more complex instrumental tasks. The commonest used informant measures are the Blessed Dementia Scale (page 40), the Cleveland Scale for Activities of Daily Living (page 143) and the Functional Assessment Staging (FAST; page 164). The Blessed Dementia Scale has been validated against pathological diagnosis, and includes both ADL and Instrumental Activities of Daily Living (IADL) measures but nothing on selection of clothing. It was originally validated on an inpatient population, the accompanying Blessed Information–Memory–Concentration Test (page 40) demonstrating this by including the question about identifying people (e.g. a cleaner or nurse on the ward), making it less applicable to someone living at home. The need for measures which span the whole range of cognitive impairments from mild (where IADLs are more affected) to severe (where both ADLs and IADLs are affected) is important, particularly in longitudinal studies over time where patient characteristics would be expected to change with deterioration in their clinical condition. The FAST is an advance in this area, allowing the extremes of cognitive function to be rated. Performance tests have been more recently developed which allow separate analysis of individual aspects of a task, e.g. initiation, sequencing, safety and recognition of completion [Structured Assessment of Individual Living Skills (SALES; page 156)]. Attention to physical (gross and fine motor movements) is given priority in some measures [e.g. the Performance Test of Activities of Daily Living (PADL; page 154)], and cognitive aspects of the tests are important. The majority of these tests do correlate with measures of cognitive function, validating their use in tapping disabilities associated with progressive mental impairment. The development of scales specifically for dementia has involved breaking up task performance, allowing, for example, prompting (all that may be necessary to allow a cognitively impaired person to complete a task) and help with sequencing to be rated separately. Several of the new scales have been developed by nurses and occupational therapists.

For information on the Disability Assessment for Dementia (DAD) and The Alzheimer's Disease Functional Assessment and Change Scale, please refer to Appendix 2.

Instrumental Activities of Daily Living Scale (IADL)

Reference   Lawton MP, Brody EM (1969) Assessment of older people: self-maintaining and instrumental activities of daily living. *The Gerontologist* 9: 179–86

Time taken 5 minutes
Rating by trained interviewer

Main indications

To assess the functional ability of older people in relation to activities of daily living.

Commentary

Two scales are reported in the paper: the Physical Self-Maintenance Scale (PSMS), detailing more basic self-care tasks and based on an instrument described by Lowenthal (1964), and the Instrumental Activities of Daily Living (Barrabee et al, 1955; Phillips, 1968), concerning more complex daily tasks. Validity was assessed compared with a measure of general physical health, a mental status questionnaire and a behaviour and adjustment rating scale. Inter-rater reliability was found to be 0.87 and 0.91 on two separate substudies.

Additional references

Barrabee P, Barrabee E, Finesinger J (1955) A normative social adjustment scale. *American Journal of Psychiatry* 112: 252–9.

Khan RL, Goldfarb AI, Pollock M et al (1960) The relationship of mental and physical status in institutionalized aged persons. *American Journal of Psychiatry* 117: 120–4.

Lowenthal MF (1964) *Lives in distress.* New York: Basic Books.

Phillips LG (1968) *Human adaptation and its failures.* New York: Academic Press.

Address for correspondence

M Powell Lawton
Philadelphia Geriatric Center
5301 Old York Road
Philadelphia
PA 19141
USA

Instrumental Activities of Daily Living Scale (IADL)

A   Ability to use telephone
1. Operates telephone on own initiative – looks up and dials numbers, etc   1
2. Dials a few well-known numbers   1
3. Answers telephone but does not dial   1
4. Does not use telephone at all   0

B   Shopping
1. Takes care of all shopping needs independently   1
2. Shops independently for small purchases   0
3. Needs to be accompanied on any shopping trip   0
4. Completely unable to shop   0

C   Food preparation
1. Plans, prepares and serves adequate meals independently   1
2. Prepares adequate meals if supplied with ingredients   0
3. Heats, serves and prepares meals, or prepares meals but does not maintain adequate diet   0
4. Needs to have meals prepared and served   0

D   Housekeeping
1. Maintains house alone or with occasional assistance (e.g., "heavy work domestic help")   1
2. Performs light daily tasks such as dish-washing, bedmaking   1
3. Performs light daily tasks but cannot maintain acceptable level of cleanliness   1
4. Needs help with all home maintenance tasks   1
5. Does not participate in any housekeeping tasks   0

E   Laundry
1. Does personal laundry completely   1
2. Launders small items – rinses stockings, etc   1
3. All laundry must be done by others   0

F   Mode of transportation
1. Travels independently on public transportation or drives own car   1
2. Arranges own travel via taxi, but does not otherwise use public transportation   1
3. Travels on public transportation when accompanied by another   1
4. Travel limited to taxi or automobile with assistance of another   0
5. Does not travel at all   0

G   Responsibility for own medications
1. Is responsible for taking medication in correct dosages at correct time   1
2. Takes responsibility if medication is prepared in advance in separate dosage   0
3. Is not capable of dispensing own medication   0

H   Ability to handle finances
1. Manages financial matters independently (budgets, writes checks, pays rent, bills, goes to bank), collects and keeps track of income   1
2. Manages day-to-day purchases, but needs help with banking, major purchases, etc.   1
3. Incapable of handling money   0

Physical self-maintenance scale

A   Toilet
1. Cares for self at toilet completely, no incontinence   1
2. Needs to be reminded, or needs help in cleaning self, or has rare (weekly at most) accidents   0
3. Soiling or wetting while asleep more than once a week   0
4. Soiling or wetting while awake more than once a week   0
5. No control of bowels or bladder   0

B   Feeding
1. Eats without assistance   1
2. Eats with minor assistance at meal times and/or with special preparation of food, or help in cleaning up after meals   0
3. Feeds self with moderate assistance and is untidy   0
4. Requires extensive assistance for all meals   0
5. Does not feed self at all and resists efforts of others to feed him   0

C   Dressing
1. Dresses, undresses, and selects clothes from own wardrobe   1
2. Dresses and undresses self, with minor assistance   0
3. Needs moderate assistance in dressing or selection of clothes   0
4. Needs major assistance in dressing, but cooperates with efforts of others to help   0
5. Completely unable to dress self and resists efforts of others to help   0

D   Grooming
(neatness, hair, nails, hands, face, clothing)
1. Always neatly dressed, well-groomed, without assistance   1
2. Grooms self adequately with occasional minor assistance, e.g. shaving   0
3. Needs moderate and regular assistance or supervision in grooming   0
4. Needs total grooming care, but can remain well-groomed after help from others   0
5. Actively negates all efforts of others to maintain grooming   0

E   Physical ambulation
1. Goes about grounds or city   1
2. Ambulates within residence or about one block distant   0
3. Ambulates with assistance of (check one) a ( ) cane, d ( ) walker, e ( ) wheel chair.   0
   1 ——— Gets in and out without help
   2 ——— Needs help in getting in and out
4. Sits unsupported in chair or wheelchair but cannot propel self without help   0
5. Bedridden more than half the time   0

F   Bathing
1. Bathes self (tub, shower, sponge bath) without help   1
2. Bathes self with help in getting in and out of tub   0
3. Washes face and hands only, but cannot bathe rest of body   0
4. Does not wash self but is cooperative with those who bathe him   0
5. Does not wash self and resists efforts to keep him clean   0

Interview for Deterioration in Daily Living Activities in Dementia (IDDD)

Reference Teunisse S, Derix MMA (1991) Measuring functional disability in community dwelling dementia patients: development of a questionnaire. *Tijdschrift voor Gerontologie en Geriatrie* 22: 53–9

Time taken 15 minutes (reviewer's estimate)
Rating by interview with main caregiver

Main indications

To assess activities of daily living in dementia.

Commentary

The scale covers 33 activities such as washing, dressing, and eating as well as more complex activities such as shopping, writing and answering the telephone, tasks performed equally by men and women (earlier scales of activities of daily living tended to rely more heavily on female-dominated and less complex tasks). Both the initiative to perform activities and the performance itself were evaluated. There was high internal consistency (alpha = 0.94) and two groups of items were discriminated: those related to self-care activity and those to more complex tasks. Functioning of the patient is examined in a structured verbal interview with the carer. The scoring is rated on a three-point scale: 1 where help is almost never needed or there has been no change, 2 where help is sometimes needed or when help is needed more often than previously, and 3 when help is almost always needed or help is needed much more than previously. The scoring is carried out by referring to behaviour in the last month, comparing it with how it was before the onset of the dementia. After a negative response the questioner is asked to check that the behaviour is unchanged compared with what it was like previously, and after a positive response questions are asked: "is the help really necessary?" "what happens if you don't help?" and "do you have to help more often than before?"

The original paper rated functional disability along with cognitive impairment (measured by the CAMCOG), behavioural disturbances [measured by the GIP (page 124)] and carer burden [measured by an instrument related to the Zarit Burden Interview (page 239)]. Inter-relationships were found in 30 mild to moderately impaired patients with dementia. Functional disability was strongly related to cognitive deterioration and behavioural disturbances, and moderately related to burden experienced by carers. Since 1991, the IDDD has been translated into several languages and a paper-and-pencil version has been used in the measurement of treatment effects.

Additional reference

Teunisse S, Derix MMA, van Crevel H (1991) Assessing the severity of dementia: patient and caregiver. *Archives of Neurology* 48: 274–7.

Address for correspondence

S Teunisse
Psychology Department
William Guild Building
King's College
University of Aberdeen
Aberdeen AB24 2UB
UK

Interview for Deterioration in Daily Living Activities in Dementia (IDDD)

1.	*Do you have to tell her that she should wash herself (take the initiative to wash herself; not only washing of hands or face, but also washing of whole body)?*	1	2	3	8	9
2.	*Do you have to assist her in washing (finding face cloth, soap; soaping and rinsing of the body)?*	1	2	3	8	9
3.	*Do you have to tell her that she should dry herself (take the initiative to dry herself, for example looking or fetching for the towel)?*	1	2	3	8	9
4.	*Do you have to assist her in drying (drying individual body-parts)?*	1	2	3	8	9
5.	*Do you have to tell her that she should dress herself (take the initiative to dress herself, for example walking to the wardrobe)?*	1	2	3	8	9
6.	*Do you have to assist her in dressing herself (putting on individual clothes in right order)?*	1	2	3	8	9

7.	Do you have to assist her in doing up her shoes, using zippers or buttons?	1	2	3	8	9
8.	Do you have to tell her that she should brush her teeth or comb her hair?	1	2	3	8	9
9.	Do you have to assist her in brushing her teeth?	1	2	3	8	9
10.	Do you have to assist her in combing her hair?	1	2	3	8	9
11.	Do you have to tell her that she should eat (take the initiative to eat; in case eating is elicited by others, it should be asked if she would take the initiative spontaneously)?	1	2	3	8	9
12.	Do you have to assist her in preparing a slice of bread?	1	2	3	8	9
13.	Do you have to assist her in carving meat, potatoes?	1	2	3	8	9
14.	Do you have to assist her in drinking or eating?	1	2	3	8	9
15.	Do you have to tell her that she should use the lavatory (take the initiative to go to the lavatory when necessary)?	1	2	3	8	9
16.	Do you have to assist her in using the toilet (undressing herself, using toilet, using closet paper)?	1	2	3	8	9
17.	Do you have to assist her in finding her way in the house (finding different rooms)?	1	2	3	8	9
18.	Do you have to assist her in finding her way in familiar neighbourhood outside the house?	1	2	3	8	9
19.	Does she – as often as before – take the initiative shopping (take the initiative to figure out what is needed)?	1	2	3	8	9
20.	Do you have to assist her in shopping (finding her way in the shops; getting goods in needed quantity)?	1	2	3	8	9
21.	Do you – or the shop-assistant – have to tell her that she should pay?	1	2	3	8	9
22.	Do you – or the shop-assistant – have to assist her in paying (knowing how much she should pay and how much should be reimbursed)?	1	2	3	8	9
23.	Is she – as often as before – interested in newspaper, book or post?	1	2	3	8	9
24.	Do you have to assist her in reading (understanding written language)?	1	2	3	8	9
25.	Do you have to assist her in writing a letter or card, or completing a form (writing of more than one sentence)?	1	2	3	8	9
26.	Does she – as often as before – start a conversation with others?	1	2	3	8	9
27.	Do you have to assist her in expressing herself verbally?	1	2	3	8	9
28.	Does she – as often as before – pay attention to conversation by other people?	1	2	3	8	9
29.	Do you have to assist her in understanding spoken language?	1	2	3	8	9
30.	Does she – as often as before – take the initiative to use the phone (both answering the phone and calling someone)?	1	2	3	8	9
31.	Do you have to assist her in using the phone (both answering the phone and calling someone)?	1	2	3	8	9
32.	Do you have to assist her in finding things in the house?	1	2	3	8	9
33.	Do you have to tell her to put out gas or coffee machine?	1	2	3	8	9

Rating:

1 = (nearly) no help needed/no change in help needed
2 = sometimes help needed/help more often needed
3 = (nearly) always help needed/help much more often needed
8 = no evaluation possible
9 = not applicable

Reproduced (with permission from the American Medical Association) from Teunisse S et al. (1991) Assessing the severity of dementia: patient and caregiver. *Archives of Neurology*, **48**, 274–7. Copyright 1991. American Medical Association.

Barthel Index

Reference Mahoney FI, Barthel DW (1965) Functional evaluation: the BARTHEL index. *Maryland State Medical Journal* 14: 61–5

Time taken 5 minutes
Rating by informant

Main indications

Assessment of physical disability in elderly people.

Commentary

The Barthel Index represents probably the oldest and most widely used scale to assess physical disability in elderly patients in general. It is often used in studies in psychiatry. Its reliability has been assessed thoroughly in four ways: by self-report, by a trained nurse, and by two independent skilled observers. Agreement was generally present in over 90% of situations. Validity, reliability, sensitivity and clinical utility are all excellent, and have been reviewed (Wade and Collin, 1988). Explicit guidelines for rating have been suggested for the scale (Novak et al, 1996), and Wade and Collins have suggested an amended scoring system of 20.

Additional references

Collin C, Wade DT, Davis S et al (1988) The Barthel ADL Index: a reliability study. *International Disability Studies* 10: 61–3.

Novak S, Johnson J, Greenwood R (1996) Barthel revisited: making guidelines work. *Clinical Rehabilitation* 10: 128–34.

Wade DT, Collin C (1988) The Barthel ADL Index: a standard measure of physical disability? *International Disability Studies* 10: 64–7.

Barthel Index

		With help	Independent
1.	Feeding (if food needs to be cut up = help)	5	10
2.	Moving from wheelchair to bed and return (includes sitting up in bed)	5–10	15
3.	Personal toilet (wash face, comb hair, shave, clean teeth)	0	5
4.	Getting on and off toilet (handling clothes, wipe, flush)	5	10
5.	Bathing self	0	5
6.	Walking on level surface	10	15
	(if unable to walk, propel wheelchair)	0*	5*
7.	Ascend and descend stairs	5	10
8.	Dressing (includes tying shoes, fastening fasteners)	5	10
9.	Controlling bowels	5	10
10.	Controlling bladder	5	10

A score of 100 indicates independence in activities of daily living.

Mahoney FI, Barthel DW. Functional Evaluation: The BARTHEL Index. *Maryland State Medical Journal* 1965; **14**(2): 61–5. Used with permission.

Functional Activities Questionnaire (FAQ)

Reference   Pfeffer RI, Kurosaki TT, Harrah CH, Chance JM, Filos S (1992) Measurement of functional activities in older adults in the community. *Journal of Gerontology* **37**: 323–9

Time taken 10 minutes (reviewer's estimate)
Rating by clinician

Main indications

For the assessment of functional capacity in older people, with or without dementia.

Commentary

The rationale for the scale was to provide operational descriptions of various levels of function, independent of education, socioeconomic status and intelligence. The Functional Activities Questionnaire (FAQ) was validated on a study of 195 adults aged over 60 with normal or very mild dementia and, after a screening test for cognitive impairment and depression, they were rated on three cognitive scales: the Mini-Mental State Examination (MMSE; page 34), the Symbol Digit Test and Subtest B of the Raven's Progressive Colour Matrices. The FAQ is rated on a seven-point scale, 1 being normal and 7 being severely incapacitated and helpless. Comparisons were made with the Instrumental Activities of Daily Living Scale (IADL; page 128). Inter-rater reliability was excellent, with correlation = 0.97, and correlation with the IADL was 0.72. The scale showed high sensitivity and specificity (0.85 and 0.81) in distinguishing between demented and non-demented people.

Address for correspondence

RI Pfeffer
Department of Neurology
University of California at Irving Medical Center
101 City Drive South
Orange
CA 92668
USA

Functional Activities Questionnaire (FAQ)

Functional capacity level	Descriptive title	Description	Residual mental function estimate (%)
1	Normal	Fully independent with no restriction: No cognitive impairment. Either no assistance or advice is required in the 10 areas of daily activities, IADL, or activities of daily living (ADL), or this does not deviate from an established life-long pattern (e.g., utilization of an accountant or business advisor).	100
2	Questionably affected: uncertain status	Qualified independence: (a) participant or alternate informant report less skill or greater difficulty than formerly in 10 areas of daily activities or IADL, but independent of others. Only compensation, if any, is self-imposed (e.g., notes, reminder) or (b) study staff observe minor word-finding problems, minimal impairment of immediate recall of recent events, questionable problem with spatial orientation in unfamiliar surroundings, but normally oriented to person, place, and date (± 1 day).	90
3	Mildly affected	Definite but mild restriction in normal activities or independence: Another supervises or advises in two or more of 10 formerly mastered areas of daily activities, or one or more areas of IADL, but participant still carries out activity. Example: requires very explicit or written directions to drive out of neighborhood, guidance in balancing checkbook but still handles own money. Alternatively, significant difficulty with activity, but spouse tolerates performance they described as substandard. Probably could not be gainfully employed, but lives independently and normally with slight environmental modification or intervention, such as one to three visits per week from friend/relative or redistribution of spouse's responsibilities.	75
4	Moderately affected	Require assistance in IADL, but carry out a portion of this function (e.g., writes own checks or pays at supermarket but another balances check book, submits medical bills, drives them to appointments or accompanies on bus. More severely affected persons in this category need intermittent supervisor (two times weekly reminders) in ADL (e.g., coordinating items of apparel, missed areas in shaving or makeup) but perform the function. Requires active external intervention for "normal" home life, but takes care of basic personal needs.	60
5	Moderately severely affected	Half or more of IADL (e.g., shopping, laundry, handling money, making appointments, transport, dispensing medication) are performed by other. Require three times weekly assistance with toilette, although may participate in dressing and feed themselves. Most are spontaneously ambulatory. Requires major readjustments of family routine, adult daycare, or variable degress of attendant assistance; they may be placed in nursing homes.	40
6	Severely affected	Requires major, daily assistance in ADL (dressing, feeding, using toilet) and total assistance with IADL. Any ambulation with assistance. Initiates almost no activity other than for feeding, toilet, comfort. Institutional care is usual.	25
7	Severely incapacitated: helpless	Totally dependent. Mute, wheelchair, or bedfast. Almost all are institutionalized and require a higher level of nursing care than available outside most acute/rehabilitation hospitals.	10

Reproduced from *Journal of Gerontology*, Vol. 37, no. 3, pp. 323–9, 1992. Copyright © The Gerontological Society of America.

Daily Activities Questionnaire (DAQ)

Reference   Oakley F, Sunderland T, Hill JL, Phillips SL, Makahon R, Ebner JD (1991) The Daily Activities Questionnaire: a functional assessment for people with Alzheimer's disease. *Physical and Occupational Therapy in Geriatrics* 10: 67–81

Time taken   15 minutes (reviewer's estimate)

Rating   from caregiver

Main indications

An objective clinical research measure of activities in daily living (ADLs) in people with Alzheimer's disease.

Commentary

The Daily Activities Questionnaire (DAQ) consists of 12 visual analogue scales (100 mm lines ranging from totally dependent to totally independent). The domains assessed are money management, cooking, shopping, recreation, home care, phone use, dressing, grooming, bathing, walking, sleeping, feeding, toileting and a global measure. The paper described significant differences in 32 patients with Alzheimer's disease and 18 normal controls. Inter-rater reliability (intraclass correlation coefficients) were all significant, with the exception of the items on recreation, walking and toileting. There were significant correlations between the severity of illness and ADLs. Normal controls were able to fill in their own questionnaire.

Address for correspondence

Francis Oakley
Occupational Therapy Service
NIH
Bethesda MD
USA

Examples of visual analogue scales and clinical questions from the Daily Activities Questionnaire (DAQ)

Dressing		*When dressing:*
Totally dependent	*Totally independent*	*Dresses without assistance* *0*
		May occasionally need some supervision or direction to dress *1*
Cooking		
Totally dependent	*Totally independent*	*Usually needs much supervision or direction to dress* *2*
		Must be physically dressed by another *3*
Money management		*If 1, 2, or 3 describe assistance provided:* ————————
Totally dependent	*Totally independent*	—— ————————————————————————
		Not applicable. Why? ————————————————

Reproduced with permission from *Physical and Occupational Therapy in Geriatrics*, 1991, The Haworth Press.

Bristol Activities of Daily Living Scale

Reference   Bucks RS, Ashworth DL, Wilcock GK, Siegfried K (1996) Assessment of activities of daily living in dementia: development of the Bristol Activities of Daily Living Scale. *Age and Ageing* **25**: 113–20

Time taken 15 minutes (reviewer's estimate)
Rating by carer

Main indications

Assessment of activities of daily living in patients with dementia either in the community or on clinical research trial.

Commentary

The scale was designed specifically for use in patients with dementia, and consists of 20 daily living abilities. Face validity was measured by way of carer agreement that the items were important, construct validity was confirmed by principal components analysis, concurrent validity by assessment with observed performance and good test/rest reliability. Three phases in the design of the scale were described. Anyone designing a scale should read this to serve as a model of clarity.

Additional reference

Patterson MB, Mack JL, Neundorfer MM et al (1992) Assessment of functional ability in Alzheimer's disease: a review and preliminary report on the Cleveland Scale for Activities of Daily Living. *Alzheimer Disease and Associated Disorders* **6**: 145–63.

Address for correspondence

GK Wilcock
Department of Care of the Elderly
Frenchay Hospital
Bristol BS16 1LE
UK

Bristol Activities of Daily Living Scale

1. Food
a. Selects and prepares food as required [ ]
b. Able to prepare food if ingredients set out [ ]
c. Can prepare food if prompted step by step [ ]
d. Unable to prepare food even with prompting and supervision [ ]
e. Not applicable [ ]

2. Eating
a. Eats appropriately using correct cutlery [ ]
b. Eats appropriately if food made manageable and/or uses spoon [ ]
c. Uses fingers to eat food [ ]
d. Needs to be fed [ ]
e. Not applicable [ ]

3. Drink
a. Selects and prepares drinks as required [ ]
b. Can prepare drinks if ingredients left available [ ]
c. Can prepare drinks if prompted step by step [ ]
d. Unable to make a drink even with prompting and supervision [ ]
e. Not applicable [ ]

4. Drinking
a. Drinks appropriately [ ]
b. Drinks appropriately with aids, beaker/straw etc. [ ]
c. Does not drink appropriately even with aids but attempts to [ ]
d. Has to have drinks administered (fed) [ ]
e. Not applicable [ ]

5. Dressing
a. Selects appropriate clothing and dresses self [ ]
b. Puts clothes on in wrong order and/or back to front and/or dirty clothing [ ]
c. Unable to dress self but moves limbs to assist [ ]
d. Unable to assist and requires total dressing [ ]
e. Not applicable [ ]

6. Hygiene
a. Washes regularly and independently [ ]
b. Can wash self if given soap, flannel, towel, etc. [ ]
c. Can wash self if prompted and supervised [ ]
d. Unable to wash self and needs full assistance [ ]
e. Not applicable [ ]

7. Teeth
a. Cleans own teeth/dentures regularly and independently [ ]
b. Cleans teeth/dentures if given appropriate items [ ]
c. Requires some assistance, toothpaste on brush, brush to mouth, etc. [ ]
d. Full assistance given [ ]
e. Not applicable [ ]

8. Bath/shower
a. Bathes regularly and independently [ ]

b.	Needs bath to be drawn/shower turned on but washes independently	[ ]	

15. Telephone

a. Uses telephone appropriately, including obtaining correct number [ ]

b. Needs bath to be drawn/shower turned on but washes independently [ ]

c. Needs supervision and prompting to wash [ ]

d. Totally dependent, needs full assistance [ ]

e. Not applicable [ ]

9. Toilet/commode

a. Uses toilet appropriately when required [ ]

b. Needs to be taken to the toilet and given assistance [ ]

c. Incontinent of urine or faeces [ ]

d. Incontinent of urine and faeces [ ]

e. Not applicable [ ]

10. Transfers

a. Can get in/out of chair unaided [ ]

b. Can get into a chair but needs help to get out [ ]

c. Needs help getting in and out of a chair [ ]

d. Totally dependent on being put into and lifted from chair [ ]

e. Not applicable [ ]

11. Mobility

a. Walks independently [ ]

b. Walks with assistance, i.e. furniture, arm for support [ ]

c. Uses aids to mobilize, i.e. frame, sticks etc. [ ]

d. Unable to walk [ ]

e. Not applicable [ ]

12. Orientation – time

a. Fully orientated to time/day/date etc. [ ]

b. Unaware of time/day etc but seems unconcerned [ ]

c. Repeatedly asks the time/day/date [ ]

d. Mixes up night and day [ ]

e. Not applicable [ ]

13. Orientation – space

a. Fully orientated to surroundings [ ]

b. Orientated to familiar surroundings only [ ]

c. Gets lost in home, needs reminding where bathroom is, etc. [ ]

d. Does not recognize home as own and attempts to leave [ ]

e. Not applicable [ ]

14. Communication

a. Able to hold appropriate conversation [ ]

b. Shows understanding and attempts to respond verbally with gestures [ ]

c. Can make self understood but difficulty understanding others [ ]

d. Does not respond to or communicate with others [ ]

e. Not applicable [ ]

15. Telephone

a. Uses telephone appropriately, including obtaining correct number [ ]

b. Uses telephone if number given verbally/visually or predialled [ ]

c. Answers telephone but does not make calls [ ]

d. Unable/unwilling to use telephone at all [ ]

e. Not applicable [ ]

16. Housework/gardening

a. Able to do housework/gardening to previous standard [ ]

b. Able to do housework/gardening but not to previous standard [ ]

c. Limited participation even with a lot of supervision [ ]

d. Unwilling/unable to participate in previous activities [ ]

e. Not applicable [ ]

17. Shopping

a. Shops to previous standard [ ]

b. Only able to shop for 1 or 2 items with or without a list [ ]

c. Unable to shop alone, but participates when accompanied [ ]

d. Unable to participate in shopping even when accompanied [ ]

e. Not applicable [ ]

18. Finances

a. Responsible for own finances at previous level [ ]

b. Unable to write cheque but can sign name and recognizes money values [ ]

c. Can sign name but unable to recognize money values [ ]

d. Unable to sign name or recognize money values [ ]

e. Not applicable [ ]

19. Games/hobbies

a. Participates in pastimes/activities to previous standard [ ]

b. Participates but needs instruction/supervision [ ]

c. Reluctant to join in, very slow, needs coaxing [ ]

d. No longer able or willing to join in [ ]

e. Not applicable [ ]

20. Transport

a. Able to drive, cycle or use public transport independently [ ]

b. Unable to drive but uses public transport or bike etc [ ]

c. Unable to use public transport alone [ ]

d. Unable or unwilling to use transport even when accompanied [ ]

e. Not applicable [ ]

Rating:

Tick only 1 box per activity. Answer with respect to last 2 weeks
Score: a = 0, b =1, c = 2, d = 3, e = 0

Reprinted from Bucks RS, Ashworth DL, Wilcock GK, Siegfried K (1996) Assessment of activities of daily living in dementia: development of the Bristol Activities of Daily Living Scale. *Age and Ageing*, **25**: 113–20. By kind permission of Oxford University Press.

Direct Assessment of Functional Status (DAFS)

Reference   Loewenstein DA, Amigo E, Duara R, Guterman A, Hurwitz D, Berkowitz N, Wilkie F, Weinberg G, Black B, Gittelman B, Eisdorfer C (1989) A new scale for the assessment of functional status in Alzheimer's disease and related disorders. *Journal of Gerontology* **44: 114–21**

Time taken 25 minutes (reviewer's estimate)
Rating by trained interviewer

Main indications

Direct assessment of functional capacities in Alzheimer's disease and other disorders.

Commentary

The Direct Assessment of Functional Status (DAFS) consists of a number of domains: time orientation; transportation; financial skills; shopping skills; eating skills; and dressing/grooming skills. Inter-rater reliability revealed kappa values of over 0.9 for all the domains, and test/retest reliability was also excellent, with all kappa values 0.86 or above. Correlations were described between the scale and the Blessed Dementia Scale (page 40) which were highly significant.

Address for correspondence

David A Loewenstein
Wien Center for Alzheimer's Disease
Mount Sinai Medical Center
Miami Beach
USA

Direct Assessment of Functional Status (DAFS)

I. Time Orientation (16 points)

A. Telling Time	Correct (2 points)	Incorrect (0 points)
(Use large model of a clock)		
3:00	_____	_____
8:00	_____	_____
10:30	_____	_____
12:15	_____	_____

B. Orientation to Date	Correct (2 points)	Incorrect (0 points)
What is the date?	_____	_____
What day is it today?	_____	_____
What month are we in?	_____	_____
What year are we in	_____	_____

II. Communication (14 points) (Using a pushbotton telephone) (If at any point the patient dials, picks up, or hangs up the phone, he/she is given credit for items tapping these specific subskills.)

A. Using the Telephone	Correct (1 point)	Incorrect (0 points)
Dial Operator (0)	_____	_____
Dial number from book	_____	_____
Dial number presented orally	_____	_____
Dial number written down	_____	_____
Pick up receiver	_____	_____
Ability to dial	_____	_____
Hang up phone	_____	_____
Correct sequence across all previous trials	_____	_____

B. Preparing a Letter for Mailing	Correct (1 point)	Incorrect (0 points)
Fold in half	_____	_____
Put in envelope	_____	_____
Seal envelope	_____	_____
Stamp envelope	_____	_____
Address (has to be exact duplicate of examiner's copy)	_____	_____
Return address (has to put correct address in upper lefthand corner)	_____	_____

III. Transportation (13 points)
(Patient has to correctly identify a driver's correct response to these road signs.)

	Correct (1 point)	Incorrect (0 points)
Stop	_____	_____
Yield	_____	_____
One way	_____	_____
No right turn	_____	_____
Green light	_____	_____
Yellow light	_____	_____
Red light	_____	_____
No "U" turn	_____	_____
Railroad crossing	_____	_____
Do not enter	_____	_____
Double yellow line	_____	_____
Passing line	_____	_____
Speed limit	_____	_____

At this point the examiner should instruct the patient that he/she will be going to a grocery store in 10 minutes and that the patient will be asked to pick out four grocery items from memory. Patient is given each grocery item, repeats it and again is asked to commit the list of four grocery items to memory.

IV. Financial (21 points) (Lay out one $10 bill, three $1 bills, one $5 bill, 3 quarters, 2 dimes, 1 nickel, 3 pennies.) Subskills include making change for grocery items.

	Correct (1 point)	Incorrect (0 points)
A. Identifying Currency		
Identify penny	___	___
Identify nickel	___	___
Identify dime	___	___
Identify quarter	___	___
Identify dollar bill	___	___
Identify $5 bill	___	___
Identify $10 bill	___	___

		Correct (1 point)	Incorrect (0 points)
B. Counting Change			
Lay out			
1–$10 bill	6 cents	___	___
1–$5 bill	102 cents (in change)	___	___
3–$1 bill	$6.73	___	___
3–quarters	$12.17	___	___
2–dimes		___	___
1–nickel		___	___
3–pennies		___	___

	Correct (1 point)	Incorrect (0 points)
C. Writing a Check		
Signature	___	___
Pay to order of	___	___
Written amount	___	___
Numeric amount	___	___
Date (location) (Does not have to be correct)	___	___

	Correct (1 point)	Incorrect (0 points)
D. Balancing a Checkbook		
Amount A ($500–$350) correct $150	___	___
Amount B ($323–$23.50) correct $299.50	___	___
Amount C ($21.75–$3.92) correct $17.83	___	___

V. Shopping (16 points) Patients told to look over the 20 grocery items and asked to select the four which were presented to him/her 10 minutes earlier.

	Correct (2 points)	Incorrect (0 points)
A. Memory for Grocery Items		
Orange juice	___	___
Soup	___	___
Cereal	___	___
Tuna fish	___	___

All of the items selected by the patient on the previous test are put back and the patient is given a written grocery list.

	Correct (2 points)	Incorrect (0 points)
B. Selecting Groceries Given a Written List		
Milk	___	___
Crackers	___	___
Eggs	___	___
Laundry detergent	___	___

	Correct (2 points)	Incorrect (0 points)
C.		
Correct change	___	___

Give the patient a $5 bill and say the bill is $2.49. Put the money out in front of them (currency from the Financial Subskills Test) and ask them to count out the change they should receive.

VI. Grooming (14 points)
The patient is taken to the bathroom and asked to:

	Correct (2 points)	Incorrect (0 points)
Take cap off toothpaste	___	___
Put toothpaste on brush	___	___
Turn on water	___	___
Brush teeth	___	___
Dampen wash cloth	___	___
Put soap on cloth	___	___
Clean face	___	___
Turn off water	___	___
Brush hair	___	___
Put on coat	___	___
Button	___	___
Tie	___	___
Zip	___	___

VII. Eating (10 points)
(Place eating utensils in front of patient.)

	Correct (2 points)	Incorrect (0 points)
Fork	___	___
Knife	___	___
Spoon	___	___
Pour water	___	___
Drink from glass	___	___

Activities of Daily Living (ADL) Index

Reference Sheikh K, Smith DS, Meade TW, Goldenberg E, Brennan PJ, Kinsella G (1979) Repeatability and validity of a modified Activities of Daily Living (ADL) Index in studies of chronic disability. *International Rehabilitation Medicine* 1: 51–8

Time taken 10 minutes (reviewer's estimate)
Rating by observer

Main indications

Assessment of activities of daily living function in chronic disability – modified to be sufficiently repeatable and valid.

Commentary

This is a 17-item scale tested on a number of different groups of patients. Inter-rater reliability and test/retest reliability were assessed in hospital and home settings, the relationship between the score and the size of the cerebral lesion was determined, and the score was compared with the patient's own perception of disability. Inter-rater reliability was 0.986 (over 2000 paired observations). Test/retest reliability (340 observations) was excellent, and the other substudies confirmed the validity of the scale.

ADL Index (Activity items)

Transfer from floor to chair	Using lavatory (simulated)
Transfer from chair to bed	Continence (bladder and bowel control)
Walking indoors	Grooming (brushing hair or shaving)
Walking outdoors	Brushing teeth (simulated)
Ascending a flight of stairs	Preparing for making tea
Descending a flight of stairs	Making tea
Dressing (overgarments)	Using taps (ordinary sink taps)
Washing (simulated)	Feeding (simulated)
Bathing (simulated)	

Score as follows:

1 = Performed without assistance (physical aids allowed)
2 = Performed greater part without assistance; some verbal or physical assistance required
3 = Complete inability to perform, even with assistance, or refusal to perform even if deemed able
Minimum score = 17, indicating no apparent handicap.
If totally unable to carry out any activity even with help then would score 51.

International Rehabilitation Medicine, **1**, 51–58, 1979. Reprinted by permission of Taylor & Francis.

Cleveland Scale for Activities of Daily Living (CSADL)

Reference   Patterson MB, Mack JL, Neundorfer MM, Martin RJ, Smyth KA, Whitehouse PJ (1992)
Assessment of functional ability in Alzheimer disease: a review and a preliminary report on the
Cleveland Scale for Activities of Daily Living. *Alzheimer Disease and Associated Disorders* 6: 145–63

Time taken 25 minutes (reviewer's estimate)

Rating from primary caregiver by nurse, clinician or trained interviewer

Main indications

Assessment of activities of daily living (ADLs) in Alzheimer's disease.

Commentary

The Cleveland Scale for Activities of Daily Living (CSADL) was designed specifically to reflect changes in the nature and extent of the broad spectrum of functional difficulties seen in individuals with Alzheimer's disease. Some 113 patients diagnosed as having Alzheimer's disease were assessed with the scale, and it was compared with the Blessed Dementia Scale (page 40) and the Mini-Mental State Examination (MMSE; page 34). The scale consists of 66 items in 16 domains of everyday activities, including both physical and instrumental ADLs, and represented all the physical and instrumental activities included in the Older Americans Resources and Services (OARS), the Functional Assessment Questionnaire (Duke University, 1978) plus several items suggested by Pfeffer in the Functional Activities Questionnaire (FAQ; page 134), as well as other items assessing more complex activities such as hobbies, communication skills and social behaviour. Within each domain, activities are broken down into several components. In the paper, five basic ADL domains were examined: bearing, dressing, eating, toileting and hygiene. Descriptions were given of the proportion of rating according to dependency level. Rating of individual items and intercorrelations of the items within each domain. The usefulness of the CSADL and its improved sensitivity of the detection of basic ADL functions were discussed.

Additional reference

Duke University Center for the Study of Aging (1978) *Multidimensional function assessment: the OARS methodology.* 2nd edition. Durham, NC: Duke University.

Address for correspondence

MB Patterson
Department of Neurology
University Hospitals of Cleveland
2074 Abington Road
Cleveland
OH 44106
USA

Cleveland Scale for Activities of Daily Living (CSADL)

Bathing – initiates bath
    prepares bath
    gets in/out
    cleans self

Toileting – controls urination
    controls bowels
    recognizes need
    eliminates at toilet
    rearranges clothes

Personal hygiene and appearance – initiates grooming
    washes hands/face
    brushes teeth
    combs hair

Dressing – initiates dressing
    selects clothes
    puts on garments
    fastens clothing

Medications

Eating – eats at appropriate intervals
    eats at appropriate time
    feeds self
    acceptable manners

Meal preparation
Mobility
Shopping
Travel
Hobbies, personal interests, employment
Housework/home maintenance
Telephone
Money management
Communication skills
Social behavior

Score as follows:

0 = Activities carried out effectively and fully independent. Normal; 1 = Generally independent, sometimes needs direction/assistance; 2 = Usually requires direction and/or assistance but independent in some situations/occasions; 3 = Completely dependent on others for direction/assistance

Cognitive Performance Test

Reference   Burns T, Mortimer JA, Merchak P (1994) Cognitive performance test: a new approach to functional assessment in Alzheimer's disease. *Journal of Geriatric Psychiatry and Neurology* 7: 46–54.

Time taken 45 minutes
Rating by trained interviewer

Main indications

Assessment of functional capacity in dementia.

Commentary

The Cognitive Performance Test claims to be different from other similar tests in that, rather than focusing on the ability to perform specific tasks, the emphasis is on the degree to which deficits in information processing compromise activities. Seventy-seven patients with mild to moderate Alzheimer's disease were studied. Inter-rater reliability was 0.91 and test retest reliability over 4 weeks was 0.89. Validity was assessed by comparison with the Mini-Mental State Examination (MMSE; page 34) and the Instrumental Activities of Daily Living Scale (IADL; page 128). Correlations with these scales were 0.67, 0.64 and 0.49 respectively. The scale strongly predicted the rate of institutionalization over a 4 year follow up period.

The scale is rated on 6 ordinal levels, profoundly disabled (level 1) and normal functioning (level 6).

Address for correspondence

Theressa Burns
Veterans Affairs Medical Center
1 Veterans Drive
Minneapolis
MN 55417
USA

Cognitive Performance Test

Initial Directions for Tasks

Dress: This test has to do with getting dressed. I want you to get dressed as if you were going outside on a cold, rainy day. You can use any of the things here. There are men's and women's things. Get dressed over your own clothes for going outside on a cold, rainy day.

Shop: I'd like to see how you do with money when you're shopping. I want you to buy a belt. Here is a wallet with some money in it. Choose a belt that fits you and one that you can pay for with the money in the wallet; then pay me the exact amount for the belt.

Toast: This next test has to do with preparing food. Make one slice of toast, then put some butter and jam on it. The supplies are on this table.

Phone: This next test has to do with using the phone. I'd like you to use the phone to find out the cost of one gallon of white paint.

Wash: Here are the directions for the next test; listen carefully. I want you to clean your hands as if you had been working outside in the yard. Take what you need from this box and use whatever you need in this room.

Travel: I want to see how well you're able to get from one place to another. This is a map of the hallways in this area. See if you can find this particular set of stairs. We are standing here. Follow the map to these stairs and point them out to me.

Source: Burns T, Mortimer JA, Merchak P (1994) Cognitive Performance Test: a new approach to functional assessment in Alzheimer's disease, *Journal of Geriatric Psychiatry and Neurology* **7**: 46–54.

Present Functioning Questionnaire (PFQ) and Functional Rating Scale (FRS)

Reference   Crockett D, Tuokko H, Koch W, Parks R (1989) The assessment of everyday functioning using the Present Functioning Questionnaire and the Functional Rating Scale in elderly samples. *Clinical Gerontologist* 8: 3–25

Time taken PFQ: 20 minutes (reviewer's estimate)
FRS: 15 minutes (reviewer's estimate)
Rating PFQ: informant-based
FRS: ideally a multidisciplinary assessment

Main indications
Estimation of everyday functioning in elderly patients.

Commentary
The Functional Rating Scale (FRS) assesses information in eight areas: memory; social/community/occupational; home/hobbies; personal care; language skills; problem solving; affect; and orientation. The Present Functioning Questionnaire (PFQ) collates reported problems in five areas: personality; everyday tasks; language skills; memory functioning; and self-care. Subjects were chosen who were either normal volunteers living in the community or refer-rals to an Alzheimer's disease clinic. A reliability study confirmed high internal consistency for the scales, with an ability to differentiate between groups of subjects.

Additional reference
Tuokko T, Crockett D, Beattie B et al (1986) The use of rating scales to assess psycho-social functioning in demented patients. Paper presented at the International Neuropsychological Society Annual Meeting. Denver, CO.

Address for correspondence
D Crockett
Division of Psychology
Department of Psychiatry
University of British Columbia
Vancouver BC
V6T 2A1

Present Functioning Questionnaire (PFQ)

Personality:
Being irritable or angry —
Being miserable or depressed —
Being tense or panicky —
Being apathetic —
Being agitated or hyperactive —
Being anxious or afraid —
Stating that "things aren't real" —
Complaining of "upsetting thoughts" —
Being aggressive —
Being suspicious —
Being insensitive to others' feelings —
Showing inappropriate smiles or laughter —
Showing decreased hobby involvement —
Talking to imaginery others —
Exhibiting inappropriate sexual activities —

Everyday tasks:
Problems performing household tasks —
Problems handling money —
Problems shopping —
Problems finding their way inside a house or building —
Problems finding their way around familiar streets —
Problems recognizing surroundings —
Problems recognizing the date or day of week —
Problems recognizing the time of day —
Awakening at night and thinking it is day —
Problems reading (except as caused by poor vision) —
Problems performing job —
Problems driving a car (if could before) —

Language skills:
Problems finding words to express him/herself —
Losing his/her vocabulary —
Problems pronouncing words —
Problems understanding others —
More frequently slurring words —
Problems clipping ends of words or sentences —
More frequently stuttering —

Problems finding names for common objects —
Problems forming any intelligible speech —

Memory functions:
Problems remembering previous actions on the same day —
Problems remembering past life events —
Asking questions repeatedly (despite answers) —
Problems recognizing faces of old friends or family —
Problems recognizing names of old friends or family —
Problems remembering newly introduced persons —
Problems leaving stove burners, water taps & light switches turned on —
Problems maintaining a train of thought —
Problems concentrating —
Problems remembering where he/she placed objects —
Increasingly frustrated over problems of remembering or thinking —
Increasingly defensive about problems remembering —
Problems remembering important personal dates —
Seemingly unaware of important current events —
Does not know own name —

Self-care functions:
Eating messily with spoon only —
Eating messily with spoon and with solid foods —
Has to be fed by someone else —
Problems dressing, e.g. occasional misplaced buttons —
Problems dressing, e.g. puts on clothes in wrong sequence —
Problems dressing, e.g. unable to dress self —
Problems with occasionally wetting bed —
Problems with frequently wetting bed —
Double incontinent —
Does not wash him/herself enough —
Must be bathed by someone else —
Grooming (combing of hair, etc.) inadequate —
Must be groomed by someone else —
Needs constant supervision in caring for self —

Functional Rating Scale (FRS)

	Healthy (1)	Questionable (2)	Mild (3)	Moderate (4)	Severe (5)
Memory	No deficit or inconsistent forgetfulness evident only on clinical interview	Variable symptoms reported by patient or relative; seemingly unrelated to level of functioning	Memory losses which intefere with daily living; more apparent for recent events	Moderate memory loss; only highly learned material retained, new material rapidly lost	Severe memory loss; unable to recall relevant aspects of current life; very sketchy recall of past life
Social/community and occupational	Neither patient nor relatives aware of any deficit	Variable levels of functioning reported by patient or relatives; no objective evidence of deficits in employment or social situations	Patient or relative aware of decreased performance in demanding employment or social settings; appears normal to casual inspection	Patient or relative aware of ongoing deterioration; does not appear normal to objective observer; unable to perform job; little independent functioning outside home	Marked impairment of social functioning; no independent functioning outside home
Home and hobbies	No changes noted by patient or relative	Slightly decreased involvement in house-hold tasks and hobbies	Engages in social activities in the home but definite impairment on some household tasks; some complicated hobbies and interests abandoned	Only simple chores/hobbies preserved; most complicated hobbies/interests abandoned	No independent involvement in home or hobbies
Personal care	Fully capable of self-care	Occasional problems with self-care reported by patient/relatives or observed	Needs prompting to complete tasks adequately (i.e. dressing, feeding, hygiene)	Requires supervision in dressing, feeding, hygiene and keeping track of personal effects	Needs constant supervision and assistance with feeding, dressing, or hygiene, etc.
Language skills	No disturbance of language report by patient or relative	Subjective complaint of, or relative reports, language deficits; usually limited to word finding or naming	Patient or relative reports variable disturbances of such skills as articulation or naming; occasional language impairment evident during examination	Patient or relative reports consistent language disturbance, language disturbance evident on examination	Severe impairment of receptive and/or expressive language; production of unintelligible speech
Problem solving and reasoning	Solves everyday problems adequately	Variable impairment of problems solving, similarities, differences	Difficulty in handling complex problems	Marked impairment on complex problem solving tasks	Unable to solve problems at any level; trial and error behavior often observed
Affect	No change in affect reported by patient or relative	Appropriate concern with respect to symptomatology	Infrequent changes in affect (e.g. irritability) reported by patient or relative; would appear normal to objective observer	Frequent changes in affect reported by patient or relative; noticeable to objective observer	Sustained alterations of affect; impaired contact with reality observed or reported
Orientation	Fully oriented	Occasional difficulties with time relationships	Marked difficulty with time relationships	Usually disoriented to time and often to place	Oriented only to person or not at all

Reproduced with kind permission from Dr H Tuokko.

Rapid Disability Rating Scale – 2 (RDRS-2)

Reference Linn MW, Linn BS (1982) The Rapid Disability Rating Scale – 2. *Journal of the American Geriatrics Society* 30: 378–82

Time taken 10 minutes (reviewer's estimate)

Rating anyone who knows the subject, preferably with one training session

Main indications

To assess disability in elderly people.

Commentary

The Rapid Disability Rating Scale (version 2) (RDRS-2) is a revision of the original scale described in 1967 (Linn, 1967). Changes were made, along with the clinical use of the instrument, over the preceding 15 years. In the main the changes were increasing the point rating from three to four, the emphasis was shifted to current activities and present behaviour (with the inference that it would then be more sensitive to change), and items were added about mobility, toileting and adaptive tasks. Global items relating to confusion and depression were also added. The scale measures 18 variables from none (=1) to severe (=4), giving a range of scores from 18 to 72. Elderly people living in the community with minimum disability would have a score of around 22, hospitalized elderly patients 32, and those in nursing homes 36. Some 100 patients were rated by two nurses independently, with intraclass correlation coefficients of between 0.62 and 0.98 and test/retest reliability (Pearson product moment correlations) of between 0.58 and 0.96. On factor analysis 120 institutionalized patients revealed the factors described in the scale – assistance with activities of daily living, degree of disability and degree of special problems. Validity was assessed by comparing ratings with independent physician ratings but self-report was used on health and mortality. An assessment over time was also made suggesting the scale is sensitive to change.

Additional reference

Linn MW (1967) A Rapid Disability Rating Scale. *Journal of the American Geriatrics Society* 15: 211.

Address for correspondence

MW Linn
Director, Social Science Research
Veterans Administration Medical Center
1201 Northwest 16th Street
Miami
FL 33125
USA

Rapid Disability Rating Scale – 2 (RDRS-2)

Directions: Rate what the person does to reflect current behavior. Circle one of the four choices for each item. Consider rating with any aids or prostheses normally used. None = completely independent or normal behavior. Total = that person cannot, will not, or may not (because of medical restriction) perform a behavior or has the most severe form of disability or problem.

Assistance with activities of daily living

Eating	None	A little	A lot	Spoon-feed; intravenous tube
Walking (with cane or walker if used)	None	A little	A lot	Does not walk
Mobility (going outside and getting about with wheelchair, etc., if used)	None	A little	A lot	Is housebound
Bathing (include getting supplies, supervising)	None	A little	A lot	Must be bathed
Dressing (include help in selecting clothes)	None	A little	A lot	Must be dressed
Toileting (including help with clothes, cleaning, or help with ostomy, catheter)	None	A little	A lot	Use bedpan or unable to care for ostomy/catheter
Grooming (shaving for men, hairdressing for women, nails, teeth)	None	A little	A lot	Must be groomed
Adaptive tasks (managing money/possessions; telephoning; buying newspaper, toilet articles, snacks)	None	A little	A lot	Cannot manage

Degree of disability

Communication (expressing self)	None	A little	A lot	Does not communicate
Hearing (with aid if used)	None	A little	A lot	Does not seem to hear
Sight (with glasses, if used)	None	A little	A lot	Does not see
Diet (deviation from normal)	None	A little	A lot	Fed by intravenous tube
In bed during day (ordered or self-initiated)	None	A little (<3 hrs)	A lot	Most/all of time
Incontinence (urine/feces, with catheter or prosthesis, if used)	None	Sometimes	Frequently (weekly +)	Does not control
Medication	None	Sometimes	Daily, taken orally	Daily; injection; (+ oral if used)

Degree of special problems

Mental confusion	None	A little	A lot	Extreme
Uncooperativeness (combats efforts to help with care)	None	A little	A lot	Extreme
Depression	None	A little	A lot	Extreme

Rating:

1 = none to 4 = severe
Score totals range from 18 (no disability) to 72 (most severe disabilities)

Reproduced, with permission, from Linn MW, Linn BS (1982) The Rapid Disability Rating Scale – 2. *Journal of the American Geriatrics Society,* Vol. 30, no. 6, pp. 378–82.

Functional Dementia Scale (FDS)

Reference   Moore JT, Bobula JA, Short TB, Mischel M (1983) A Functional Dementia Scale. *The Journal of Family Practice* **16**: 499–503

Time taken 15 minutes (reviewer's estimate)

Rating by carers

Main indications

An instrument used by families to monitor functional disability in dementia.

Commentary

The Functional Dementia Scale (FDS) contains 20 items in three subscales: activities of daily living, orientation and affect. The instrument was designed starting with 38 items in a pilot study which underwent further refinement. Cluster analysis reduced the number of items to 20, the final version being tested for reliability and validity.

Inter-rater reliability was assessed on 40 patients, with agreement on over 80% of items. Test/retest reliability was 0.88, as was concurrent validity measured by existing cognitive tests, the Short Portable Mental Status Questionnaire (SPMSQ; page 56) and the SET Test (page 58).

Address for correspondence

James T Moore
Duke-Watts Family Medicine Program
407 Crutchfield Street
Durham
NC 27704–2799
USA

Functional Dementia Scale (FDS)

1. Has difficulty in completing simple tasks on own, e.g., dressing, bathing, doing arithmetic
2. Spends time either sitting or in apparently purposeless activity
3. Wanders at night or needs to be restrained to prevent wandering
4. Hears things that are not there
5. Requires supervision or assistance in eating
6. Loses things
7. Appearance is disorderly if let to own devices
8. Moans
9. Cannot control bowel function
10. Threatens to harm others
11. Cannot control bladder function
12. Needs to be watched so doesn't injure self, e.g., by careless smoking, leaving the stove on, falling
13. Destructive of materials around him, e.g., breaks furniture, throws food trays, tears up magazines
14. Shouts or yells
15. Accuses others of doing him bodily harm or stealing his possessions when you are sure the accusations are not true
16. Is unaware of limitations imposed by illness
17. Becomes confused and does not know where he/she is
18. Has trouble remembering
19. Has sudden changes of mood, e.g., gets upset, angered, or cries easily
20. If left alone, wanders aimlessly during the day or needs to be restrained to prevent wandering

Rating:
1 = None little of the time
2 = Some of the time
3 = Good part of the time
4 = Most/all of the time

Performance Test of Activities of Daily Living (PADL)

Reference Kuriansky J, Gurland B (1976) The Performance Test of Activities of Daily Living. *International Journal of Aging and Human Development* 7: 343–52

Time taken 20 minutes (reviewer's estimate)
Rating by experienced interviewer

Main indications

To measure the self-care capacity of old-age psychiatry patients.

Commentary

The Performance Test of Activities of Daily Living (PADL) scale is a measure of actual performance on a series of activities in daily living functions, thus overcoming the drawback of the subjective nature of self or observer reports. Some 16 activities were measured on a total of 96 patients, 48 each in New York and London as part of the US/UK project (Copeland et al, 1976). Inter-rater reliability was 0.90 and face and content validity were apparent.

Additional reference

Copeland JRM, Kelleher MJ, Kellett JM et al (1976) A semi-structured clinical interview for the assessment of diagnosis and mental state in the elderly: the Geriatric Mental State Schedule. I. Development and reliability. *Psychological Medicine* **6**: 451–9.

Performance Test of Activities of Daily Living (PADL)

Tasks

Task requests

		Props to be used
1.	Drink from a cup	Cup
2.	Use a tissue to wipe nose	Tissue box
3.	Comb hair	Comb
4.	File nails	Nail file
5.	Shave	Shaver
6.	Lift food onto spoon and to mouth	Spoon with candy on it
7.	Turn faucet on and off	Faucet
8.	Turn light switch on and off	Light switch
9.	Put on and remove a jacket with buttons	Jacket
10.	Put on and remove a slipper	Slipper
11.	Brush teeth, including removing false ones	Toothbrush
12.	Make a phone call	Telephone
13.	Sign name	Paper and pen
14.	Turn key in lock	Keyhole and key
15.	Tell time	Clock
16.	Stand up and walk a few steps and sit back down	

Sample items

Activity	Preparation	Interviewer instructions	Patient performance	Rating
Eating	Place candy on spoon and put spoon on flat surface in front of patient	"Show me how you eat"	Grasps spoon by handle	0 1 9
			Keep spoon horizontal	0 1 9
			Keeps candy balanced on spoon	0 1 9
			Aims at mouth	0 1 9
			Touches spoon to mouth	0 1 9
Grooming	Place comb on table in front of patient	"Show me how you comb your hair"	Takes comb in hand	0 1 9
			Grasps comb properly	0 1 9
			Brings comb to hair	0 1 9
			Makes combing motions	0 1 9
Dressing	Give patient jacket with sleeves	"Put this jacket on for me and then take it off"	Takes hold of jacket	0 1 9
			Slips one arm in jacket	0 1 9
			Pulls jacket over shoulders and back	0 1 9
			Slips other arm into sleeve	0 1 9
			Frees one arm	0 1 9
			Frees other arm	0 1 9
			Removes jacket from body	0 1 9

Reproduced from Kuriansky J, Gurland B (1976) The Performance Test of Activities of Daily Living. *International Journal of Aging and Human Development* **7**: 343–52, published by Baywood Publishing Co.

Structured Assessment of Independent Living Skills (SALES)

Reference   Mahurin RK, DeBettignieis and Pirozzolo FJ (1991) Structured assessment of independent living skills: preliminary report of a peformance measure of functional abilities in dementia. *Journal of Gerontology* 46: 58–66

Time taken 60 minutes (reviewer's estimate)

Rating by trained interviewer

Main indications

Assessment of everyday activities affected in dementia.

Commentary

The Structued Assessment of Independent Living Skills (SALES) score is divided into a motor score (the addition of the 4 scales: fine motor skills, gross motor skills, dressing skills and eating skills) with a cognitive score representing the addition of expressive language, receptive language, time and orientation and money-related skills. Social interaction and mental activities are rated separately. SALES is divided into 10 subscales, each with 5 items rated on a 3-point scale giving a maximum score of 150 points. A number of neuropsychological tests were carried out to act as markers of validity. The scale was administered to 18 patients with Alzheimer's disease and 18 controls. Test/retest for the total score was 0.81. Inter-rater reliability was 0.99. There were significant differences between the findings on the patients with Alzheimer's disease and the normal controls. Total score was correlated with the Mini-Mental State Examination (MMSE; page 34), the Global Deterioration Scale (page 166) and IQ test. There was no relation with the Geriatric Depression Scale (page 2).

Address for correspondence

Roderick K Mahurin
Alzheimer's Disease Research Center
Baylor College of Medicine
Department of Neurology
6550 Fannin – Suite 1801
Houston TX 77030
USA

Structured Assessment of Independent Living Skills (SALES)

Name: Date:

Age: Sex: Handedness: Education: Examiner:

Diagnosis:
Note: If patient is unable to complete task, assign maximum time of 60" unless otherwise indicated

MOTOR TASKS

Fine Motor Skills	Time	Score

1. Picks up coins   0=drops two 1=drops one 2=slow 3=normal (8")
2. Removes wrappers   0=needs assistance 1=tears one or more 2=slow 3=normal (35")
3. Cuts with scissors 0=can't cut 1=off line 2=slow 3=normal (32")
4. Folds letter and places in envelope 0=can't fold 1=doesn't fit 2=slow 3=normal (16")
5. Uses key in lock 0=can't insert 1=can't unlock 2=slow 3=normal (13")
   Subtotal:

Gross Motor Skills	Time	Score

1. Stands up from sitting 0=unable 1=uses arms of chair 2=slow 3=normal (2")
2. Opens and walks through door 0=unable 1=needs door held open
   2=slow 3=normal (5")
3. Regular gait 0=unable 1=assistive device 2=slow 3=normal (6")
   Time 1) __ 2) __ Mean __ Steps 1) __ 2) __ Mean __
4. Tandem gait 0=unable, steps off 4 or more times 1=steps off 2–3 times
   2=slow (1 step off allowed) 3=normal (9")
   Time 1) __ 2) __ Mean __ Steps off line 1) __ 2) __ Mean __
5. Transfers object across room   0=drops 1=inaccurate placement 2=slow 3=normal (6")
   Time 1) __ 2) __ Mean __
   Subtotal:

Dressing Skills	Time	Score

1. Puts on shirt (maximum=120")   0=can't put on or button 1=misaligned
   2=slow 3=normal (86")
2. Buttons cuffs of shirt   0=unable 1=one cuff 2=slow 3=normal (45")
3. Puts on jacket   0=can't put on 1=needs help with zipper 2=slow 3=normal (27")
4. Ties shoelaces   0=unable/wrong feet 1=knot comes undone 2=slow 3=normal (9")
5. Puts on gloves   0=unable 1=one hand 2=slow 3=normal (21")
   Subtotal:

Eating Skills	Time	Score

1. Drinks from glass 0=unable 1=spits 2=slow 3=normal (3")
2. Transfers food with spoon 0=unable 1=drops 2=slow 3=normal (11")
3. Cuts with fork and knife 0=unable 1=drops 2=slow 3=normal (16")
4. Transfers food with fork 0=unable 1=drops 2=slow 3=normal (16")
5. Transfers liquid with spoon 0=unable 1=spills 2=slow 3=normal (13")
   Subtotal:

Total Motor Time _____   Total Motor Score _____

COGNITIVE TASKS

Expressive Language	Score

1. Quality of expression 0=severe < 25% 1=moderate 25–90% 2=mild 90-99% 3=intact
2. Repetition 0=no items 1=1 item 2=2 items 3=all 3 items
3. Object naming 0=3 or less 1=4 items 2=5 items 3=all 6 items
4. Writes legible note 0=illegible 1=1 item 2=2 items 3=all 3 items
5. Completes application form 0=3 or less 1=4 items 2=5 items 3=all 6 items
   Subtotal:

Scale is continued overleaf

Receptive language

Score

1. *Reads and follows printed instructions 0=none 1=1 item 2=2 items 3=all 3 items*
2. *Understands written material 0=none 1=1-4 items 2=5 items 3=all 6 items*
    Article 1: Correct 1) __ 2) __ 3)
    Article 2: Correct 1) __ 2) __ 3)
3. *Understands common signs 0=none 1=1 item 2=2 items 3=all 3 items*
4. *Follows verbal directions 0=none 1=1 item 2=2 items 3=3 items*
    1)Touch shoulder 2)Hands on table, close eyes 3)Draw circle, hand pencil, fold paper
5. *Identifies named objects 0=none 1=1 item 2=2 items 3=all 3 items*
    Subtotal:

Time and Orientation

Score

1. *States time on clock (6:14) 0=off over 1 hour 1=off within 1 hour 2=off 10 minutes*
    3=correct within 1 minute
2. *Calculates time interval (until 7:30) 0=off 1 hour 1=off within 1 hour 2=off within 15 minutes*
    3=correct within 1 minute
3. *States time of alarm setting (8:15) 0=off 1 hour 1=off within 1 hour 2=off within 15 min*
    3=correct within 1 minute
4. *Locates current date on calendar 0=incorrect month 1=correct month*
    2=correct week 3=correct date
5. *Correctly reads calendar 0=none 1=1 item 2=2 items 3=all 3 items*
    1) Fridays 2) Day of 15th 3) 2nd Monday
    Subtotal:

Money-Related Skills

Score

1. *Counts money 0=none 1=1 item 2=2 items 3=all 3 items*
    1) 35 cents __ 2) 95 cents __ 3) $1.41 __
2. *Makes change 0=none 1=1 item 2=2 items 3=all 3 items*
    1) ($75 from $1.00)=S.25 __ 2) ($41 from $.50)=$.09 __
    3) ($2.79 from $5.00)=$2.21 __
3. *Understands monthly utility bill 0=none 1=1 item 2=2 items 3=all 3 items*
    1) (Light Co.) __ 2) ($38.46) __ 3) (3/6/87) __
4. *Writes check 0=2 or less 1=3 items 2=4 items 3=all 5 items*
    1)Date 2)Payee 3)Numerical amount 4)Written amount 5)Signature
5. *Understands chequebook 0=none 1=1 item 2=2 items 3=all 3 items*
    1)Checks on August 11 2)Check #355 3)Balance ($440.40)
    Subtotal:

Total Cognitive Score ___

Instrumental Activities

Score

1. *Uses telephone book 0=none 1=1 item 2=2 items 3=all 3 items*
2. *Dials telephone number 0=cannot handle phone 1=misdials number*
    2=needs help to read 3=correctly reads and dials
3. *Understands medication label 0=none 1=1 item 2=2 items 3=all 3 items*
4. *Opens medication container 0=can't open two 1=can't open one 2=needs cue 3=normal*
5. *Follows simple recipe 0=unable 1=1 step 2=2 steps 3=all 3 steps*

    Subtotal:

Social Interaction

Score

1. *Responds to greeting and farewell 0=none 1=1 item 2=2 items 3=all 3 items*
2. *Responds to request for information 0=none 1=1 item 2=2 items 3=all 3 items*
3. *Responds to social directives 0=none 1=1 item 2=2 items 3=all 3 items*
4. *Requests needed information 0=none 1=1 item 2=2 items 3=all 3 items*
5. *Understanding non-verbal expression 0=none 1=1 item 2=2 items 3=all 3 items*

    Subtotal:

GRAND TOTAL SCORE _____

Direct Assessment of Activities of Daily Living in Alzheimer's Disease

Reference   Skurla E, Roger JC, Sunderland T (1988) Direct assessment of activities of daily living in Alzheimer's disease. *Journal of the American Geriatrics Society* 36: 97–103

Time taken 19.4 minutes

Rating by direct observation

Main indications

Assessment of activities of daily living by using a direct measure of self-care.

Commentary

Nine patients with Alzheimer's disease and nine matched normal controls were assessed using the four experimental tasks of dressing, meal preparation, telephoning and purchasing. Verbal prompts were given as necessary to help to initiate a task, as were visual and physical prompting. Each type of prompt was repeated twice. Two scores were obtained for each item. The first is a performance score rated 0–4, the second is the time required to complete each task. Significant positive correlations were found between the severity of dementia as measured by the Clinical Severity Rating and the ADL Situational Task, but a non-significant trend for a positive correlation between the latter and the test of cognitive function used the Short Portable Mental Status Questionnaire (SPMSQ; page 56). The Situational Task allowed the examiner to ascertain the nature of the impairment affecting performance and may have implications for caregiving strategies.

Performance of each subtask was scored 0–4 according to the following code: 4 = complete subtask independently; 3 = requires verbal prompting; 2 = requires verbal and visual prompting; 1 = requires verbal and physical prompting; 0 = does not complete the subtask. Maximum score for dressing is 40, for meal preparation is 36, for telephoning 44 and for purchasing 32. The subjects total raw score is then divided by the highest possible score to obtain a percentage for each ADL task. A higher percentage corresponds to better or more independent performances. Possible scores range from 0 to 152.

Direct Assessment of Activities of Daily Living in Alzheimer's Disease – ADL Situational Task

Dressing: Selecting and donning clothing for a cold, rainy day

1. Attempts to select clothing.
2. Selects appropriate clothing for weather conditions.
3. Selects adequate amount of clothing for weather.
4. Selects clothing of approximate size.
5. Attempts to put on clothing.
6. Puts on clothing in correct order.
7. Puts clothing on right side out and front forward.
8. Puts on reasonable layers of clothing.
9. Puts shoes on correct feet.
10. Buttons or snaps coat or sweater correctly.

Meal Preparation: Making a cup of instant coffee

1. Attempts to read the directions.
2. Puts an adequate amount of water in the pot.
3. Places pot on burner.
4. Turns burner on to correct temperature.
5. Opens jar.
6. Measures reasonable amount of coffee, sugar, and cream into cup.
7. Removes water from heat when hot and pours it into cup.
8. Uses caution around hot burner and pot.
9. Turns off burner.

Telephoning: Calling to find out pharmacy hours

1. Attempts to use phone book.
2. Uses alphabetized headings to find pharmacies.
3. Selects number from appropriate category.
4. Picks up the receiver before dialing.
5. Holds receiver correctly.
6. Attempts to dial the number.
7. Dials the number correctly.
8. Begins conversation when connection is made.
9. Asks appropriate questions to find out pharmacy hours.
10. Reports correct information.
11. Places receiver down correctly.

Purchasing: Using money to purchase a snack and gloves

1. Attempts to select a snack.
2. Selects an edible item for a snack.
3. Attempts to pay for snack.
4. Pays with the correct amount of change.
5. Attempts to select gloves.
6. Selects gloves that are the appropriate size.
7. Attempts to pay for the gloves.
8. Pays correct amount of money.

Refined ADL Assessment Scale (RADL)

Reference Tappen R (1994) Development of the refined ADL assessment scale for patients with Alzheimer's and related disorders. *Journal of Gerontological Nursing* 20: 36–41.

Time taken 20 minutes
Rating by nurses

Main indications

Designed specifically for patients with Alzheimer's disease in the middle and later stages of the illness.

Commentary

The Refined ADL Assessment Scale (RADL) is composed of 14 separate tasks within 5 selected ADL areas (toileting, washing, grooming, dressing and eating). Each task is broken down into its component steps, the number of steps ranging from 5 to 21. The amount of time and help needed to complete the task is recorded. Reliability on 28 patients was between 50% and 90% without training and up to 100% agreement among nurse raters scoring a videotaped stimulation. Validity of the instrument was assessed by comparison with existing ADL scales [PSMS; page 129, and the Performance Test of Activities of Daily Living (PADL; page 154)]. Correlations were moderate.

Additional References

Beck C (1988) Measurement of dressing performance in persons with dementia. *American Journal of Alzheimer's care and Related Disorders and Research* 3(3): 21–5.

Warzak WJ, Kilburn J (1990) A behavioral approach to activities of daily living. In Tupper DE, Cicerone KD (eds), *The neuropsychology of everyday life: Assessment and basic competences.* Boston: Kluwer Academic, 285–305.

Wiener JM, Hanley RJ, Clark R et al (1990) Measuring the activities of daily living: Comparisons across national surveys. *Journal of Gerontology* 45: S229–37.

Address for correspondence

Ruth Tappen
School of Nursing
University of Miami
PO Box 248153 (5801 Red Road)
Coral Gables
FL 33124
USA

Sample Subscale from the Refined ADL Assessment Scale (RADL): Wash Hands

Given: Person standing or sitting at wheelchair-height sink. Bar of soap and paper towels at sink. Initial cue: "Now, wash your hands."

	Unassisted 6	Verbal Prompt 5	Nonverbal Prompt 4	Physical Guiding 3	Full Assist (Attempt Made) 2	Full Assist (No Attempt Made) 1	N/A*
Walk to sink							
Turn on water							
Place both hands in water							
Get soap							
Put soap on hands							
Put soap down							
Rub hands together							
Rinse hands							
Turn off water							
Get paper towel							
Dry hands							
Drop towel in wastebasket							
Leave bathroom							

Time to complete this action: _____ minutes.

*The N/A column (Not Applicable) is used only if the particular step is not necessary.

- Toileting: entering bathroom, using toilet facilities;
- Washing: washing hands, washing face;
- Grooming: brushing teeth, combing hair;
- Dressing: putting on pants, putting on shirt or blouse, putting on shoes; and
- Eating: cutting food, using a fork, using a spoon, drinking from a glass or cup, using a napkin.

Each of these tasks is broken down into its component steps. The number of steps ranges from 5 to 21 for a given task. The amount of time it takes the individual to complete each task is also recorded.

On the RADL, the cognitively impaired person's ability to perform each component step is rated in terms of the amount of assistance needed to complete the step successfully, ranging from unassisted to full assistance (Wiener et al, 1990).

Using a series similar to the one described by Beck (1988) and Warzak and Kilburn (1990), the individual is rated as having completed each step unassisted, with only a verbal prompt, with verbal and nonverbal prompts, with physical guiding, or with full assistance. Full assistance is rated as having been done with or without an attempt to perform the behavior. These five levels of assistance are defined as follows:

- Unassisted: done without further action on the part of the caregiver after initial cue;
- Verbal prompt: spoken directions only from caregiver;
- Nonverbal prompt: gestures, demonstration of correct behavior by caregiver;
- Physical guiding: caregiver provided some assistance with the behavior but patient participates in carrying out the step; and
- Full assistance: patient unable to contribute to carrying out the step (note whether the patient attempted the behavior).

Reproduced, with permission, from Tappen R (1994) Development of the refined ADL assessment scale for patients with Alzheimer's and related disorders. *Journal of Gerontological Nursing* 36–41.

Bayer Activities of Daily Living Scale (B-ADL)

Reference Hindmarch I, Lehfeld H, Jongh P (1998) *Dementia and Geriatric Cognitive Disorders* 9 (Suppl. 2): 20–6.

Time taken 20 minutes (reviewer's estimate)
Rating by caregiver

Main indications

Assessment of activities of daily living in people with mild to moderate dementia.

Commentary

The B-ADL scale was developed because of the need to measure changes in activities of daily living in the early stages of dementia. Sponsored by the pharmaceutical company Bayer, this scale was developed following an international series of field studies. One hundred and forty-one informant and 63 self-rated questionnaires were tested, and only those items sensitive to changes in early dementia and those without a significant gender of cultural bias were removed. Twenty-one items remained and a further four were added after the end of the pilot study, giving a total of 25 questions. The two introductory questions evaluate everyday activities, questions 3–20 assess direct problems in relation to specific tasks of everyday living, and the final five items relate to cognitive functions. The scoring is on a 10-point scale by asking the caregiver to draw a line through one of the appropriate circles marked 1–10. A global score is computed by summing the total score and dividing it by the number of answered items with a figure rounded to two decimal places, giving a total score of between 1.00 and 10.00. Further tests are underway to establish the reliability and validity of the scale.

Additional References

Erzigkeit H, Overall J, Stemmler M et al (1995) Assessing behavioural changes in anti-dementia therapy: perspectyives of an international ADL project. In Bergener M, Brocklehurst J, Finkel S (eds), *Ageing, Health and Healing.* New York: Springer 1995, pp. 359–74.

Lehfeld H, Reisberg B, Finkel S et al (1997) Informant rated activities of daily living assessments. *Alzheimer's Disease and Associated Disorders* 1 (Suppl 4), S39–44.

Bayer Activities of Daily Living Scale (B-ADL)

Does the person have difficulty

1. ...managing his/her everyday activities?
2. ...taking care of him/herself?
3. ...taking medication without supervision?
4. ...with personal hygiene?
5. ...observing important dates or events
6. ...concentrating on reading?
7. ...describing what he/she has just seen or heard?
8. ...taking part in a conversation?
9. ...using the telephone?
10. ...taking a message for someone else?
11. ...going for a walk without getting lost?
12. ...shopping?
13. ...preparing food?
14. ...correctly counting out money?
15. ...understanding his/her personal financial affairs?
16. ...giving directions if asked the way?
17. ...using domestic appliances?
18. ...finding his/her way in an unfamilar place?
19. ...using transportation?
20. ...participating his/her leisure activities?
21. ...continuing with the same task after a brief interruption?
22. ...doing two things at the same time?
23. ...coping with unfamiliar situations?
24. ...doing things safely?
25. ...performing a task when under pressure?

Instructions
The questions above are about everyday activities with which the patient might have difficulty. The frequency of occurrence of these difficulties are rated on a scale of 1–10 – with a rating of 1 indicating that the difficulty never arises and 10 indicating that it always arises. If the question is not applicable to the patient, or if the patient's experience of the difficulty is in anyway unclear, then these responses must be recorded too – as 'not applicable' and 'unknown' respectively. An example of this scoring is shown below:

	not applicable	unknown	SCORE
never ①②③④⑤⑥⑦⑧⑨⑩ always	☐	☐	☐

Reproduced with permission of S. Karger AG, Basel.

Global assessments/ quality of life

These are useful in describing, in broad terms, the severity of dementia. This can be of use in looking at a population and may be useful for measuring change. The assumption behind some of these tests is that dementia progresses in an orderly and linear form. This is clearly inaccurate, but there is still some use in identifying whether patients are mild, moderate or severely demented. The Clinical Dementia Rating (CDR; page 168) is the simplest scale, and is constructed from six domains, whereas the Global Deterioration Scale (GDS; page 166) emphasizes the signs and symptoms of dementia in the later stages of the illness. The Sandoz Clinical Assessment – Geriatric (SCAG; page 188) includes a seven-point severity rating scale after 18 questions covering a wide variety of features of dementia. The Hierarchic Dementia Scale (page 183) also rates global severity, but there has not been as much published work on it and functional and social capacity are not included. Some measures mix a variety of features together [e.g. the Mattis Dementia Scale (page 186), the Dementia Rating Scale (page 176), the GBS Scale (page 177), the PAMIE Scale (page 180), the Stockton Geriatric Rating Scale (page 182), the SCAG and the Psychogeriatric Dependency Rating Scales (PGDRS; page 174)].

Quality of life (QOL) is a difficult area to discuss because of the inherent problems in defining the term and the fact that it invariably means different things to different people. It is generally accepted that QOL in dementia is multi-faceted and one should try to individualize it. The concept of QOL for patients has been broekn down into four domains: two objective and two subjective. Behavioural competence encompasses activities of daily living, cognitive performance and social behaviour, all of which can be measured. The second objective measure is the envionment, and scales such as the Social Care Environment Scale can evaluate the surroundings of a patient and rate them according to a set standard. The two subjective measures are the person's evaluation of their own environment in specific domains (e.g. housing, income, children, work) and finally a global measure of their evaluation of their own self within that environment. These two latter judgements are hard to sustain in the presence of significant cognitive impairment. As such, many of the measures in this book could be regarded as contributing to an overall QOL assessment which could be inferred from the absence of many of the disabilities measured in the scales. Specific measures of QOL

are included which attempt to summarize the concept but, in themselves, are probably not useful unless combined with other assessments of the self and the environment. The Quality of Life in Alzheimer's Disease: Patient and Caregiver Report (QOL-AD; page 288) attempts to measure QOL specifically in dementia. It is brief and addresses both the patient and the carer. Generic measures of QOL should be used with caution, although the scale described by Blau (Quality of Life in Dementia; page 280) has been used to show change in trials of drugs for Alzheimer's disease.

Global measures of change have become increasingly popular in drug trials, with the basic underlying assumption being that clinicians can detect a change in patients based on an interview without the need for formal scales. This is an inherently reasonable assumption, on which most of medicine is based. The first scale of this type was the Clinicians' Global Impression of Change (CGIC; page 170), in which patients were rated on a seven-point scale from very much improved to very much worse. This proved relatively insensitive to change, and structuring of the instruments began, driven in part by the pharmaceutical industry's attempt to provide a clinically meaningful assessment of real life change rather than relying on a change of a few points on a cognitive rating scale. This structuring spawned a number of scales (page 170), including the CIBIC and the CIBIC plus 9, in which information from an informant was provided in addition to the clinician interview. This structuring is helpful, but the downside is that the measures simply change into more rating scales rather than capturing the clinician's view of the patient. The CIBI has probably been most frequently tested and used in the recently published Aricept trials.

With the understandable emphasis on outcomes, it has become fashionable to look at changes over time in patients with cognitive impairment. Outcomes can be thought of as changes in a particular scale or scales, many of which were not designed to be sensitive to change but are used in that way in any case. Second (and easier to measure), are outcomes which are predetermined endpoints of disease such as admission to institutional care, progression to a predefined level of disability (such as the emergence of incontinence) or to a defined degree of dementia severity (say CDR 3 on the Clinical Dementia Rating). These are in addition to the ultimate outcome measure – death.

Functional Assessment Staging (FAST)

Reference   Reisberg B (1988) Functional assessment staging (FAST). *Psychopharmacology Bulletin* 24: 653–9

Time taken 2 minutes (once all the information is gathered)
Rating by clinician, after interview with informant

Main indications

Assessment of funtional change in ageing and dementia.

Commentary

The Functional Assessment Staging (FAST) is a rating scale which can be used as part of the Global Deterioration Scale (GDS; page 166). It rates functional change in 7 major stages with a total of 16 successive stages and substages. Reliability of the FAST has been demonstrated with intra-class correlations of above 0.85. Concurrent validity has been assessed against the GDS and a number of neuropsychological tests (Reisberg et al, 1994). It has been shown that functional detriments in Alzheimer's disease proceed in a hierarchial ordinal pattern reflecting the FAST stages (Sclan and Reisberg, 1992). A particular advantage of the FAST is that it identifies a total of 11 substages according to the later stages of the GDS and so is particularly useful in the detailed staging and substaging of severe Alzheimer's disease.

Additional references

Reisberg B (1986) Dementia: a systematic approach to identifying reversible causes. *Geriatrics* 41: 30–46

Reisberg B et al (1994) Dementia staging in chronic care populations. *Alzheimer Disease and Associated Disorders* 8: S188–S205.

Sclan S, Reisberg B (1992) FAST in Alzheimer's disease; reliability, validity and ordinality. *International Psychogeriatrics* 4 (suppl 1): 55–69.

Address for correspondence

Barry Reisberg
Department of Psychiatry
Aging and Dementia Research Center
NYU Medical Center
550 First Avenue
NY 10016
USA

Functional Assessment Staging (FAST)

Yes	Months[1]	No.		
__	_____	__	1.	No difficulties, either subjectively or objectively.
__	_____	__	2.	Complains of forgetting location of objects; subjective work difficulties.
__	_____	__	3.	Decrease job functioning evident to coworkers; difficulty in traveling to new locations.
__	_____	__	4.	Decreased ability to perform complex tasks (e.g., planning dinner for guests; handling finances; marketing)
__	_____	__	5.	Requires assistance in choosing proper clothing.
__	_____	__	6a.	Difficulty putting clothing on properly.
__	_____	__	6b.	Unable to bathe properly; may develop fear of bathing.
__	_____	__	6c.	Inability to handle mechanics of toileting (i.e., forgets to flush, doesn't wipe properly).
__	_____	__	6d.	Urinary incontinence.
__	_____	__	6e.	Fecal incontinence.
__	_____	__	7a.	Ability to speak limited (1 to 5 words a day).
__	_____	__	7b.	All intelligible vocabulary lost.
__	_____	__	7c.	Nonambulatory.
__	_____	__	7d.	Unable to sit up independently.
__	_____	__	7e.	Unable to smile.
__	_____	__	7f.	Unable to hold head up.

TESTER: _____ COMMENTS: _____

Note: Functional staging score = Highest ordinal value. [1]Number of months FAST stage deficit has been noted.

Reproduced from Reisberg B (1988) Functional assessment staging (FAST). *Psychopharmacology Bulletin* **24**: 653–9.

Global Deterioration Scale (GDS)

Reference   Reisberg B, Ferris SH, de Leon MJ, Crook T (1982) The Global Deterioration Scale (GDS) for assessment of primary degenerative dementia. *American Journal of Psychiatry* 139: 1136–9

Time taken 2 minutes (once information has been collected)
Rating by clinician

Main indications

A staging instrument indicating deterioration in dementia.

Commentary

The Global Deterioration Scale (GDS) is the main part of a clinical rating system called the Global Deterioration Scale Staging System. Three independent measures are included in the Staging System: the GDS, the Brief Cognitive Rating Scale (BCRS; page 52) and the Functional Assessment Staging measure (FAST; page 164). The GDS is made up of detailed clinical descriptions of seven major clinically distinguishable stages, ranging from normal cognition to very severe dementia. Concurrent validity of the GDS has been demonstrated by a highly significant correlation between ratings and other neuropsychological tests such as the Mini-Mental State Examination (MMSE; page 34) (Reisberg et al, 1988). Content validity of the GDS was demonstrated independently by developing a 30-item questionnaire which, following a principal components analysis, clustered naturally into stages corresponding with GDS descriptions (Overall et al, 1990).

Inter-rater and test/retest reliability has been demonstrated regularly at over 0.90 in terms of both test/retest and inter-rater reliability (Reisberg et al, 1996). It has a wide number of uses as a staging measure in descriptive and intervention studies.

Additional references

Overall J, Scott J, Rhodes H, Lesser J (1990) Empirical scaling of the stages of cognitive decline in senile dementia. *Journal of Geriatric Psychiatry and Neurology* 3: 212–20.

Reisberg B, Ferris S, Schulman E et al (1986) Longitudinal course of normal aging and progressive dementia of the Alzheimer's type: a prospective study of 106 subjects over a 3.6 year mean interval. *Progress in Neuro-psychopharmacology and Biological Psychiatry* 10: 571–8.

Reisberg B et al (1988) Stage specific behavioural cognitive and in vivo changes in community residing subjects with AAMI and AD. *Drug Development Research* 15: 101–4.

Reisberg B et al (1993) Clinical stages of normal ageing in Alzheimer's disease: the GDS staging system. *Neuroscience Research Communications* 13: 551–4.

Reisberg B et al (1996) Overview of methodologic issues for pharmacologic trials in mild, moderate and severe Alzheimer's disease. *International Psychogeriatrics* 8: 159–93.

Address for correspondence

Barry Reisberg
Department of Psychiatry
Aging and Dementia Research Center
NYU Medical Center
550 First Avenue
NY 10016
USA

Global Deterioration Scale (GDS)

1. No subjective complaints of memory deficit. No memory deficit evident on clinical interview.

2. Subjective complaints of memory deficit, most frequently in following areas:
   (a) forgetting where one has placed familiar objects.
   (b) forgetting names one formerly knew well.

3. Earliest clear-cut deficits.

   Manifestations in more than one of the following areas:
   (a) patient may have gotten lost when travelling to an unfamiliar location.
   (b) co-workers become aware of patient's relatively poor performance.
   (c) word and/or name finding deficit become evident to intimates.
   (d) patient may read a passage or book and retain relatively little material.
   (e) patient may demonstrate decreased facility remembering names upon introduction to new people.
   (f) patient may have lost or misplaced an object of value.
   (g) concentration deficit may be evident on clinical testing.

4. Clear-cut deficit on careful clinical interview.
   Deficit manifest in following areas:
   (a) decreased knowledge of current and recent events.
   (b) may exhibit some deficit in memory of one's personal history.
   (c) concentration deficit elicited on serial subtractions.
   (d) decreased abilty to travel, handle finances, etc.

   Frequently no deficit in following areas:
   (a) orientation to time and place.
   (b) recognition of familiar persons and faces.
   (c) ability to travel to familiar locations.

5. Patient can no longer survive without some assistance.

   Patient is unable during interview to recall a major relevant aspect of their current life, e.g.:
   (a) their address or telephone number of many years.
   (b) the names of close members of their family (such as grandchildren).
   (c) the name of the high school or college from which they graduated.

6. May occasionally forget the name of the spouse upon whom they are entirely dependent for survival.
   Will be largely unaware of all recent events and experiences in their lives.
   Retain some knowledge of their surroundings; the year, the season, etc.
   May have difficulty counting by 1s from 10, both backward and sometimes forward.

   Will require some assistance with activities of daily living:
   (a) may become incontinent.
   (b) will require travel assistance but occasionally will be able to travel to familiar locations.

   Diurnal rhythm frequently disturbed.
   Almost always recall their own name.
   Frequently continue to be able to distinguish familiar from unfamiliar persons in their environment.

   Pesonality and emotional changes occur. These are quite variable and include:
   (a) delusional behavior, e.g. patients may accuse their spouse of being an imposter; may talk to imaginary figures in the environment , or to their own reflection in the mirror.
   (b) obsessive symptoms, e.g. person may continually repeat simple cleaning activities.
   (c) anxiety symptoms, agitation, and even previously non-existent violent behavior may occur.
   (d) cognitive abulia, e.g. loss of willpower because an individual cannot carry a thought long enough to determine a purposeful course of action.

7. All verbal abilities are lost over the course of this stage.
   Early in this stage words and phrases are spoken but speech is very circumscribed.
   Later there is no speech at all – only grunting.

   Incontinent; requires assistance toileting and feeding.

   Basic psychomotor skills (e.g. ability to walk) are lost with the progression of this stage.
   The brain appears to no longer be able to tell the body what to do.
   Generalized and cortical neurologic signs and symptoms are frequently present.

Source: *American Journal of Psychiatry*, Vol. 139, pp. 1136–1139, 1982. Copyright 1982, the American Psychiatric Association. Reprinted by permission. The GDS is copyrighted. Copyright © 1983 by Barry Reisberg, M.D. All rights reserved.

Clinical Dementia Rating (CDR)

Reference Hughes CP, Berg L, Danziger WL, Coben LA, Martin RL (1982) A new clinical scale for the staging of dementia. *British Journal of Psychiatry* 140: 566–72; updated by Morris J (1993) The CDR: current version and scoring rules. *Neurology* 43: 2412–3.

Time taken the scale is usually completed in the setting of a detailed knowledge of the individual patient. As such, much of the information will already have been gathered, either as part of normal clinical practice or as part of a research study. If a separate interview is carried out, about 40 minutes is needed to gather the relevant information.

Rating by a clinician using information gathered as part of clinical practice

Main indications

A global measure of dementia.

Commentary

The Clinical Dementia Rating (CDR) has now become one of the gold standards of global ratings of dementia in trials of patients with Alzheimer's disease. Six domains are assessed: memory; orientation; judgement and problem solving; community affairs; home and hobbies; and personal care. CDR ratings are 0 for healthy people, 0.5 for questionable dementia and 1, 2 and 3 for mild, moderate and severe dementia as defined in the scale. The total CDR rating is made from the sum of boxes which represents an aggregate score of each individual's areas. Inter-rater reliability was excellent (correlation coefficient 0.89). The original study included 58 healthy controls and 59 people with dementia. A number of different scales were used in an interview with the spouse and subject, taking about 90 minutes in total. The Blessed Dementia Scale (page 40) (Blessed et al, 1968), the Face–Hand Test (FHT; page 68) (Zarit et al, 1978) and the Short Portable Mental Status Questionnaire (SPMSQ; page 56) were used, and highly significant correlation was found between these tests and the final CDR rating.

The reliability of the CDR has been further established (Berg et al, 1988). Longitudinal data are available on its use (e.g. Berg et al, 1992; Galasko et al, 1995) and it has been validated against neuropathological information (Morris et al, 1988).

Additional references

Berg L, Miller J, Baty A et al (1992) Mild senile dementia of Alzheimer type. *Annals of Neurology* **31**: 242–9.

Berg L, Miller JP, Storandt M et al. (1988) Mild senile dementia of the Alzheimer type: 2. Longitudinal assessment. *Annals of Neurology* **23**: 497–84.

Blessed G, Tomlinson B, Roth M (1968) The association between quantative measures and dementia and senile change in the cerebral grey matter of elderly subjects. *British Journal of Psychiatry* **114**: 797–811.

Burke W, Miller P, Rueben E et al (1988) Reliability of the Washington University Clinical Dementia Rating. *Archives of Neurology* **45**: 31–2.

Galasko D, Edland S, Morris J et al (1995) The consortium to establish a registry for Alzheimer's disease. Part 11. Clinical milestones in patients with Alzheimer's disease followed over 3 years. *Neurology* **45**: 1451–5.

Morris J, McKeel D, Fulling K et al (1988) Validation of clinical diagnostic criteria for Alzheimer's disease. *Annals of Neurology* **24**: 17–22.

Pfeiffer E (1975) A short portable mental state questionnaire for the assessment of organic brain deficit in elderly patients. *Journal of the American Geriatrics Society* **23**: 433–41.

Zarit S, Miller N, Khan R (1978) Brain function, intellectual impairment and education in the aged. *Journal of the American Geriatrics Society* **26**: 58–67.

Address for correspondence

J Morris
Memory and Aging Project
Washington University School of Medicine
660 South Euclid Avenue
PO Box 8111
St Louis
MO 63110
USA

Clinical Dementia Rating (CDR)

	Impairment				
	None **0**	**Questionable** **0.5**	**Mild** **1**	**Moderate** **2**	**Severe** **3**
Memory	No memory loss or slight inconstant forgetfulness	Consistent slight forgetfulness; partial recollection of events; "benign" forgetfulness	Moderate memory loss; more marked for recent events; defect interferes with everyday activities	Severe memory loss; only highly learned material retained; new material rapidly lost	Severe memory loss; only fragments remain
Orientation	Fully oriented	Fully oriented except for slight difficulty with time relationships	Moderate difficulty with time relationships; oriented for place at examination; may have geographic disorientation elsewhere	Severe difficulty with time relationships; usually disoriented to time, often to place	Oriented to person only
Judgment and Problem Solving	Solves everyday problems and handles business and financial affairs well; judgment good in relation to past performance	Slight impairment in solving problems, similarities, and differences	Moderate difficulty in handling problems, similarities, and differences; social judgment usually maintained	Severely impaired in handling problems, similarities, and differences; social judgment usually impaired	Unable to make judgments or solve problems
Community Affairs	Independent function at usual level in job, shopping, and volunteer and social groups	Slight impairment in these activities	Unable to function independently at these activites although may still be engaged in some; appears normal to casual inspection	No pretense of independent function outside home Appears well enough to be taken to functions outside a family home	Appears too ill to be taken to functions outside a family home
Home and Hobbies	Life at home, hobbies, and intellectual interests well maintained	Life at home, hobbies, and intellectual interests slightly impaired	Mild but definite impairment of function at home; more difficult chores abandoned; more complicated hobbies and interests abandoned	Only simple chores preserved; very restricted interests, poorly maintained	No significant function in home
Personal Care	Fully capable of self-care		Needs prompting	Requires assistance in dressing, hygiene, keeping of personal effects	Requires much help with personal care; frequent incontinence

Rating:
Score only as decline from previous usual level due to cognitive loss, not impairment due to other factors

Reproduced from the *British Journal of Psychiatry*, Hughes CP, Berg L, Danziger WL, Coben LA, Martin RL (1982) A new clinical scale for the staging of dementia. Vol. 140, pp. 566–72. © 1982 Royal College of Psychiatrists. Reproduced with permission.

Clinicians' Global Impression of Change

Reference   Guy W (ed) (1976) Clinical Global Impressions (CGI). In: *ECDEU Assessment Manual for Psychopharmacology.* US Department of Health and Human Services, Public Health Service, Alcohol Drug Abuse and Mental Health Administration, NIMH Psychopharmacology Research branch, 218–22.

Time taken varies: 10–40 minutes
Rating by trained rater

Main indications
Global ratings.

Commentary
These measures depend on the ability of a clinician to detect change. By definition, they are global ratings of a patient's clinical condition, and inevitably draw information from a wide variety of sources. These scales have been used extensively in clinical trials of anti-dementia drugs, and assess change from a specified baseline. Only minimal conditions are provided, and the rating is made by choosing and response. The various scales are summarized in the table.

Additional references
Knopman D et al (1994) The Clinician Interview-Based Impression (CIBI): a clinician's global change rating scale in Alzheimer's disease. *Neurology* 44: 2315–21.

Schneider LS, Olin JT (1996) Clinical global impressions in Alzheimer's clinical trials. *International Psychogeriatrics* 8: 277–88.

Schneider LS et al (1997) Validity and reliability of the Alzheimer's Disease co-operative study – clinical global impression of change. *Alzheimer Disease Associated Disorders* 11: S22–32.

Selected Global Impressions of Change scales used in clinical trials

Clinicians' Global Impression of Change (CGIC) (Guy, 1976)
- Also used as a general term for various impressionistic measures, rated by the clinician, based on interviews with or without a collateral source, with or without reference to mental status examination, and with or without reference to cognitive assessment results
- Rated on 7 points: 1 = very much improved; 2 = much improved; 3 = minimally improved; 4 = no change; 5 = minimally worse; 6 = much worse; 7 = very much worse.

FDA Clinicians' Interview-Based Impression of Change (CIBIC)
- FDA modifications to the CGIC suggested that clinical change should be patient interview only
- Access to other sources of information is prevented to minimize bias and maintain independence. During a 10-minute interview, the clinician should systematically assess the domains ordinarily considered part of a clinical examination.
- Rationale: if an experienced clinician can perceive clinical change on the basis of an interview, then such change is likely to be clinically meaningful.
- Various constructions have been made by different companies.

Clinicians' Interview-Based Impression of Change – Plus (CIBIC+)
- A CIBIC as described above except conducted by interviewing both the patient and informant has come to be known as CIBIC+.

CIBI (Parke–Davis) (Schneider and Olin, 1997; Knopman et al, 1997)
- Thorough interviews of the patient and caregiver by a clinician experienced in managing AD patients, require that 8 specific itemss be addressed, including

assessment of mental status.
- A follow-up interview solely with the patient prior to making a change rating.
- Rating is made on a 7-point ordinal scale similar to the CGIC.
- Interviewer is required to assess patient's history, strengths and weaknesses, language, behaviors sensitive to change, motivation, activities of daily living, and anything else of apparent importance.

ADCS-CGIC (Schneider et al, 1997)[1]
- Assesses 15 areas under the domains of cognition, behavior, and social and daily functioning.
- Using a form as a guideline, both patient and caregiver are interviewed; order is not specified.
- Under each area is a list of sample probes and space for notes. There are few requirements for the interviews – an assessment of mental status must be made; clinicians are not permitted to ask about side effects, nor to discuss the patient's functioning with others.
- Change rating is made on the 7-point CGIC scale.

NYU CIBIC+
- Relatively more structured than the previous instruments, requiring separate interviews with the patient to assess cognition and with the caregiver to assess functional activities.
- Uses elements of previously validated assessments of cognition, daily functional activities, and behavior.
- Additional descriptors are provided for the 7-point scale so that for a 1-point minimal rating, change must be 'detectable'; for a 2-point moderate rating, change must be 'clearly apparent', and for a 3-point marked rating, change must be 'dramatic'.

From Schneider LS (1997) An overview of rating scales used in dementia reseaerch, *Alzheimer Insights* – Special Edition, pp. 8–14.

[1]For further information, please refer to Appendix 2 at the end of this book.

Crichton Royal Behavioural Rating Scale (CRBRS)

Reference Robinson RA (1961) Some problems of clinical trials in elderly people. *Gerontologia Clinica* **3**: 247–57

Time taken 10–15 minutes (reviewer's estimate)
Rating by informant

Main indications
For the assessment of psychogeriatric patients.

Commentary
The original paper by Robinson was a description of a scale used in clinical practice. It contains no data but is a masterpiece of clinical description. The Crichton Royal Behavioural Rating Scale (named after Crichton Royal Hospital in Dumfries, Scotland) has been used in a number of different studies and is available in a self-completed version or one to be used with informants (Wilkin and Thompson, 1989). The main scale items are: mobility, memory, orientation, communication, co-operation, restlessness, dressing, feeding, bearing and continence. A confusion subscale has been described which is the sum of the memory orientation and communication scales, and has been found separately to be a reliable and easy method to identify the presence of dementia (Vardon and Blessed, 1986). Validity has been shown to be good when compared to cognitive tests, and construct validity and internal consistence have also been measured (Wilkin and Thompson, 1989). Inter-rater reliability is excellent (Cole, 1989).

Additional references
Cole M (1989) Inter-rater reliability of the Crichton Geriatric Behaviour Rating Scale. *Age and Ageing* **18**: 57–60.

Vardon VM, Blessed G (1986) Confusion ratings and abbreviated mental test performance: a comparison. *Age and Ageing* **15**: 139–44.

Wilkin D, Thompson C (1989) Crichton Royal Behavioural Rating Scale. In *User's guide to dependency measures in elderly people. Social Services Monographs.* Sheffield: University of Sheffield.

Crichton Royal Behavioural Rating Scale (CRBRS)

Score	1 Mobility	2 Orientation	3 Communication	4 Co-operation	5 Restlessness
1	Fully ambulant (including stairs)	Complete	Always clear and retains information	Actively co-operative	None
2	Usually independent (not stairs)	Orientated in ward and identifies persons correctly	Can indicate needs. Can understand simple verbal directions. Can deal with simple information	Passively co-operative	Intermittent
3	Walks with supervision	Misidentifies persons and surroundings but can find way about	Understands simple verbal and non-verbal information but does not indicate needs	Requires frequent encouragement and/or persuasion	Persistent by day
4	Walks with artificial aids or under careful supervision	Cannot find way to bed or to toilet without assistance	Cannot understand simple verbal or non-verbal information but retains some expressive ability	Rejects assistance and shows some independent but poorly directed activity	Persistent by day with frequent nocturnal restlessness
5	Bedfast or mainly so, Chairfast	Lost	No effective contact	Completely resistive or withdrawn	Constant

6 Dressing	7 Feeding	8 Cotinence	9 Sleep	10 Objective	11 Mood Subjective
Dresses correctly unaided	Feeds correctly unaided at appropriate times	Fully continent	Normal (hypnotic not required)	Normal and stable affective response and appearance	Well-being or euphoria
Dressing imperfect but adequate	Feeds adequately with minimum supervision	Nocturnal incontinence unless toileted. Occasional accident (urine or faeces)	Requires occasional hypnotic; or occasionally restless	Fair affective response; or not always appropriate or stable	Self-reproachful, listless, dejected, indecisive, lacks interest. (Not completely well though no specific complaints)
Dressing adequate with minimum supervision	Does not feed adequately unless continually supervised	Continent by day if regularly toileted	Sleeps well with regular hypnotic; or usually restless for a period every night	Marked blunting or impairment of mood or inappropriateness of affect	Marked somatic or hypochondriacal concern. Preoccupation
Dressing inadequate unless continually supervised	Defective feeding because of physical handicap or poor appetite	Urinary incontinence in spite of regular toileting	Occasionally disturbed in spite of regular standard hypnotic	Emotional lability or incontinence of affect. Retarded, lacks spontaneity but can respond	Severe retardation or agitation. Marked withdrawal though responds to questioning
Unable to dress or retain clothing because of mental impairment	Unable to feed because of mental impairment	Regularly/ frequently doubly incontinent	Disturbed even with heavier sedation	Hallucinations or nihilistic delusions of guilt or somatic dysfunction	Suicidal or death wishes. Mute, or agitated to the point of incoherence

Reproduced with permission of S. Karger AG, Basel.

Psychogeriatric Dependency Rating Scales (PGDRS)

Reference   Wilkinson IM, Graham-White J (1980) Psychogeriatric Dependency Rating Scales (PGDRS). A method of assessment for use by nurses. *British Journal of Psychiatry* 137: 558–65

Time taken 20 minutes (reviewer's estimate)
Rating by staff

Main indications

Measure of dependency in elderly patients.

Commentary

The rationale behind the development of the Psychogeriatric Dependency Rating Scales (PGDRS) was specifically to use the knowledge of nurses dealing with psychogeriatric patients in as informed a way as possible to measure orientation, behaviour and physical problems in inpatients, emphasizing the need to define dependency (i.e. nursing time demanded by the patient). Reliability and validity information were presented on over 600 patients. Inter-rater reliability was 0.61 for the orientation items, 0.48 for the behaviour and 0.58 for the physical items. The scales have good face validity and reliability validated against independent judgements of nursing time demanded against diagnosis. A shorter version of the scales was also devised.

Psychogeriatric Dependency Rating Scales (PGDRS)

1. Orientation

Yes	No	
☐	☐	Name in full
☐	☐	Age (years)
☐	☐	Relatives—recognize
☐	☐	Realtives—name
☐	☐	Staff—recognize
☐	☐	Staff—name
☐	☐	Bedroom
☐	☐	Dining room
☐	☐	Bathroom
☐	☐	Belongings

2. Behaviour

N	O	F	
☐	☐	☐	Disruptive
☐	☐	☐	Manipulating
☐	☐	☐	Wandering
☐	☐	☐	Socially Objectionable
☐	☐	☐	Demanding Interaction
☐	☐	☐	Communication Difficulties
☐	☐	☐	Noisy
☐	☐	☐	Active Aggression
☐	☐	☐	Passive Aggression
☐	☐	☐	Verbal Aggression
☐	☐	☐	Restless
☐	☐	☐	Destructive—Self
☐	☐	☐	Destructive (Property)
☐	☐	☐	Affect—Elated
☐	☐	☐	Delusions/Hallucinations
☐	☐	☐	Speech Content

3. Physical

Hearing
- ☐ Full
- ☐ Slight
- ☐ Severe
- ☐ Deaf

Visual
- ☐ Full
- ☐ Slight
- ☐ Severe
- ☐ Blind

Speech
- ☐ Full
- ☐ Slight
- ☐ Severe
- ☐ Dumb

Mobility
- ☐ Full
- ☐ Stairs
- ☐ Aids
- ☐ Assistance
- ☐ Chairfast
- ☐ Bedfast

Dressing
- ☐ Full
- ☐ Verbal
- ☐ Partial
- ☐ Assistance

Personal Hygiene

Verbal guidance		Physical assistance
☐	Oral	☐
☐	Washes	☐
☐	Cleans*	☐
☐	Hair	☐
☐	Bath entry	☐
	*after toileting	

N	O	F	
☐	☐	☐	Requires Toiletting
☐	☐	☐	Urine—Day
☐	☐	☐	Urine—Night
☐	☐	☐	Faeces—Day
☐	☐	☐	Faeces—Night
☐	☐	☐	Feeding

Special Physical Disabilities: (specify)

Rating:

N = Never
O = Occasionally = 2/5 days or less
F = Frequently = 3/5 days or more

Reproduced from the *British Journal of Psychiatry*, Wilkinson IM, Graham-White J (1980) Psychogeriatric Dependency Rating Scales (PGDRS). A method of assessment for use by nurses. Vol. 137, pp. 558–65. © 1980 Royal College of Psychiatrists. Reproduced with permission.

Dementia Rating Scale

Reference   Lawson JS, Rodenburg M, Dykes JA (1977) A Dementia Rating Scale for use with psychogeriatric patients. *Journal of Gerontology* 32: 153–9

Time taken 20–25 minutes (reviewer's estimate)
Rating by observer

Main indications

Evaluation of global functioning in dementia.

Commentary

The Dementia Rating Scale is a 27-item scale rated on a simple yes/no response. Inter-rater reliability was 0.95. Test/retest reliability was above 0.59 (depending on time lapse), and internal consistency was assessed using split half reliability and found to be 0.86. A factor analysis revealed eight factors, four accounting for 50% of the variance. The scale was able to differentiate between patients with organic and functional illness.

Dementia Rating Scale

1. Disorientation to place
    (Where are you now? If the patient fails to reply or gives irrelevant reply—Are you in a school, a church, a hospital or a house? Only the alternative "hospital" earns a zero score.)
2. Disorientation to people
    (Ability to distinguish staff from patients scores zero.)
3. Disorientation to time
    (Year.)
4. Disorientation to time
    (Month.)
5. Disorientation to time
    (Day.)
6. Disorientation to time of day
    (Morning, afternoon, evening. Consider meals—lunch and supper as cut-off points.)
7. Disorientation to inside surroundings
    (Inability to find bathroom.)
8. Disorientation to own age
    (Within five years earns zero score.)
9. Loss of personal identity
    (Patient does not know whom he is.)
10. Eating
    (Inability to feed himself without assistance for reasons other than physical illness.)
11. Dressing
    (Inability to dress himself without assistance for reasons other than physical illness.)
12. Incontinence
    (Incontinence of urine during the day.)
13. Sleep
    (Repeat of PRN hypnotic required.)
14. Wandering
    (Patient roams aimlessly though the hospital or ward.)
15. Motor restlessness
    (Pacing or agitated behavior for other than physical reasons.)
16. Slowing of motor function
    (For other than physical reasons.)
17. Motor perseveration
    (Purposeless repetition of a movement.)
18. Verbal perseveration
    (Purposeless repetition of a syllable, word or phase.)
19. Echopraxia
    (Copies the movement of others.)
20. Echoalia
    (Copies verbal utterances of others.)
21. Emotional lability
    (Inappropriate and sudden change of emotional expression.)
22. Catastrophic reaction
    (Affect of inappropriate intensity in response to inconsequential events.)
23. Aggression
24. Inability to write own name
    (Cannot sign name for other than physical reasons.)
25. Inability to read
    (Cannot read "The grass is green" for other than physical reasons.)
26. Linguistic expression
    (Noticeable difficulty in word finding or object naming.)
27. Understanding
    (Inability to understand spoken word.)

Rating:
Score "1" if pathology is present; otherwise score "0"

GBS Scale

Reference   Gottfries CG, Bråne G, Steen G (1982) A new rating scale for dementia syndromes. *Gerontology* 28: 20–31

Time taken 30 minutes
Rating by trained observer

Main indications

To rate the degree of physical inactivity, impairment of intellectual and emotional capacities and mental symptoms common in dementia.

Commentary

The GBS Scale is divided into four subscales in order to estimate the motor, intellectual and emotional functions and symptom characteristics of the dementia syndromes. Its aim is that information is collected for a quantitative measure of dementia rather than a diagnosis. The reliability of the scale was tested on 100 patients and found to be between 0.83 and 0.93. Validity was from correlation with another geriatric rating scale (the Gottfries–Gottfries Scale, quoted by the authors).

Address for correspondence

CG Gottfries
Department of Psychiatry and Neurochemistry
St Jörgens Hospital
S-422 03 Hisings Backa
Sweden

GBS Scale

MOTOR FUNCTIONS

1. Motor insufficiency in undressing and dressing
2. Motor insufficiency in taking food
3. Impaired physical activity
4. Deficiency of spontaneous activity
5. Motor insufficiency in managing personal hygiene
6. Inability to control bladder and bowel

INTELLECTUAL

1. Impaired orientation in space
2. Impaired orientation in time
3. Impaired personal orientation
4. Impaired recent memory
5. Impaired distant memory
6. Impaired wakefulness
7. Impaired concentration
8. Inability to increase tempo
9. Absentmindedness
10. Longwindedness
11. Distractability

EMOTIONAL FUNCTIONS

1. Emotional blunting
2. Emotional lability
3. Reduced motivation

DIFFERENT SYMPTOMS COMMON IN DEMENTIA

1. Confusion
2. Irritability
3. Anxiety
4. Agony
5. Reduced mood
6. Restlessness

Instructions: *Assess the condition of the patient as it has been during the most recent period, using the following questionnaire (__ weeks __ days). For each question the patient can score 0, 2, 4 or 6 points. Mark with a cross the alternative answer which in your view corresponds to the condition of the patient. If the condition of the patient does not correspond to any one of the defined alternatives but lies somewhere between them, mark alternative 1, 3 or 5. For three vairables, it is also possible to mark 9 = patient not testable. By repeated ratings – do it every day at the same time.*

Geriatric Rating Scale (GRS)

Reference   Plutchik R, Conte H, Lieberman M, Bakur M, Grossman J, Lehrman N (1970) Reliability and validity of a scale for assessing the functioning of geriatric patients. *Journal of the American Geriatrics Society* 18: 491–500

Time taken 20–25 minutes (reviewer's estimate)
Rating by observer, no special training needed

Main indications

The assessment of behavioural problems and ability of geriatric patients.

Commentary

The Geriatric Rating Scale (GRS) was developed after identification of key areas by professionals and review of existing scales, in particular the Stockton Geriatric Rating Scale (page 182). The study was carried out on 281 inpatients, data being obtained on 207. Inter-rater reliability was 0.87, and validity was assessed by the ability of the individual items to differentiate between the 30 highest ranking and 30 lowest ranking subjects in terms of overall functioning in comparing the results with non-geriatric patients. Independent ratings by clinicians confirmed the accuracy of the scale in evaluating functioning of patients.

Geriatric Rating Scale (GRS)

1. When eating, the patient requires.
2. The patient is incontinent.
3. When bathing or dressing, the patient needs.
4. The patient will fall from his bed or chair unless protected by side rails.
5. With regard to walking, the patient.
6. The patient's vision, with or without glasses, is.
7. The patient's hearing is.
8. With regard to sleep, the patient.
9. During the day, the patient sleeps.
10. With regard to restless behavior at night, the patient is.
11. The patient's behavior is worse at night than in the daytime.
12. When not helped by other people, the patient's appearance is.
13. The patient masturbates or exposes himself publicly.
14. The patient is confused (unable to find his way around the ward, loses his possessions, etc.).
15. The patient knows the names of.
16. The patient communicates in any manner (by speaking, writing, or gestering) well enough to make himself easily understood.
17. The patient reacts to his own name.
18. The patient plays games, has hobbies, etc.
19. The patient reads books or magazines on the ward.
20. The patient will begin conversations with others.
21. The patient is willing to do things asked of him.
22. The patient helps with chores on the ward.
23. Without being asked, the patient physically helps other patients.
24. With regard to friends on the ward, the patient.
25. The patient talks with other people on the ward.
26. The patient has a regular work assignment.
27. The patient is destructive of materials around him (breaks furniture, tears up magazines, etc.)
28. The patient disturbs other patients or staff by shouting or yelling.
29. The patient steals from other patients or staff members.
30. The patient **verbally** threatens to harm other patients or staff.
31. The patient **physically** tries to harm other patients or staff.

Patients are scored on a scale of 0–2, with 0 indicating never, none or no, and 2 indicating often, many or extremely

Reproduced from Plutchik R, Conte H, Lieberman M, Bakur M, Grossman J, Lehrman N, Reliability and validity of a scale for assessing the functioning of geriatric patients. *Journal of the American Geriatrics Society*, Vol. 18, no. 6, pp. 491–500.

PAMIE Scale

Reference   Gurel L, Linn MW, Linn BS (1972) Physical and mental impairment-of-function evaluation in the aged: the PAMIE Scale. *Journal of Gerontology* 27: 83–90

Time taken 45 minutes
Rating by a nurse familiar with the patient

Main indications

The quantitative description of behaviours in geriatric patients and those with mental illness.

Commentary

The PAMIE Scale was developed to meet the need for an instrument which would allow a comprehensive behavioural evaluation of the disabilities of a heterogeneous group of patients going from hospital to nursing home care. The instrument was based on two previous scales, the Self-Care Inventory (SCI) (Gurel and Davis, 1967), which looked at the areas of ambulation, feeding, dressing, toileting and bathing; and the 43-item Patient Evaluation Scale (PES) (Gurel, 1968), which looked at particular dimensions such as impairment in ambulation, self-care, dependency, verbal hostility, bedfastness, sensory motor impairment, mental disorganization and co-opera-

tion. The PAMIE Scale focused on information from both these scales, but also included deteriorated appearance, withdrawal and apathy, anxiety, depression and paranoia. Factor analysis revealed 10 factors (self-care, irritability, confusion, anxiety-depression, bedridden-moribund, behavioural deterioration, paranoid ideas, psychomotor disability, withdrawal-apathy, mobility) plus a special items section. Validation was with the Cumulative Illness Rating Scale.

Additional references

Gurel L (1968) Community resources and VA outplacement. In *Proceedings of 13th Annual Conference VA Cooperative Studies in Psychiatry*. Denver, April 1968. Washington DC: Veterans Administration, 85–9.

Gurel L, Davis JE Jr (1967) A survery of self-care dependency in psychiatric patients. *Hospital and Community Psychiatry* 18: 135–8.

PAMIE Scale

1. **Which of the following best fits the patient?**
   Has no problem in walking
   Slight difficulty in walking, but manages. May use cane
   Great difficulty in walking, but manages. May use crutches or stroller
   Uses wheelchair to get around by himself
   Uses wheelchair pushed by others
   Doesn't get around much, mostly or completely bedfast, or restricted to chair

2. **As far as you know, has the patient had one or more strokes (C.V.A.)**
   No stroke
   Mild stroke(s)
   Serious stroke(s)

3. **Which of the following best fits the patient?**
   In bed all almost all day
   More of the waking day in bed, than out of bed
   About half of the waking day in bed, and about half out of bed
   More of the waking day out of bed than in bed
   Out of bed all or almost all day

4.	Eats a regular diet	YES	NO
5.	Is given bed baths	YES	NO
6.	Gives sarcastic answers	YES	NO
7.	Takes a bath/shower without help or supervision	YES	NO
8.	Leaves his clothes unbuttoned	YES	NO
9.	Is messy in eating	YES	NO
10.	Is irritable and grouchy	YES	NO

11. Keeps to himself	YES	NO
12. Say he's not getting good care and treatment	YES	NO
13. Resists when asked to do things	YES	NO
14. Seems unhappy	YES	NO
15. Doesn't make much sense when talks to you	YES	NO
16. Acts as though he has a chip on his shoulder	YES	NO
17. Is IV or tube fed once a week or more	YES	NO
18. Has one or both hands/arms missing or paralyzed	YES	NO
19. Is cooperative	YES	NO
20. Is toileted in bed by catheter and/or enema	YES	NO
21. Is deaf or practically deaf, even with hearing aid	YES	NO
22. Ignores what goes on around him	YES	NO
23. Knows who he is and where he is	YES	NO
24. Gives the staff a "hard time"	YES	NO
25. Blames other people for his difficulties	YES	NO
26. Says, without good reason, that he's being mistreated or getting a raw deal	YES	NO
27. Gripes and complains a lot	YES	NO
28. Says other people dislike him, or even hate him	YES	NO
29. Says he has special or superior abilities	YES	NO
30. Has hit someone or been in a fight in last six months	YES	NO
31. Eats without being closely supervised or encouraged	YES	NO
32. Says he's blue and depressed	YES	NO
33. Isn't interested in much of anything	YES	NO
34. Has taken his clothes off at the wrong time or place during the last six months	YES	NO
35. Makes sexually suggestive remarks or gestures	YES	NO
36. Objects or gives you an argument before doing what he's told	YES	NO
37. Is distrustful and suspicious	YES	NO
38. Looks especially neat and clean	YES	NO
39. Seems unusually restless	YES	NO
40. Says he's going to hit people	YES	NO
41. Receives almost constant safety supervision (for careless smoking, objects in mouth)	YES	NO
42. Looks sloppy	YES	NO
43. Keeps wandering off the subject when you talk with him	YES	NO
44. Is noisy, talks very loudly	YES	NO
45. Does things like brush teeth, comb hair, and clean nails without help or urging	YES	NO
46. Has shown up drunk or brought a bottle on the ward	YES	NO
47. Cries for no obvious reason	YES	NO
48. Says he would like to leave the hospital	YES	NO
49. Wets or soils once a week or more	YES	NO
50. Has trouble remembering things	YES	NO
51. Has one or both feet/legs missing or paralyzed	YES	NO
52. Walks flight of steps without help	YES	NO
53. When needed, takes medication by mouth	YES	NO
54. Is easily upset when little things go wrong	YES	NO
55. Uses the toilet without help or supervision	YES	NO
56. Conforms to hospital routine and treatment program	YES	NO
57. Has much difficulty in speaking	YES	NO
58. Sometimes talks out loud to himself	YES	NO
59. Chats with other patients	YES	NO
60. Is shaved by someone else	YES	NO
61. Seems to resent it when asked to do things	YES	NO
62. Dresses without any help or supervision	YES	NO
63. Is often demanding	YES	NO
64. When left alone, sits and does nothing	YES	NO
65. Says others are jealous of him	YES	NO
66. Is confused	YES	NO
67. Is blind or practically blind, even with glasses	YES	NO
68. Decides things for himself, like what to wear, items from canteen (or canteen cart), etc	YES	NO
69. Swears, uses vulgar or obscene words	YES	NO
70. When you try to get his attention, acts as though lost in a dream world	YES	NO
71. Looks worried and sad	YES	NO
72. Most people would think him a mental patient	YES	NO
73. Shaves without any help or supervision, other than being given supply	YES	NO
74. Yells at people when he's angry or upset	YES	NO
75. Is dressed or has his clothes changed by someone	YES	NO
76. Gets own tray and takes it to eating place	YES	NO
77. Is watched closely so he doesn't wander	YES	NO

Stockton Geriatric Rating Scale

Reference   Meer B, Baker JA (1966) The Stockton Geriatric Rating Scale. *Journal of Gerontology* 21:
392–403

Time taken 10–15 minutes

Rating by nurse carer

Main indications

Rating of needs based on behaviour and physical and mental functioning.

Commentary

The Stockton Geriatric Rating Scale was designed to assess behaviour of a geriatric patient in a hospital set-ting. The original paper also wished to describe the significant dimensions of the behaviour of patients on a long-stay ward. Over 1000 patients in the Stockton State Hospital were assessed using the scale, and a factor analysis was carried out identifying four factors: physical disability, apathy, communication failure and socially irritating behaviour. Inter-rater reliability of the four factors ranged from 0.7 (communication failure) to 0.88 (physical disability). Validity has been assessed according to outcome.

Stockton Geriatric Rating Scale

1. The patient will fall from his bed or chair unless protected by side rails or soft ties (day or night).
2. The patient helps out on the ward (other than a regular work assignment).
3. The patient understands what you communicate to him (you may use speaking, writing, or gesturing).
4. The patient is objectionable to other patients **during the day** (loud or constant talking, pilfering, soiling furniture, interfering in affairs of others).
5. Close supervision is necessary to protect the patient, due to feebleness, from other patients.
6. The patient keeps self occupied in constructive or useful activity (works, reads, play games, has hobbies, etc.).
7. The patient communicates in any manner (by speaking, writing, or gesturing).
8. The patient engages in repetitive vocal sounds (yelling, moaning, talking, etc.) which are directed to no one in particular or to everyone.
9. When bathing or dressing, the patient requires.
10. The patient socializes with other patients.
11. The patient knows his own name.
12. The patient threatens to harm other patients, staff, or people outside the hospital **either** verbally (e.g. "I'll get him") **or** physically (e.g. raising of fist).
13. The patient is able to walk.
14. The patient, without being asked, physically helps one or more patients in various situations (pushing wheel chair, helping with food tray, assisting in shower, etc.).
15. The patient wants to go home or leave the hospital.
16. The patient is objectionable to other patients **during the night** (loud or constant talking, pilfering, soiling furniture, interfering in affairs of others, wandering about, getting into some other patient's bed, etc.).
17. The patient is incontinent of urine and/or feces (day or night).
18. The patient takes the initiative to **start** conversations with others (exclude side remarks not intended to open conversations).
19. The patient **accuses** others (patients, staff, or people outside the hospital) of doing him bodily harm or stealing his personal possessions (if you are **sure** the accusations are true, rate zero; otherwise rate one or two).
20. The patient is able to feed himself.
21. The patient has a regular work assignment.
22. The patient is destructive of materials around him (breaks furniture, tears up magazines, sheets, clothes, etc.).

Patients are scored on a scale of 0–2, with 0 indicating never, none or no, and 2 indicating often, many or extremely

Hierarchic Dementia Scale

Reference   Cole MG, Dastoor DP, Koszycki D (1983) The Hierarchic Dementia Scale. *Journal of Clinical Experimental Gerontology* **5: 219–34**

Time taken 15–30 minutes

Rating by observer

Main indications

To assess cognitive performance over a wide range of disabilities including reflexes and comprehension.

Commentary

The Hierarchic Dementia Scale allows the rapid identification of the highest level of performance for each of 20 mental functions. Being able to start at an appropriate level to that of patient allows problems arising from the presence of physical, sensory or emotional handicaps, fatigue and irritability to be overcome. Validation studies were performed on 50 patients with dementia (Alzheimer's disease and multi-infarct dementia) against the Blessed Dementia Scale (page 40) and the Crichton Royal Geriatric Rating Scale (page 171). Inter-rater reliability was 0.89 and test/retest reliability 0.84. Cronbach's alpha was 0.97. The maximum score for the whole scale is 200. A person with very mild dementia would score around 160; someone with very severe dementia scores less than 40.

Additional reference

Cole M, Dastoor D (1987) A new hierarchic approach to the management of dementia. *Psychosomatics* **28**: 258–304.

Ronnberg L, Ericsson K (1994) Reliability and validity of the Hierarchic Dementia Scale. *International Psychogeriatrics* **6**: 87–94.

Address for correspondence

Martin G Cole
St Mary's Hospital Center
3830 Avenue Lacombe
Montreal PQ
H3T 1M5
Canada

1. Orienting
10. No impairment
8. Shakes examiner's hand
6. Reacts to auditory threat
4. Reacts to visual threat
2. Reacts to tactile threat

2. Prefrontal
10. None
8. Tactile prehension
6. Cephalobuccal reflex
4. Orovisual reflex
2. Oral tactile reflex

3. Ideomotor
10. Reversed hands
9. Double rings
8. Double fingers
7. Opposed hands
6. Single ring
5. Single finger
4. Clap hands
3. Wave
2. Raise hands
1. Open mouth

4. Looking
10. Finds images
8. Searches for images
6. Grasps content of picture
4. Scans picture
2. Looks at picture

5. Ideational
10. Imaginary match and candle
9. Imaginary nail and hammer
8. Imaginary scissors
7. Imaginary comb
6. Match and candle
5. Nail and hammer
4. Scissors
3. Comb
2. Put on shoes
1. Open door

6. Denomination
10. No errors
9. Nominal aphasia—parts
8. Nominal aphasia—objects
7. Use of parts
6. Use of objects
5. Conceptual field—parts
4. Conceptual field—objects
3. Sound alike—parts
2. Sound alike—objects
1. Deformed words

7. Comprehension
   Verbal:
5. Close eyes and touch left ear
4. Clap hands three times
3. Touch your right eye
2. Touch your nose
1. Open mouth

   Written:
5. Close eyes and touch left ear
4. Clap hands three times
3. Touch your right eye
2. Touch your nose
1. Open mouth

8. Registration
10. Spoon, candle, scissors, button whistle
8. Spoon, candle, scissors, button
6. Spoon, candle, scissors
4. Spoon, candle
2. Spoon

9. Gnosis
10. Superimposed words
9. Sumperimposed images
8. Digital gnosis
7. Right-left—examiner
6. Right-left—self
5. Body parts—examiner
4. Body parts—self
3. Touch (pinch) 5 cm
2. Touch (pinch) 5 to 15 cm
1. Response to touch (pinch)

10. Reading
10. Paragraph
8. Paragraph with error(s)
6. The cat drinks milk
4. Receive
2. M

11. Orientation
10. Date
8. Month
6. Year of birth
4. Morning or afternoon
2. First name

12. Construction
10. Four blocks diagonal
8. Four blocks square
6. Two blocks diagonal
4. Two blocks square
2. Form board circle

13. Concentration
10. Serial 7s (100, 93,...)
9. Serial 3s (30, 27,...)
8. Months of year backward
7. Days of week backward
6. 93 to 85
5. 10 to 1
4. Months of year forward
3. Days of week forward
2. 1 to 10
1. Actual counting

14. Calculation
10. 43 – 17
9. 56 + 19
8. 39 – 14
7. 21 + 11
6. 15 – 6
5. 18 + 9
4. 9 – 4
3. 8 + 7
2. 2 – 1
1. 3 + 1

15. Drawing
10. Cube
9. Cube (difficulty with perspective)
8. Two rectangles
7. Circle and square
6. Rectangle
5. Square
4. Circle inside circle
3. Circle
2. Line
1. Scribble

16. Motor
10. No impairment
9. Increased muscle tone—repeated
8. Increased muscle tone—initial
7. Loss of rhythm
6. Loss of associated movements
5. Contractures of legs
4. Kyphosis
3. Vertical restriction of eye movement
2. Nonambulatory
1. Lateral restriction of eye movement

17. Remote memory
10. Amount of pension
8. Number of grandchildren
6. Year of marriage or of first job
4. Father's occupation
2. Place of birth

18. Writing
Form:
5. Flowing style
4. Loss of flow
3. Letters misshapen
2. Repetition or substitution of letters
1. Scribble

Content:
5. No error
4. Word substitution
3. Missing preposition
2. Missing verb or noun
1. Missing 3 or 4 words

19. Similarities
10. Airplane—bicycle
8. Gun—knife
6. Cat—pig
4. Pants—dress
2. Orange—banana

20. Recent memory
10. All five
8. Any four
6. Any three
4. Any two
2. Any one

Reprinted from Cole MG, Dastoor DP, Koszycki D, *Journal of Experimental Gerontology*, **5**, 219–234, by courtesy of Marcel Dekker Inc.

Mattis Dementia Rating Scale

Reference   Mattis S (1976) Mental status examination for organic mental syndrome in the elderly patient. In: Bellak L, Karasu T, eds. *Geriatric psychiatry: a handbook for psychiatrists and primary care physicians.* New York: Grune & Stratton, 77–101

Time taken 30–45 minutes

Rating by structured interview

Main indications

For the neuropsychological assessment of patients with dementia.

Commentary

The Mattis Dementia Rating Scale is a standardized neuropsychological test battery that provides a global measure of dementia on five subscales. Its advantage is that it assesses a range of cognitive abilities and is able to monitor change in dementia. Cognitive deficits which are affected early in Alzheimer's disease are assessed, as are tests likely to be affected in other dementias (e.g. attention and initiation in subcortical dementia). This makes the scale particularly well-suited for comparisons of neuropsychological differences between different types of dementia. Rosser and Hodges (1994) found that patients with Alzheimer's disease were more impaired on memory subtests whereas patients with subcortical disease (Huntington's disease and progressive supranuclear palsy) were more impaired on the initiation/perseveration subtest. A score of less than 100 out of the total of 144 indicates moderate dementia.

Additional reference

Rosser A, Hodges J (1994) The Dementia Rating Scale in Alzheimer's disease, Huntington's disease and progressive supranuclear palsy. *Journal of Neurology* 241: 531–6.

Address for correspondence

NFER-Nelson

Darville House

2 Oxford Road East

Windsor

Berks SL4 1DF

UK

Mattis Dementia Rating Scale (DRS): constitution and scores of the five subtests

Attention subtest			*Conceptualization subtests*	
Digit span (forwards and backwards)	8		Similarities	8
Two-step commands	2		Inductive reasoning	3
One-step commands	2		Detection of different item	3
Imitation of commands	4		Multiple choice similarities	8
Counting A's	6		Identities and oddities	16
Counting randomly arranged A's	5		Create a sentence	1
Read a word list	4			(39)
Match figures	4			
	(37)		*Memory subtest*	
			Recall a sentence (I)	4
Initiation subtest			Recall a self-generated sentence (II)	3
Fluency for supermarket items	20		Orientation (e.g. date, place)	9
Fluency for clothing items	8		Verbal recognition	5
Verbal repetition (e.g. bee, key, gee)	2		Figure recognition	4
Double alternating movements	3			(25)
Graphomotor (copy alternating figures)	4			
	(37)		Total score	144
Construction subtest				
Copy geometric designs	6			

This scale is available from NFER Nelson.

Sandoz Clinical Assessment – Geriatric (SCAG)

Reference Shader RI, Harmatz JS, Salzman C (1974) A new scale for clinical assessment in geriatric populations: Sandoz Clinical Assessment – Geriatric (SCAG). *Journal of the American Geriatrics Society* 22: 107–13

Time taken 15–20 minutes (reviewer's estimate)
Rating by anyone familiar with the patient; training is required

Main indications

Assessment of psychopathology in older people.

Commentary

The Sandoz Clinical Assessment – Geriatric (SCAG) represents one of the early scales for the assessment of older people based on the assumption that many similar scales used for geriatric psychopharmacologic research are not used specifically with the elderly (Salzman et al, 1972). The original study was described in two parts. One was on 51 geriatric subjects (25 volunteers and 26 hospital inpatients) where the SCAG was rated against an existing measure, the Mental Status Examination Record (Spitzer and Endicott, 1971). The second was an assessment of inter-rater reliability on eight subjects by four psychiatrists. The first study showed good differentiation using the SCAG scale between four groups of individuals: health, minimum dementia, depression and severe dementia. Good separation was found between the groups. Inter-rater reliability resulted in an average intraclass correlation coefficient of 0.75.

Additional references

Salzman C, Kochansky GE, Shader IR (1972) Rating scales for geriatric psychopharmacology – a review. *Psychopharmacology Bulletin* 8: 3.

Spitzer R, Endicott IJ (1971) An integrated group of forms for automated psychiatric case records. *Archives of General Psychiatry* 24: 540.

Address for correspondence

Richard I Shader
Department of Pharmacology and Experimental Therapeutics
Tufts University School of Medicine
136 Harrison Avenue
Boston
MA 02111
USA

Sandoz Clinical Assessment – Geriatric (SCAG)

1. CONFUSION: Lack of proper association for surroundings, persons and time not with it. Slowing of thought processes and impaired comprehension, recognition and performance; disorganization. Rate on patient's response and on reported episodes since last interview.
2. MENTAL ALERTNESS: Reduction of attentiveness, concentration , responsiveness, alcrity, and clairty of thought, impairment of judgement and ability to make decisions. Rate on structured questions and response at interview.
3. IMPAIRMENT OF RECENT MEMORY: Reduction in ability to recall recent events and actions of importance to the patient, e.g. visits by members of family, content of meals, notable environmental changes, personal activities. Rate on structured pertinent questions and not on reported performance.
4. DISORIENTATION: Reduced awareness of place and time, identification of persons including self. Rate on response to questions at interview only.
5. MOOD DEPRESSION: Dejected, despondent, helpless, hopeless, preoccupation with defeat or neglect by family or friends, hypochondriacal concern, functional somatic complaints, early waking. Rate on patient's statements, attitude and behavior.
6. EMOTIONAL LABILITY: Instability and inappropriateness of emotional response, e.g. laughing or crying or other undue positive or negative response to non provoking situations as the interviewer sees them.
7. SELF CARE: Impairment of ability to attend to personal hygiene, dressing, grooming, eating and getting about. Rate on observation of patient at and outside interview situation and not on statements of patients.
8. ANXIETY: Worry, apprehension, overconcern for present or future, fears, complaints of functional somatic symptoms, e.g. headache, dry mouth, etc. Rate on patient's own subjective experience and on physical signs, e.g. trembling, sighing, sweating, etc. if present.
9. MOTIVATION INITIATIVE: Lack of spontaneous interest in initiating or completing task, routine duties and even attending to individual needs. Rate on observed behavior rather than patient's statements.
10. IRRITABILITY (Cantankerousness): Edgy, testy, easily frustated, low tolerance threshold to aggravation and stress or challenging situations. Rate on patient's statements and general attitude at interview.
11. HOSTILITY: Verbal aggressiveness, animosity, contempt, quarrelsome, assaultive. Rate on impression at interview and patient's observed attitude and behavior towards others.
12. BOTHERSOME: Frequent unnecessary requests for advice or assistance, interference with others, restlessness. Rate on behavior at and outside the interview situation.
13. INDIFFERENCE TO SURROUNDINGS: Lack of interest in everyday events, pastimes and environment where interest previously existed, e.g. news, TV, heat, cold, noise. Rate on patient's statements and observed behavior during and outside the interview situation.
14. UNSOCIABILITY: Poor relationships with others, unfriendly, negative reaction to social and communal recreational activities, aloof. Rate on observed behavior and not patient's own impression.
15. UNCOOPERATIVENESS: Poor compliance with instructions or requests for participation. Performance with ill-grace, resentment or lack of consideration for others. Rate on attitudes and responses at interview and observed behavior outside interview situation.
16. FATIGUE: Sluggish, listless, tired, weary, worn out, bushed. Rate on patient's statements and observed responses to normal daily activities outside interview situation.
17. APPETITE (Anorexia): Disinclination for food, inadequate intake, necessity for dietary supplements, loss of weight. Rate on observed attitude towards eating, food intake encouragement required and loss of weight.
18. DIZZINESS: In addition to true vertigo, dizziness in this context includes spells of uncertainty of movement and balance, subjective sensations in the head apart from pain, e.g., lightheadedness. Rate on physical examination as well as patient's subjective experience.
19. OVERALL IMPRESSION OF PATIENT: Considering your total clinical experience and knowledge of the patient, indicate the patient's status at this time, taking into account physical, psychic and mental functioning.

Rating:
1 = not present
2 = very mild
3 = mild
4 = mild to moderate
5 = moderate
6 = moderatly severe
7 = severe

Reproduced from Shader RI, Harmatz JS, Salzman C, A new scale for clinical assessment in geriatric populations: Sandoz Clinical Assessment – Geriatric (SCAG). *Journal of the American Geriatrics Society*, Vol. 22, no. 3, pp. 107–113.

Comprehensive Psychopathological Rating Scale (CPRS)

Reference Bucht G, Adolfsson R (1983) The Comprehensive Psychopathological Rating Scale in patients with dementia of Alzheimer type and multiinfarct dementia. *Acta Psychiatrica Scandinavica* **68**: 263–70

Time taken 20 minutes (reviewer's estimate)
Rating by clinician

Main indications

The assessment of neuropsychiatric features of dementia in patients with Alzheimer's disease and multi-infarct dementia.

Commentary

The Comprehensive Psychopathological Rating Scale (CPRS) is an extensive scale measuring a wide range of symptoms and signs. A subscale of items commonly seen in dementia was taken from the larger scale and two additional items – recent memory and long-term memory – were added. A three-point severity rating scale was used on 18 patients with Alzheimer's disease and 20 with multi-infarct dementia.

Additional reference

Åsberg M, Perris CP, Schalling D et al (1978) The CPRS – development and applications of a psychiatric rating scale. *Acta Psychiatrica Scandinavica* (**Suppl**): 271.

Address for correspondence

G Bucht
Umea Dementia Research Group
Department of Geriatric Medicine and Geriatric Psychiatry
University Hospital
Umea
Sweden

Comprehensive Psychopathological Rating Scale (CPRS)

Reported items		Observed items	
1.	Sadness	41.	Apparent sadness
2.	Elation	42.	Elated mood
4.	Hostile feelings	43.	Hostility
5.	Inability to feel	44.	Labile emotional response
6.	Pessimistic thoughts	47.	Sleepiness
7.	Suicidal thoughts	48.	Distractability
14.	Lassitude	50.	Perplexity
15.	Fatiguability	52.	Disorientation
16.	Concentration difficulties	55.	Specific speech defects
17.	Failing memory	58.	Perseveration
19.	Reduced sleep	59.	Overactivity
20.	Increased sleep	60.	Slowness of movement
24.	Aches and pains	61.	Agitation
26.	Loss of sensation or movement	62.	Involuntary movements
31.	Ideas of persecution	64.	Mannerisms and postures
38.	Other auditory hallucinations	65.	Hallucinatory behaviour
40.	Other hallucinations	66.	Global rating of illness
		68.	Recent memory
		69.	Long-term memory

Scaling from 0 to 3 on all items. Use of half-steps recommended

Progressive Deterioration Scale (PDS)

Reference DeJong R, Osterlund OW, Roy GW (1989) Measurement of quality-of-life changes in patients with Alzheimer's disease. *Clinical Therapeutics* 11: 545–54

Time taken 10–15 minutes (based on interview lasting 90 minutes)
Rating by a carer

Main indications

Assesses changes in the quality of life of patients with Alzheimer's disease.

Commentary

The need for measures to assess the effects of medication on quality of life prompted the development of the Progressive Deterioration Scale (PDS), which involved three steps: step 1 – interviews with caregivers detailing particular facets of the disease which affected quality of life; step 2 – testing and preparation of questionnaires using the factors which were found to discriminate between various stages of Alzheimer's disease as characterized by the Global Deterioration Scale (GDS; page 166) leading to a final version; and step 3 – validation of the final version on a different group of patients and measures of reliability. The 27 items came from a number of different content areas.

Content areas for questionnaire items that differentiate Global Deterioration Scale stages in Alzheimer's disease:

- Extent to which patient can leave immediate neighbourhood.
- Ability to travel distances safely alone.
- Confusion in familiar settings.
- Use of familiar household implements.
- Participation/enjoyment of leisure/cultural activities.
- Extent to which patient does household chores.
- Involvement in family finances, budgeting, etc.
- Interest in doing household tasks.
- Travel on public transportation.
- Self-care and routine tasks.
- Social function/behaviour in social settings.

The scale achieved 95% accuracy in discriminating between normal controls and patients with Alzheimer's disease and an overall 80% accuracy in discriminating between controls and patients with early, middle and late Alzheimer's disease. Coefficients of reliability ranged from 0.92 to 0.95. Test/retest reliability was generally significant at 0.80.

Address for correspondence

Richard DeJong
Parke-Davis Pharmaceuticals Research Division
Warner-Lambert Company
Ann Arbor
MI
USA

Summary of content areas for the Progressive Deterioration Scale (PDS)

- *Extent to which patient can leave immediate neighbourhood.*
- *Ability to safely travel distances alone.*
- *Confusion in familiar settings.*
- *Use of familiar household implements.*
- *Participation/enjoyment of leisure/cultural activities.*
- *Extent to which patient does household chores.*
- *Involvement in family finances, budgeting, etc.*
- *Interest in doing household tasks.*
- *Travel on public transportation.*
- *Self-care and routine tasks.*
- *Social function/behaviour in social settings.*

Chapter 3

Global mental health assessments

There are some situations in which a global rating of symptoms is required in elderly patients without any particular reason to suspect or to be looking for a specific diagnosis such as depression or dementia. These measures may be useful in the setting of general practice where a relatively quick global assessment may help in pointing toward the need for a further assessment for depression or dementia. They can also be very useful in nursing and residential home care where a global rating of a resident (or group of residents) is necessary. The Sandoz Clinical Assessment – Geriatric (SCAG; page 188) and the Brief Psychiatric Rating Scale (BPRS; page 194) are early examples of this type of scale. Later ones include the Neurobehavioral Rating Scale (NRS; page 96), the Global Assessment of Psychiatric Symptoms (GAPS; page 198), the Multidimensional Observation Scale for Elderly Subjects (MOSES; page 206) (Helmes et al, 1987) and the Crichton Royal Behaviour Rating Scale (CRBRS; page 171). The SCAG, NRS and CRBRS are discussed in Chapter 2 in view of their association with dementia. More lengthy interviews are the Geriatric Mental State Schedule (GMSS; page 200) and, derived from that, the Comprehensive Assessment and Referral Evaluation schedule (CARE; page 212), which itself has a shortened version, and the two subscales of the depression and cognitive impairment items codified in the Brief Assessment Schedule. The GMSS is used predominantly outside the USA, and has a diagnostic algorithm (AGECAT) allowing computerized diagnoses.

The Canberra Interview for the Elderly (page 201), the Structured Interview for the Diagnosis of the Alzheimer's Type and Multi-infarct Dementia and Dementias of other Aetiology (SIDAM; page 197), the Cambridge Mental Disorders of the Elderly Examination (CAMDEX; page 208) and the Pittsburgh Agitation Scale (PAS; page 112) are relatively lengthy interviews similar to the GMSS and CARE.

The NRS, SCAG, CRBRS and MOSES have sections which are relevant to people with mild to moderate cognitive impairment and would be of use where a high risk of impairment is thought to be present, while the BPRS and GAPS are more general. There is evidence that the SCAG and BPRS are sensitive to measure change. Therefore, if a drug trial or change in service were planned, these would be the instruments of choice.

Brief Psychiatric Rating Scale (BPRS)

Reference Overall JE, Gorham DR (1962) The Brief Psychiatric Rating Scale. *Psychological Reports* 10: 799–812

Time taken 18 minutes
Rating by trained interviewer

Main indications

A rapid assessment of global psychiatric symptomatology particularly suited to the evaluation of patient change.

Commentary

The Brief Psychiatric Rating Scale (BPRS) is a 16-item, 7-point ordered category rating scale which has been developed through previous versions (Gorham and Overall, 1960). The questions are completed in 2 or 3 minutes following the interview. The ratings are divided into those based on observation of the patient (tension, emotional withdrawal, mannerisms and posturing, motor retardation and unco-operativeness) and all the others based on verbal report. Product moment correlation tested inter-rater reliability, and this varied from 0.56 to 0.87 for the 16-item scale. Data were presented to allow a "total pathology" score using independent ratings from 20 psychiatrists.

Additional references

Gorham DR, Overall JE (1960) Drug action profiles based upon an abbreviated psychiatric rating scale. *Journal of Nervous and Mental Disease* **132**: 528–35.

Gorham DR, Overall JE (1961) Dimensions of change in psychiatric symptomatology. *Diseases of the Nervous System* **22**: 576–80.

Address for correspondence

JE Overall
Department of Psychiatry and Behavioral Sciences
University of Texas Medical School at Houston
PO Box 20708
Houston
TX 77225
USA

Brief Psychiatric Rating Scale (BPRS)

Directions: Draw a circle around the term under each symptom which best describes the patient's present condition.

1. SOMATIC CONCERN – Degree of concern over present bodily health. Rate the degree to which physical health is perceived as a problem by the patient, whether complaints have realistic basis or not.

   Not present   Very mild   Mild   Moderate   Moderate, severe   Severe   Extremely severe

2. ANXIETY – Worry, fear, or over-concern for present or future. Rate solely on the basis of verbal report of patient's own subjective experiences. Do not infer anxiety from physical signs or from neurotic defense mechanisms.

   Not present   Very mild   Mild   Moderate   Moderate, severe   Severe   Extremely severe

3. EMOTIONAL WITHDRAWAL – Deficiency in relating to the interviewer and the interview situation. Rate only degree to which the patient gives the impression of failing to be in emotional contact with other people in the interview situation.

   Not present   Very mild   Mild   Moderate   Moderate, severe   Severe   Extremely severe

4. CONCEPTUAL DISORGANIZATION – Degree to which the thought processes are confused, disconnected or disorganized. Rate on the basis of integration of the verbal products of the patient; do not rate on the basis of the patient's subjective impression of his own level of functioning.

   Not present   Very mild   Mild   Moderate   Moderate, severe   Severe   Extremely severe

5. GUILT FEELINGS – over-concern or remorse for past behavior. Rate on the basis of the patient's subjective experiences of guilt as evidenced by verbal report with appropriate affect; do not infer guilt feelings from depression, anxiety, or neurotic defenses.

   Not present   Very mild   Mild   Moderate   Moderate, severe   Severe   Extremely severe

6. TENSION – Physical and motor manifestations of tension, "nervousness", and heightened activation level. Tension should be rated solely on the basis of physical signs and motor behavior and not on the basis of subjective exprinces of tension reported by the patient.

    Not present   Very mild   Mild   Moderate   Moderate, severe   Severe   Extremely severe

7. MANNERISMS AND POSTURING – Unusual and unnatural motor behavior, the type of motor behavior which causes certain mental patients to stand out in a crowd of normal people. Rate only abnormality of movements; do not rate simple heightened motor activity here.

    Not present   Very mild   Mild   Moderate   Moderate, severe   Severe   Extremely severe

8. GRANDIOSITY – Exaggerated self-opinion, conviction of unusual ability or powers. Rate only on the basis of patient's statements about himself or self-in-relation-to-others, not on the basis of his demeanor in the interview situation.

    Not present   Very mild   Mild   Moderate   Moderate, severe   Severe   Extremely severe

9. DEPRESSIVE MOOD – Despondency in mood, sadness. Rate only degree of despondency; do not rate on the basis of inferences concerning depression based upon general retardation and somatic complaints.

    Not present   Very mild   Mild   Moderate   Moderate, severe   Severe   Extremely severe

10. HOSTILITY – Animosity, contempt, belligerence, disdain for other people outside the interview situation. Rate solely on the basis of the verbal report of feelings and actions of the patient toward others; do not infer hostility from neurotic defenses, anxiety nor somatic complaints. (Rate attitude toward interviewer under "uncooperativeness".)

    Not present   Very mild   Mild   Moderate   Moderate, severe   Severe   Extremely severe

11. SUSPICIOUSNESS – Belief (delusional or otherwise) that others have now, or have had in the past, malcious or discriminatory intent toward the patient. One the basis of verbal report, rate only those suspicions which are currently held whether they concern past or present circumstances.

    Not present   Very mild   Mild   Moderate   Moderate, severe   Severe   Extremely severe

12. HALLUCINATORY BEHAVIOR – Perceptions without normal external stimulus correspondence. Rate only those experiences which are reported to have occurred within the last week and which are described as distinctly different from the thought and imagery processes of normal people.

    Not present   Very mild   Mild   Moderate   Moderate, severe   Severe   Extremely severe

13. MOTOR RETARDATION – Reduction in energy level evidenced in slowed movements and speech, reduced body tone, decreased number of movements. Rate on the basis of observed behavior of the patient only; do not rate on basis of patient's subjective impression of own energy level.

    Not present   Very mild   Mild   Moderate   Moderate, severe   Severe   Extremely severe

14. UNCOOPERATIVENESS – Evidences of resistance, unfriendliness, resentment, and lack of readiness to cooperate with the interviewer. Rate only on the basis of the patient's attitude and responses to the interviewer and the interview situation; do not rate on basis of reported resentment or uncooperativeness outside the interview situation.

    Not present   Very mild   Mild   Moderate   Moderate, severe   Severe   Extremely severe

15. UNUSUAL THOUGHT CONTENT – Unusual, odd, strange, or bizarre thought content. Rate here the degree of unusualness, not the degree of disorganization of thought processes.

    Not present   Very mild   Mild   Moderate   Moderate, severe   Severe   Extremely severe

16. BLUNTED AFFECT – Reduced emotional tone, apparent lack of normal feeling or involvement.

    Not present   Very mild   Mild   Moderate   Moderate, severe   Severe   Extremely severe

Overall JE, Gorham DR "The Brief Psychiatric Rating Scale." *Psychological Reports*, 1962, **10**, 799–812. © Southern Universities Press.

Relative's Assessment of Global Symptomatology (RAGS)

Reference   Raskin A, Crook T (1988) Relative's assessment of global symptomatology (RAGS). *Psychopharmacology Bulletin* 24: 759–63

Time taken 15 minutes (reviewer's estimate)
Rating by observer, no training required

Main indications

Specifically designed for use by a close relative or friend of a patient to assess his or her behaviour in the community.

Commentary

This is a 21-item scale assessing psychiatric symptoms and behaviour. It emerges from a series of papers reflecting analyses of psychopathology at interview (Raskin et al, 1967, 1969; Shulterbrandt et al, 1974). The RAGS was administered to 456 individuals. Construct validity was shown by successful discrimination of 14 of the 21 RAGS items in distinguishing patients with senile dementia from other groups. It correlated with ratings on a mood scale and a memory scale of other self-administered instruments. A "total pathology" score can be derived by reversing the score for item 2.

Additional references

Raskin A (1985) Validation of a battery of tests designed to assess psychopathology in the elderly. In Burrows GD, Norman TR, Dennerstein L, eds. *Clinical and pharmaco-logical studies in psychiatric disorders.* London: John Libbey, 337–43.

Raskin A, Schulterbrandt JG, Reatig N et al (1967) Factors of psychopathology in interview, ward behavior and self-report ratings of hospitalized depressives. *Journal of Consulting and Clinical Psychology* **31**: 270–8.

Raskin A, Schuterbrandt JG, Reatig N et al (1969) Replication of factors of psychopathology in interview, ward behavior and self-report ratings of hospitalized depressives. *Journal of Nervous and Mental Disease* **148**: 87–98.

Schulterbrandt JG, Raskin A, Reatig N (1974) Further replications of factors of psychopathology in the interview, ward behavior and self-report ratings of hospitalized depressed patients. *Psychological Reports* **34**: 23–32.

Address for correspondence

Allen Raskin
7658 Water Oak Point Road
Pasadena
MD 21122
USA

Relative's Assessment of Global Symptomatology (RAGS)

To what extent does he or she:

1. Need help in caring for personal needs and appearance?
2. Participate in social and recreational activities?
3. Appear depressed, blue, or despondent?
4. Appear tense, anxious, and inwardly distressed?
5. Display irritability, annoyance, impatience, or anger?
6. Appear suspicious of people?
7. Report peculiar or strange thoughts or ideas?
8. Appear to be hearing or seeing things that are not there?
9. Show mood swings or changes?
10. Appear excited or "high" emotionally?
11. Have difficulty in sleeping at night?
12. Appear slowed-down, fatigued, and lacking in energy?
13. Lack motor coordination?
14. Have difficulty speaking?
15. Express concern with own bodily health?
16. Appear inattentive?
17. Appear confused, perplexed, or otherwise seem to be having difficulty organizing his/her thoughts?
18. Seem disoriented?
19. Appear forgetful?
20. Appear agitated?
21. Show variability in mental functioning?

Score:
1 = Not at all; 2 = A little; 3 = Moderately; 4 = Quite a bit; 5 = Extremely

Structured Interview for the Diagnosis of the Alzheimer's Type and Multi-infarct Dementia and Dementias of other Aetiology (SIDAM)

Reference   Zaudig M, Mittelhammer J, Hiller W, Pauls A, Thora C, Morinigo A, Mombour W (1991) SIDAM – a structured interview for the diagnosis of dementia of the Alzheimer type, multi-infarct dementia and dementias of other aetiology according to ICD-10 and DSM-III-R. *Psychological Medicine* 21: 225–36

Time taken 30 minutes

Rating by clinician addressed to the patient and carer

Main indications

A structured interview for the diagnosis of dementia according to ICD-10 and DSM-III-R criteria.

Commentary

The Structured Interview for the Diagnosis of the Alzheimer's Type and Multi-infarct Dementia and Dementias of other Aetiology (SIDAM) was constructed primarily to differentiate patients with dementia from non-demented individuals according to the DSM-III-R and ICD-10 criteria. The SIDAM is divided into the following sections: (1) a brief semi-structured clinical overview with the patient or information concerning aspects of the subject's past and present medical history; (2) a cognitive examination [when scored separately, this is designated the SISCO, with a range of 0–55 (no cognitive impairment)]; all items of the Mini-Mental State Examination (MMSE; page 34) are contained in the SISCO; (3) a structured schedule for the recording of clinical judgement in relation to the aetiology of dementia and differentiation from other psychiatric conditions; (4) a severity grading for dementia; (5) a list of present and past medical disorders; (6) a summary sheet; (7) a diagnostic algorithm. Sixty subjects underwent the reliability study, with measures of test/retest reliability with agreements of over 95% and very good kappa values for all subtypes of dementia, the lowest being for multi-infarct dementia (0.64).

Address for correspondence

M Zaudig
Psychosomatic Hospital
Schuetzemstreet 16
86949 Windach
Germany

Global Assessment of Psychiatric Symptoms (GAPS)

References   Raskin A, Gershon S, Crook TH, Sathananthan G, Ferris S (1978) The effects of hyperbaric and normobaric oxygen on cognitive impairment in the elderly. *Archives of General Psychiatry* 35: 50–6

Raskin A, Crook T (1988) Global Assessment of Psychiatric Symptoms (GAPS). *Psychopharmacology Bulletin* 24: 721–5

Time taken   approximately 15–20 minutes (reviewer's estimate)
Rating   by trained observers

Main indications
A global assessment of psychiatric symptoms for use in older people, designed to detect change.

Commentary
The Global Assessment of Psychiatric Symptoms (GAPS) is a 19-item abbreviated version of a larger inventory used in a study of the effects of hyperbaric oxygen in older people (Raskin et al, 1978): the Observer Rated Inventory of Psychic and Somatic Complaints – Elderly, modelled after the Brief Psychiatric Rating Scale (BPRS; page 194). The GAPS has been administered to 509 people over the age of 60 in institutions in the USA and 290 normal elderly control subjects. Intraclass correlation coefficients ranged from 0.43 to 0.72. Mean differences on the scale calculated across different diagnostic groups showed successful differentiation between the groups. Raskin (1985) produced validity measures of the GAPS showing correlations between both independent measures of memory and depression and self-report.

Additional reference
Raskin A (1985) Validation of a battery of tests designed to assess psychopathology in the elderly. In Burrows GD, Norman TR, Dennerstein L, eds. *Clinical and pharmacological studies in psychiatric disorders*. London: John Libbey, 337–43.

Address for correspondence
Allen Raskin
7658 Water Oak Point Road
Pasadena
MD 21122
USA

Global Assessment of Psychiatric Symptoms (GAPS)

To what extent does the patient:

1. Appear sloppy or unkempt in appearance?
2. Lack motor coodination?
3. Appear slowed-down, fatigued and lacking in energy?
4. Have difficulty speaking?
5. Appear confused, perplexed, or otherwise seem to be having difficulty organizing his/her thoughts?
6. Seem disoriented?
7. Appear inattentive?
8. Appear forgetful?
9. Appear friendly or sociable?
10. Display irritability, annoyance; impatience, or anger?
11. Appear depressed, blue, or despondent?
12. Appear tense, anxious and inwardly distressed?
13. Appear agitated?
14. Appear suspicious of people?
15. Report peculiar or strange thoughts or ideas?
16. Appear to be hallucinating?
17. Appear excited or "high" emotionally?
18. Complain of difficulty in sleeping at night?
19. Express concern with bodily health?

Score:
1 = Not at all
2 = A little
3 = Moderately
4 = Quite a bit
5 = Extremely

Reproduced from Raskin A, Crook T (1988) Global Assessment of Psychiatric Symptoms (GAPS). *Psychopharmacology Bulletin* **24**: 721–5.

Psychogeriatric Assessment Scales (PAS)

Reference   Jorm AF, MacKinnon AJ, Henderson AS, Scott R, Christensen H, Korten AE, Cullen JS, Mulligan R (1995) The Psychogeriatric Assessment Scales: a multidimensional alternative to categorical diagnoses of dementia and depression in the elderly. *Psychological Medicine* 25: 447–60

Time taken 10 minutes (reviewer's estimate)
Rating by trained lay interviewer or clinician, after familiarization with the manual

Main indications

The Psychogeriatric Assessment Scales (PAS) provide an assessment of the clinical changes seen in dementia and depression. It is easy to administer, can be used by lay interviewers and is intended for use in research and service evaluation.

Commentary

The PAS has the benefits of assessing both dementia and depression. There are three scales derived from an interview with the subject (cognitive impairment, depression and stroke) and three from an interview with an informant (cognitive decline, behavioural change and stroke). The scales cover the clinical domain as defined in ICD-10 and DSM-III-R and are based on the Canberra Interview for the Elderly (CIE; page 201). The results are described using data from three samples – two clinical samples and one population sample, the latter having about 1000 peo-ple and the two others about 60. Five factors emerged from the principal components analysis of each item: cognitive decline, cognitive impairment, behaviour change, stroke and depression. Internal consistency ranged from 0.58 to 0.86, test/retest correlations between 0.47 and 0.66, and validity was proven against other mood and cognitive scales.

Additional reference

Jorm AF, MacKinnon AJ, Christensen H et al (1997) The Psychogeriatric Assessment Scales (PAS): further data on psychometric properties and validity from a longitudinal study of the elderly. *International Journal of Geriatric Psychiatry* 12: 93–100.

Address for correspondence

AF Jorm
NH and MRC Social Psychiatry Research Unit
The Australian National University
Canberra
ACT 0200
Australia

Geriatric Mental State Schedule (GMSS)

References   Copeland JRM, Kelleher MJ, Kellett JM, Gourlay AJ, Gurland BJ, Fleiss JL, Sharpe L (1976) A semi-structured clinical interview for the assessment of diagnosis of mental state in the elderly: the Geriatric Mental State Schedule. I. Development and reliability. *Psychological Medicine* 6: 439–49

Gurland BJ, Fleiss JL, Goldberg K, Sharpe L, Copeland JRM, Kelleher MJ, Kellett JM (1976) A semi-structured clinical interview for the assessment of diagnosis of mental state in the elderly: the Geriatric Mental State Schedule. II. A factor analysis. *Psychological Medicine* 6: 451–9

Time taken   40–45 minutes
Rating   by trained interviewer

Main indications

Assessment of psychopathology in elderly people.

Commentary

The Geriatric Mental State Schedule (GMSS) is one of the most widely used and respected assessment instruments for measuring a wide range of psychopathology in elderly people both in institutionalized settings and, more importantly, in community settings. It is based on the Present State Examination (Wing et al, 1974) and the Psychiatric Status Schedule (Spitzer et al, 1970), and consists of a number of detailed questions concerning psychopathology and behaviour in the last month. Literature on the GMSS is extensive, and a number of different factors can be derived from the results. The instrument was used in the original US/UK project (Cowan et al, 1975), and there is a computerized algorithm of proven reliability and validity, the AGECAT (Copeland et al, 1986). A history and aetiology schedule is also available. The GMSS can conveniently be given via a laptop computer ,and it has been translated into a number of different languages.

Additional references

Copeland JRM, Kelleher MJ, Kellett JM et al (1975) Cross-national study of diagnosis of the mental disorders: a comparison of the diagnoses of elderly psychiatric patients admitted to mental hospitals serving Queens County, New York, and the former Borough of Camberwell, London. *British Journal of Psychiatry* 126: 11–20.

Copeland JRM, Dewey ME, Griffiths-Jones HM (1986) A computerized psychiatric diagnostic system and case nomenclature for elderly subjects: GMS and AGECAT. *Psychological Medicine* 16: 89–99.

Cowan DW, Copeland JRM, Kelleher MJ et al (1975) Cross-national study of diagnosis of the mental disorders: a comparative psychometric assessment of elderly patients admitted to mental hospitals serving Queens County, New York, and the former Borough of Camberwell, London. *British Journal of Psychiatry* 126: 560–70.

Spitzer RL, Endicott J (1969) DIAGNO II: further developments in a computer program for psychiatric diagnosis. *American Journal of Psychiatry* 125: 12–21.

Spitzer RL, Endicott J, Fleiss JL et al (1970) Psychiatric Status Schedule: a technique for evaluating psychopathology and impairment in role functioning. *Archives of General Psychiatry* 23: 41–55.

Spitzer RL, Fleiss JL (1974) A re-analysis of the reliability of psychiatric diagnosis. *British Journal of Psychiatry* 125: 341–7.

Wing JK, Cooper JE, Sartorius N (1974) *The measurement and classification of psychiatric symptoms: an instruction manual for the PSE and Catego program.* Cambridge: Cambridge University Press.

Factors derived from the Geriatric Mental State Schedule (GMSS)

1. Depression
2. Anxiety
3. Impaired memory
4. Retarded speech
5. Hypomania
6. Somatic concerns
7. Observed belligerence
8. Reported belligerence
9. Obsessions
10. Drug–alcohol dependence
11. Cortical dysfunction
12. Disorientation
13. Lack of insight
14. Depersonalization–derealization
15. Paranoid delusion
16. Subjective experience of disordered thought
17. Visual hallucination
18. Auditory hallucination
19. Abnormal motor movements
20. Non-social speech
21. Incomprehensibility

Canberra Interview for the Elderly (CIE)

Reference   Henderson AS et al (1992) The Canberra Interview for the Elderly: a new field instrument for the diagnosis of dementia and depression by ICD-10 and DSM-III-R. *Acta Psychiatrica Scandinavica* 85: 105–13

Time taken 69 minutes with subjects, 37 minutes with informant (average values)
Rating designed to be administered by lay interviewers

Main indications

An instrument for identifying cases of dementia and depression for research purposes.

Commentary

An instrument was designed in which items systematically represented the elements for depression and dementia in DSM-III-R and ICD-10 diagnostic criteria. A computer algorithm of the diagnoses was then constructed, leading to a diagnosis. The Canberra Interview for the Elderly (CIE) is particularly useful for epidemiological studies and acceptable to the elderly. The instrument involves some pictorial material which could not be stored on disk and is available in booklet form. Test/rerest reliability is high and comparison with cognitive function tests and diagnostic categories (ICD-10 and DSM-III-R) is excellent.

Address for correspondence

AS Henderson
Director
NH and MRC Psychiatric Epidemiology Research Centre
The Australian National University
Canberra
ACT 0200
Australia

Canberra Interview for the Elderly (CIE)

Memory functioning
    Long-term memory
    Short-term verbal memory
    Short-term nonverbal memory
    History of deterioration

Intellectual performance
    Premorbid intelligence
    Orientation to time and place
    Vocabulary
    Similarities

Sentence verification
Verbal fluency
Phrase repetition
Object naming
Mental concentration
Copying, writing, pointing, following simple and complex commands (dyspraxia)
Perceptual identification
Perceptual motor speed and intelligence
History of deterioration

Survey Psychiatric Assessment Schedule (SPAS)

Reference   Bond J, Brooks P, Carstairs V, Giles L (1980) The reliability of a Survey Psychiatric Assessment Schedule for the elderly. *British Journal of Psychiatry* 137: 148–62

Time taken 20–30 minutes (reviewer's estimate)
Rating by qualified observer

Main indications

Intended to assess the prevalence of the whole range of psychiatric disorders affecting elderly people.

Commentary

Orignally derived from a short version of the Geriatric Mental State Schedule (GMSS; page 200) the Survey Psychiatric Assessment Schedule (SPAS) consists of 51 items divided into three groups: organic disorders (scores vary from 0 to 12), affective disorders/psychoneurosis (scores vary from 0 to 65) and schizophrenia/paranoid disorders (scores vary from 0 to 10). Cut-off points are available to indicate the severity from each of the global scores.

Additional reference

Bond J (1987) Psychiatric illness in later life. A study of the prevalance in a Scottish population. *International Journal of Geriatric Psychiatry* 2: 39–57.

Address for correspondence

John Bond
Centre for Health Services Research
University of Newcastle
21 Claremont Place
Newcastle upon Tyne
NE2 4AA
UK

Survey Psychiatric Assessment Schedule (SPAS)

1. I'd like to begin by checking that I have got a few details correct.

Both names correct	1

Could you spell your last name for me? And your first name?

Both names not correct	0

(Check against spelling of name provided from records. One minor spelling error allowed.)

No reply/don't know	0

2a. What is the full postal address here?

(Check with records)	Both number and street (or name of institution) correct	1
	Number and/or street (or name of institution) incorrect	0
	No reply/don't know	0

b.

	Town or district correct	1
	Town or district incorrect	0
	No reply/don't know	0

3. My name is .... (Give last name only) I'd like you to remember that.

Correct or almost correct	1

Can you repeat that please. (Spell and repeat name 3 times or until

Totally incorrect	0

correctly repeated. Accept only approximation to correct pronunciation).

No reply	0

4. How old were you on your last birthday? (If vague ask) About how old are you?

Same as record	1
Different from records	0
No reply/don't know	0

5. What year were you born in?

Same as records	1
Different from records	0
No reply/don't know	0

Other survey questions about general health of subject.

6. Do you remember my name? What is it? (Accept any approximation to correct pronunciation).

7. What is the date today? (Allow error of one day).

8. What month is this? (Allow error of one week, e.g. March in first week of April).

9. What year is this? (Allow error of one month, e.g. 1977 in January 1978).

10. Who is the Prime Minister?

11. Who was the Prime Minister before this?

Questions 6–11 score 1 for correct name; 0 for incorrect or no reply/don't know

I should now like to get some idea of how you yourself have been getting along lately – how your general health has been, and how you have been feeling about things. Some of the things I am now going to ask you may not apply to you but I am just making sure that everything has been mentioned. Most of the questions I shall ask you will apply to how you have been feeling in the last month.

12. Most people have some sort of worries or troubles from time to time. Have you worried a great deal about any of the following recently: money, ill health, housing, people you live with, relatives, neighbours, what people think of you, having done something wrong, not doing things properly, not being able to cope.
(If worries about any of these ask 13–15)

	Score 1 for every positive reply	**Score**
13. How often do you worry?	Never	0
	Some days	1
	Most days	2

14. When you worry about these things is it unpleasant or not?

Not unpleasant	0
Unpleasant	1

15. Can you stop yourself worrying?

Can stop	0
If I do something	1
Cannot stop worrying	2

16. Have there been times lately when you have been nervous or anxious for no good reason? Is this no more than usual or more than usual?

None	0
No more than usual	1
More than usual	2

17. **If yes at 16.** Does this happen from time to time or most of the time?

Not anxious	0
From time to time	1
Most of the time	2

18. Are you troubled with frightening dreams?

No	0
Yes	1

19. Do you wake in fear or panic?

No	0
Yes	1

20. **If yes at 18 or 19**. Does this happen occasionally, some nights or most nights?

Never	0
Occasionally	1
Some nights	2
Most nights	3

21. Do you feel tense and restless?

No	0
Yes	1

Scale is continued overleaf

22. People sometimes have fears that they know don't make sense, like being afraid of crowds or certain activities. Do you have any fears like this? For instance, do you tend to get very frightened: when you are alone; in a small room; when you are in a crowd; when you travel by bus; when you are in a shop; in open spaces; when in an enclosed space.
Probe to establish whether or not fear is reasonable.
Score 1 for only fears which are unreasonable.

	Score 1 for all unreasonable fears

23. Does this fear/these fears ever prevent you from doing things you want to do? Is there anything you can do to overcome this like taking someone with you?

No	0
Can overcome	1
Cannot overcome	2

24. Do you ever feel your heart pounding? (If yes) Is this because you get frightened or is it for some other reason?

No	0
Not frightened	1
Frightened	2

25. Do ever feel yourself trembling? (If yes) Is this because you get frightened or is it for some other reason?

No	0
Not frightened	1
Frightened	2

26. Do you ever get dizzy? (If yes) Is this because you get frightened or is it for some other reason?

No	0
Not frightened	1
Frightened	2

27. Do you ever get hot or cold all over? (If yes) Is this because you get frightened or is it for some other reason?

No	0
Not frightened	1
Frightened	2

28. Do you ever faint or lose consciousness? (If yes) Is this because you get frightened or is it for some other reason?

No	0
Not frightened	1
Frightened	2

29. Do you ever get a sinking feeling in your stomach? (If yes) Is this because you get frightened or is it for some other reason?

No	0
Not frightened	1
Frightened	2

30. Have you been depressed or miserable during the past month for no good reason? (If yes) Is this no more than usual or more than usual?

No	0
No more than usual	1
More than usual	2

31. (If yes at 30). Does this come and go or is it constant?

Come and go	0
Constant	1

32. (If yes at 30). Does it interfere with your life or not?

Does not interfere	0
Interferes	1

33. How much have you cried lately?

Not at all	0
Once or twice a month	1
More often than this	2

34. How much have you felt like crying or have wanted to cry, without actually weeping, for no good reason?

Not at all	0
Once or twice a month	1
More often than this	2

35. How do you see your future?

All right	0
Avoids thinking about it	1
Seems bleak/dark/ hopeless	2

36. Have there been times lately when you wish you were dead?

No	0
Yes	1

37. Have you had trouble sleeping?

No	0
Yes	1

38. Do you have difficulty getting off to sleep?

No	0
Yes	1

39. Do you lie awake during the night for an hour or more?

No	0
Yes	1

40. Do you wake early and lie awake?

No	0
Yes	1

41. Do you regularly take tablets to make you sleep?

Never	0
Some nights	1
Most nights	2

42. Is anyone interfering with your thoughts in a strange way which you cannot understand? (If yes) In what way?

No	0
Yes	1

43. Can other people read your thoughts in some strange way which you cannot understand? (If yes) In what way?

No	0
Yes	1

44. Do you feel people are putting thoughts into your head in some strange way which you cannot understand? (If yes) In what way?

No	0
Yes	1

45. Do you feel people are controlling your mind against your will? (If yes) In what way?

No	0
Yes	1

46. Do you get a peculiar feeling that people are taking thoughts out of your head? (If yes) In what way?

No	0
Yes	1

47. Are there people you do not trust? (If yes) Who and why don't you trust them?

No	0
Yes	1

48. Do people laugh at you and say unpleasant things about you behind your back? (If yes) What do they say?

No	0
Yes	1

49. Do you feel that people are trying to upset or harm you in any way for no good reason? (If yes) Who and how are they trying to harm you?

No	0
Yes	1

50. Do you ever see or hear something on television or on radio or in the papers which is directed at you or has a special meaning for you and nobody else? (If yes) What do you see or hear?

No	0
Yes	1

51. Do you ever think you hear a voice when there is nobody there? (If yes) Where does the voice come from? What does it say?

No	0
Yes	1

Section 1 – Additive scores derived

No organic disorder	9–12
Mild organic disorder	7–8
Severe organic disorder	0–6

Section 2 – Summate responses

Non-case	0–10
Case	11–22

Section 3 – Any positive answer indicates a possible case

Multidimensional Observation Scale for Elderly Subjects (MOSES)

Reference   Helmes E, Csapo KG, Short J-A (1987) Standardization and validation of the Multidimensional Observation Scale for Elderly Subjects (MOSES). *Journal of Gerontology* **42**: 395–405

Time taken 25 minutes (reviewer's estimate)
Rating by observers trained in the subject

Main indications

Assessment of behaviours in elderly people.

Commentary

The Multidimensional Observation Scale for Elderly Subjects (MOSES) rates different areas of functioning (multidimensional), and this overcomes the difficulties of global ratings of impairment, which are sometimes regarded as being too broad. The MOSES was developed from a longitudinal research programme which included the development of the London Psychogeriatric Rating Scale (LPRS) (Hersch et al, 1978). The MOSES was developed by empirical factor analyses of earlier instruments identifying major areas of functioning, adding questions about depression and developing specific anchor points in the ratings. The final result was a 40-item test assessing five areas of functioning (eight items each): self-care functioning, disorientated behaviour, depressed/anxious mood, irritable behaviour and withdrawn behaviour (Helmes et al, 1985).

The original paper reports the results on 2542 individuals – inter-rater reliability was acceptable (e.g. intraclass correlation coefficients ranged from 0.50 to 0.99; internal consistency was around 0.8). Validity was tested by examining 12-month follow-up and comparisons with the Zung Depression Status Inventory (Zung, 1972) and the Robertson Short Status Questionnaire (Robertson et al, 1982), the Kingston Dementia Rating Scale (Lawson et al, 1977), the PAMIE Scale (page 180) (Gurel et al, 1972) and the London Psychogeriatric Rating Scale (Hersch et al, 1978). There were significant correlations between subscales of the MOSES and the other measures proving validity.

Additional references

Gurel L, Linn MW, Linn BS (1972) Physical and mental impairment-of-function evaluation in the aged: the PAMIE scale. *Journal of Gerontology* **27**: 83–90.

Helmes E, Csapo KG, Short JA (1985) *History, development and validation of a new rating scale for the institutionalized elderly: the Multidimensional Observation Scale for Elderly Subjects (MOSES) (Bulletin No 8501).* Dept of Psychiatry, University of Western Ontario, Canada.

Lawson JS, Rodenburg M, Dykes JA (1977) A dementia rating scale for use with psychogeriatric patients. *Journal of Gerontology* **32**: 153–9.

Robertson D, Rockwood K, Stolee P (1982) A short mental status questionnaire. *Canadian Journal on Aging* **1**: 16–20.

Zung WWK (1972) The Depression Status Inventory: an adjunct to the Self-Rating Depression Scale. *Journal of Clinical Psychology* **28**: 539–43.

Address for correspondence

E Helmes
Psychology Department
London Psychiatric Hospital
Box 2532
Station A
London
Ontario N6A 4H1
Canada

Items covered in the Multidimensional Observation Scale for Elderly Subjects (MOSES)

1. Dressing
2. Bathing (Including baths and showers)
3. Grooming
4. Incontience (Of either urine of feces)
5. Using the toilet
6. Physical mobility
7. Getting in and out of bed
8. Use of restraints
9. Understanding communication
10. Talking
11. Finding way around inside
12. Recognizing staff
13. Awareness of place
14. Awareness of time
15. Memory for recent events
16. Memory for important past events
17. Looking sad and depressed
18. Reporting sadness and depression
19. Sounding sad and depressed
20. Looking worried and anxious
21. Reporting worry and anxiety
22. Crying
23. Pessimism about the future
24. Self concern
25. Co-operation with nursing care
26. Following staff requests and instructions
27. Irritability
28. Reactions to frustration
29. Verbal abuse of staff
30. Verbal abuse of other residents
31. Physical abuse of others
32. Provoking arguments with other residents
33. Preferring solitude
34. Initiating social contacts
35. Responding to social contacts
36. Friendships with other residents
37. Interest in day-to-day events
38. Interest in outside events
39. Keeping occupied
40. Helping other residents

Reproduced from *Journal of Gerontology*, Vol. 42, no. 4, pp. 395–405, 1987. Copyright © The Gerontological Society of America.

Cambridge Mental Disorders of the Elderly Examination (CAMDEX)

Reference   Roth M, Tym E, Mountjoy CQ, Huppert FA, Hendrie H, Verma S, Goddard R (1986) CAMDEX. A standardised instrument for the diagnosis of mental disorder in the elderly with special reference to the early detection of dementia. *British Journal of Psychiatry* 149: 698–709

Time taken interview with subject approximately 60 minutes. Informant section approximately 20 minutes
Rating by interview

Main indications

An interview schedule for the diagnosis and measurement of dementia in the elderly.

Commentary

The Cambridge Mental Disorders of the Elderly Examination (CAMDEX) is a structured instrument comprising eight sections. The CAMDEX is designed to provide a formal diagnosis according to operational diagnostic criteria in one of 11 categories. Normally, four types of dementia are assessed: Alzheimer's disease, multi-infarct dementia, mixed Alzheimer's and multi-infarct dementia, and dementia due to other causes – delirium (with or without depression), depression, anxiety or phobic disorders, paranoid or paraphrenic illness, and other psychiatric disorders. A five-point scale allows severity of dementia and severity of depression to be rated. The original paper describes results on 92 patients. Inter-rater reliability ranged from a median of 0.83 for the observational parts of the CAMDEX up to 0.94 for the patient interview.

With regard to clinical diagnoses of dementia, a cut-off of 79/80 on the CAMCOG (maximum = 106) yielded a result of 92% sensitivity and 96% specificity. A description of clinical diagnostic scales for Alzheimer's disease, multi-infarct dementia and depression is included.

Additional references

O'Connor D, Pollitt P, Hyde J et al (1990) The progression of mild idiopathic dementia in a community population. *Journal of the American Geriatrics Society* 39: 246–51.

O'Connor D, Pollitt P, Hyde J et al (1990) Follow-up study of dementia diagnosed in the community using the CAMDEX. *Acta Psychiatrica Scandinavica* 81: 78–82.

Address for correspondence

Felicia A Huppert
Department of Psychiatry
Level E4
Box 189
Addenbrooke's Hospital
Cambridge CB2 2QQ
UK

The Cambridge Mental Disorders of the Elderly Examination (CAMDEX)

Section A
Particulars regarding present physical and mental state, past history, family history. It starts with 3 questions: name, age and date of bith. If the answers are obtained to 2 out of 3, section A is abandoned and Section B is completed.

Section B
This is the cognitive section which includes questions allowing the Mini-Mental State Examination to be completed as well as specific cognitive items in the CAMDEX and CAMCOG scales
orientation – time place
language – comprehension (motor response, verbal response, expression, naming, definitions, repetition, spontaneous speech, reading comprehension)
memory – recall (visual and verbal), recognition, retrieval of remote and recent information.
Registration – attention and concentration.
Praxis – copy and drawing, spontaneous writing, ideational praxis, writing to dictation, idea motor praxis.
Tactile perception – calculation, abstract thinking, visual perception (famous people), object, constancy, recognition of person/function.
Passage of time.

Section C
This consists of interviewer's observation on appearance, behaviour, mood, speech, mental slowing activity and thought process, bizarre behaviour and level of consciousness.

Section D
Simple physical examination.

Section E
Results of laboratory and radiological investigations.

Section F
Medication.

Section G
Additional information.

Section H
Interview with informant.
History of present difficulty (personality, memory, general mental function, functioning everyday activities, clouding/delirium, depressed mood, sleep, paranoid features, cerebro-vascular problems).

Questions pertaining to subject's past history.
Questions pertaining to family and past history.

Nurses' Observation Scale for Geriatric Patients (NOSGER)

Reference   Spiegel R, Brunner C, Ermini-Fünfschilling D, Monsch A, Notter M, Puxty J, Tremmel L (1991) A new behavioural assessment scale for geriatric out- and in-patients: the NOSGER (Nurses' Observation Scale for Geriatric Patients). *Journal of the American Geriatrics Society* 39: 339–47

Time taken 20 minutes
Rating by nursing staff

Main indications

Assessment of behaviour and functioning in elderly patients.

Commentary

The Nurses' Observation Scale for Geriatric Patients (NOSGER) was developed from two existing scales: the Nurses' Observation Scale for Inpatient Evaluation (NOSIE; page 100) and the Geriatric Evaluation by Relative's Rating Instrument (GERRI; page 250). It was designed in view of the need to develop a useful instrument of longitudinal studies in psychogeriatrics, in particular fulfilling the requirements of the scale as follows:

(a) Applicable to institutionalized community patients covering a wide range of behaviours.
(b) Easy to use for professionals and lay people.
(c) Covering a wide range of behaviours relevant to daily function independent of sex or social class.

The new scale was limited to 30 items, assigned on the basis of content to coincide with one of six areas of assessment: memory, instrumental activities of daily living, self-care, activities of daily living, mood, social behaviour and disturbing behaviour. Three validation studies have been carried out, which are referred to in the main paper. NOSGER items were selected specifically to avoid complicated and ambiguous expression and those which relatives might find offensive – delusions and hallucination were therefore omitted, as were questions with a negative formulation. Inter-rater reliability was found in the three validation studies to be 0.7, with the exception of mood and disturbing behaviour, where they were less than 0.6. The test/retest reliability yielded values between 0.8 and 0.9. Validity was assessed using a number of other scales, with generally good results.

Address for correspondence

R Spiegel
Clinical Research CNS Department
Sandoz Pharma Ltd
402 Basle
Switzerland

Nurses' Observation Scale for Geriatric Patients (NOSGER)

1. Shaves or puts on makeup, combs hair without help.
2. Follows favourite radio or TV programmes.
3. Reports he/she feels sad.
4. Is restless during the night.
5. Is interested in what is going on around him/her.
6. Tries to keep his/her room tidy.
7. Is able to control bowels.
8. Remembers a point in conversation after interruption.
9. Goes shopping for small items (newspaper, groceries).
10. Reports feeling worthless.
11. Continues with some favourite hobby.
12. Repeats the same point in conversation over and over.
13. Appears sad or tearful.
14. Clean and tidy in appearance.
15. Runs aways.
16. Remembers names of close friends.
17. Helps others as far as physically able.
18. Goes out inappropriately dressed.
19. Is orientated when in usual surroundings.
20. When asked questions, seems quarrelsome and irritable.
21. Makes contact with people around.
22. Remembers where clothes and other things are placed.
23. Is aggressive (verbally or physically).
24. Is able to control bladder function (urine).
25. Appears to be cheerful.
26. Maintains contact with friends or family.
27. Confuses the identity of some people with others.
28. Enjoys certain events (visits, parties).
29. Appears friendly and positive in conversation with family members or friends.
30. Behaves stubbornly, does not follow instructions or rules.

Comments:

Answer with respect to last 2 weeks only
Score all as follows: All of the time
                                 Most of the time
                                 Often
                                 Sometimes
                                 Never

Comprehensive Assessment and Referral Evaluation (CARE)

Reference   Gurland D, Kuriansky J, Sharpe L, Simon R, Stiller P, Birkett P (1977) The Comprehensive Assessment and Referral Evaluation (CARE): rationale, development and reliability. *International Journal of Ageing and Human Development* 8: 9–42

Time taken 45–90 minutes

Rating by trained interviewer

Main indications

A comprehensive measure of health and social problems of older people.

Commentary

The Comprehensive Assessment and Referral Evaluation (CARE) is an assessment technique intended to assimilate information on the health and social problems of older people. The CARE is essentially a semi-structured interview guide with an inventory of defined ratings. It is comprehensive in that it covers a whole range of problems – medical, psychiatric, nutritional, social and economic. It can be administered to all groups, and is therefore useful in deciding if a person should be referred, and its scope allows it to evaluate the effectiveness of a service. The CARE covers a number of different areas of functioning outlined, and the original publication suggested (prior to a factor analysis being performed) the following dimensions: memory/disorientation; depression/anxiety; immobility/incapacity; physical/perceptual; isolation; and poor housing. The first two were indicative of psychiatric problems, the second two medical/physical problems and the last two socioeconomic problems. Reliability is presented for these dimensions in the form of intraclass correlations, and is generally good with the exception of the medical/physical ratings. Familiarity with the instrument was cited as the reason for the low scores.

Additional references

Copeland J (1976) A semi-structured clinical interview for the assessment of diagnosis and mental state in the elderly. *Psychological Medicine* 6: 451–9.

Macdonald A, Mann A, Jenkins R et al (1982) An attempt to determine the impact of four types of care upon the elderly in London by the study of matched groups. *Psychological Medicine* 12: 193–200.

Comprehensive Assessment and Referral Evaluation (CARE)

Identifying data/Dementia I: Census type data/Country of Origin/Race/Length of time spoken English

Dementia II: Error in length of residence/telephone number
General enquiries about main problems
Worry/depression/suicide/self-depreciation
Elation
Anxiety/fear of going out/infrequency of excursions
Referential and paranoid ideas
Household arrangement/loneliness
Family and friendly relationships/present and past Isolation index/closeness
Emergency assistance
Anger/family burden on subject
Obsessions/thought reading
Weight/appetite/digestion/difficulties in shopping and preparing food/dietary intake/alcohol intake
Sleep disturbance
Depersonalization

Dementia III: Subjective and objective difficulty with memory/tests or recall
Fits and faints/autonomic functions/bowel and bladder
Slowness and anergia/restlessness
Self-rating of health
Fractures and operations/medical and non-medical attention/examinations/medicines or drugs/drug addiction
Arthritis/aches and pains
Breathlessness/smoking/heart disease/hypertension/chest pain/cough/hoarseness/fevers
Limitation in mobility/care of feet/limitation of exertion/simple tests of motor function
Sores, growths, discharges/strokes/hospitalization and bed-rest
Hearing/auditory hallucinations
Vision/visual hallucinations
Hypochondriasis
Disfigurement/antisocial behavior
Loss of interests/activities list
History of depression
Organizations and religion/educational and occupational history
Work and related problems/retirement history
Income/health insurance/medical and other expenses/handling of finances/shortages
Housing facilities and related problems
Ability to dress/do chores/help needed or received
Neighborhood and crime
Overall self-rating of satisfaction/happiness/insight
Mute/stuporous/abnormalities of speech
Additional observations of subject and environment/communication difficulties

Reproduced from Gurland D, Kuriansky J, Sharpe L, Simon R, Stiller P, Birkett P (1977) The Comprehensive Assessment and Referral Evaluation (CARE): rationale, development and reliability. *International Journal of Ageing and Human Development* **8**: 9–42, published by Baywood Publishing Co.

Chapter 4

Physical examination

There are relatively few scales in this chapter. Most are directed towards the side-effects of neuroleptics, tardive dyskinesia and Parkinsonism. The recording of soft neurological signs is important in the research setting.

Cambridge Neurological Inventory

Reference   Chen EYH, Shapleske J, Luque R, McKenna PJ, Hodges JR, Calloway SP, Hymas NFS, Dening TR, Berrios GE (1995) The Cambridge Neurological Inventory: a clinical instrument for assessment of soft neurological signs in psychiatric patients. *Psychiatry Research* 56: 183–204

Time taken 20–40 minutes
Rating by trained examiner

Main indications

To identify soft neurological signs and other patterns of neurological impairment relevant to neurobiological localization and prognosis in schizophrenia and other psychiatric disorders.

Commentary

The Cambridge Neurological Inventory is a standardized inventory designed to complement the basic neurological examination. Items were drawn from other neurological scales (Quitkin et al, 1976; Walker, 1981; Tweedy et al, 1982; Buchanan and Heinrichs, 1988). The inventory required at least five practice trials before clinical use. The scale has a wider scope than others published, and is precise in using operational definitions for eliciting signs. Inter-rater reliability for most of the items is above 0.85, and was able to distinguish between patients with schizophrenia and controls.

Additional references

Buchanan RW, Heinrichs DW (1988) The Neurological Evaluation Scale (NES): a structured instrument for the assessment of neurological signs in schizophrenia. *Psychiatry Research* 27: 335–50.

Quitkin F, Rifkin A, Klein DF (1976) Neurological soft signs in schizophrenia and character disorders. *Archives of General Psychiatry* 33: 845–53.

Tweedy J, Reding M, Gracia C et al (1982) Significance of cortical disinhibition signs. *Neurology* 32: 169–73.

Walker E (1981) Attentional and neuromotor functions of schizophrenic, schizoaffectives and patients with other affective disorders. *Archives of General Psychiatry* 38: 1355–8.

Address for correspondence

Eric YH Chen
Department of Psychiatry
Univesity of Cambridge
Addenbrooke's Hospital
Cambridge CB2 2QQ
UK

Cambridge Neurological Inventory

PART 1

Speech assessment:	Articulation Aprosodic speech Unintelligible speech	Extremity examinations:	Tone, strength, reflex

PART 2
Soft sign examinations
  i.e. primitive reflexes, repetitive movement, sensory integration, finger nose test, mirror movements, left–right orientation

Eye movement assessment:	Smooth pursuit – extent, smoothness, gaze impersistence Saccadia – smoothness, blink suppression, lateral head movement
Cranial nerve assessment:	Winlang (lateralization) Glabellar tap Rapid tongue movement

PART 3
Posture and movement assessment – including catatonia, tardive dyskinesia, gait, balance

Rate as follows:
0 = Normal; 0.5 = Subthreshold; 1 = Definitely abnormal; 2 = Grossly abnormal;
9 = Missing/unable to test or lack of co-operation/comprehension

Webster Scale (and other Parkinson's Disease Scales)

Reference   Webster DD (1988) Critical analysis of the disability in Parkinson's disease. *Modern Treatment* 5: 257–82

Time taken 15–20 minutes (reviewer's estimate)
Rating by clinician

Main indications

Assessing the degree of disability in Parkinson's disease.

Commentary

The original paper is a model of clinical observation and clinical description and, while well supported by references, contains no empirical data about a patient population. The scale has been used in the assessment of dementia, e.g. Girling and Berrios (1990).

Other rating scales used in the assessment of Parkinson's disease include the Unified Parkinson's Disease Rating Scale (UPDRS) (England and Schwab, 1956; Fahn and Elton, 1987), a staging scale described by Hoehn and Yahr (1967), and the North Western University Disability Scale (Cantor et al, 1961). Other scales are available (for review, see Fahn and Elton, 1987).

Additional references

Cantor C, Torre R, Mier M (1961) A method of evaluating disability in patients with Parkinson's disease. *Journal of Nervous and Mental Disease* 133: 143–7.

England A, Schwab R (1956) Post-operative evaluation of 26 selected patients with Parkinson's disease. *Journal of the American Geriatrics Society* 4: 1219–32.

Fahn S, Elton R (1987) Unified Parkinson's Disease Rating Scale. In Fahn S, Marsden C, Goldstein M et al, eds. *Recent developments in Parkinson's disease*, Vol. 2. Macmillan Healthcare Information.

Girling D, Berrios G (1990) Extrapyramidal signs: primitive reflexes in frontal lobe function in senile dementia of the Alzheimer type. *British Journal of Psychiatry* 157: 888–93.

Hoehn M, Yahr N (1967) Parkinsonism: onset, progression and mortality. *Neurology* 17: 427–42.

Webster Scale

Bradykinesia of hands – including handwriting
0 No involvement.
1 Detectable slowing of the supination–pronation rate evidenced by beginning difficulty in handling tools, buttoning clothes, and with handwriting.
2 Moderate slowing of supination–pronation rate, one or both sides, evidenced by moderate impairment of hand function. handwriting is greatly impaired, micrographia present.
3 Severe slowing of supination–pronation rate. Unable to write or button clothes. Marked difficulty in handling utensils.

Rigidity
0 Non-detectable.
1 Detectable rigidity in neck and shoulders. Activation phenomenon is present. One or both arms show mild, negative, resting rigidity.
2 Moderate rigidity in neck and shoulders. Resting rigidity is positive when patient not on medication.
3 Severe rigidity in neck and shoulders. Resting rigidity cannot be reversed by medication.

Posture
0 Normal posture. Head flexed forward less than 4 inches.
1 Beginning poker spine. Head flexed forward up to 5 inches
2 Beginning arm flexion. Head flexed forward up to 6 inches. One or both arms raised but still below waist.
3 Onset of simian posture. Head flexed forward more than 6 inches. One or both hands elevated above the waist. Sharp flexion of hand, beginning interphalangeal extension. Beginning flexion of knees.

Upper extremity swing
0 Swings both arms well.
1 One arm definitely decreased in amount of swing.
2 One arm fails to swing.
3 Both arms fail to swing.

Gait
0 Steps out well with 18–30 inch stride. Turns aout effortlessly.
1 Gait shortened to 12–18 inch stride. beginning to strike one heel. Turn around time slowing. Requires several steps.
2 Stride moderately shortened – now 6–12 inches. Both heels beginning to strike floor forcefully.

Scale is continued overleaf

3 Onset of shuffling gait, steps less than 3 inches. Occasional stuttering-type or blocking gait. Walks on toes – turns around very slowly.

Tremor

0 No detectable tremor found.

1 Less than one inch of peak-to-peak tremor movement observed in limbs or head at rest or in either hand while walking or during finger to nose testing.

2 Maximum tremor envelope fails to exceed 4 inches. Tremor is severe but not constant and patient retains some control of hands.

3 Tremor envelope exceeds 4 inches. Tremor is constant and severe. Patient cannot get free of tremor while awake unless it is a pure cerebellar type. Writing and feeding himself are impossible.

Facies

0 Normal. Full animation. No stare.

1 Detectable immobility. Mouth remains closed. Beginning features of anxiety or depression.

2 Moderate immobility. Emotion breaks through at markedly increased threshold. Lips parted some of the time. Moderate appearance of anxiety or depression. Drooling may be present.

3 Frozen facies. Mouth open ¼ inch or more. Drooling may be severe.

Seborrhea

0 None.

1 Increased perspiration, secretion remaining thin.

2 Obvious oiliness present. Secretion much thicker.

3 Marked seborrhoea, entire face and head covered by thick secretion.

Speech

0 Clear, loud, resonant, clearly understood.

1 Beginning of hoarseness with loss of inflection and resonance. Good volume and still easily understood.

2 Moderate hoarseness and weakness. Constant monotone, unvaried pitch. Beginning of dysarthria, hesitancy, stuttering, difficult to understand.

3 Marked harshness and weakness. Very difficult to hear and to understand.

Self-care

0 No impairment.

1 Still provides full self-care but rate of dressing definitely impeded. Able to live alone and often still employable.

2 Requires help in certain critical areas, such as turning in bed, rising from chairs, etc. Very slow in performing most activities but manages by taking much time.

3 Continuously disabled. Unable to dress, feed himself, or walk alone.

Score as follows:

0 = No involvement/not detectable/not impaired

1 = Early disease

2 = Moderate disease

3 = Severe disease

Source: Webster DD (1968) Critical analysis of the disability in Parkinson's disease. *Modern Treatment* **5**: 257–82.

Tardive Dyskinesia Rating Scale (TDRS)

Reference   Simpson GM, Lee JH, Zoubok B, Gardos G (1979) A rating scale for tardive dyskinesia.
Psychopharmacology 64: 171–9

Time taken 20–25 minutes (reviewer's estimate)
Rating by clinician

Main indications

For the assessment of the nature and severity of abnormal movements in psychiatric patients. Useful for studies in older people with schizophrenia.

Commentary

The Tardive Dyskinesia Rating Scale (TDRS) is a 43-item scale consisting of the standard assessment (from absent to very severe on a six-point scale) of neurological signs in the face, neck and trunk, and extremities, and changes affecting the whole body. Inter-rater reliability is generally high, ranging between 0.55 and 1.0 using Pearson's correlation. An abbreviated dyskinesia scale is also available consisting of 13 items with similar inter-rater reliability.

Additional reference

Simpson G (1988) Tardive dyskinesia rating scale. *Psychopharmacology Bulletin* 24: 803–807.

Tardive Dyskinesia Rating Scale (TDRS)

Face

1. Blinking of eyes —
2. Tremor of eyelids —
3. Tremor of upper lip (rabbit syndrome) —
4. Pouting of the (lower) lip —
5. Puckering of lips —
6. Sucking movements —
7. Chewing movements —
8. Smacking of lips —
9. Bonbon sign —
10. Tongue protrusion —
11. Tongue tremor —
12. Choreoathetoid movements of tongue —
13. Facial tics —
14. Grimacing —
15. Other (describe) —
16. Other (describe) —

Neck and trunk

17. Head nodding —
18. Retrocollis —
19. Spasmodic torticollis —
20. Torsion movements (trunk) —
21. Axial hyperkinesia —
22. Rocking movement —
23. Other (describe) —
24. Other (describe) —

Extremities (upper)

25. Ballistic movements —
26. Choreoathetoid movements – fingers —
27. Choreoathetoid movements – wrists —
28. Pill-rolling movements —
29. Caressing or rubbing face and hair —
30. Rubbing of thighs —
31. Other (describe) —
32. Other (describe) —

Extremities (lower)

33. Rotation and/or flexion of ankles —
34. Toe movements —
35. Stamping movements – standing —
36. Stamping movements – sitting —
37. Restless legs —
38. Crossing/uncrossing legs – sitting —
39. Other (describe) —
40. Other (describe) —

Entire body

41. Holokinetic movements —
42. Akathisia —
43. Other (describe) —

Score:

1 = Absent
2 = Questionable
3 = Mild
4 = Moderate
5 = Moderately severe
6 = Very severe

Neurological Evaluation Scale (NES)

Reference   Buchanan RW, Heinrichs DW (1989) The Neurological Evaluation Scale (NES): a structured instrument for the assessment of neurological signs in schizophrenia. *Psychiatry Research* 27: 335–50

Time taken 30 minutes (reviewer's estimate)
Rating by clinician

Main indications

A structured neurological examination particularly focusing on areas of impairment found in schizophrenia.

Commentary

The Neurological Evaluation Scale (NES) was developed following an extensive search of systematic reviews and clinical studies of neurological abnormalities in patients with schizophrenia. Three functional areas were described: sensory dysfunction, motor and co-ordination, and impaired sequencing. A 28-item scale was described. Inter-rater reliability (intraclass correlations) was above 0.8 for the majority of items (reliability was also assessed by a nurse, following training lasting approximately 20 hours)

and reliability of above 0.72 was found. In 98 patients, validity was assessed by determining the ability of the scale to differentiate between patients and controls, and highly significant differences were found.

Additional reference

Heinrichs DW, Buchanan RW (1988) The significance and meaning of neurological signs in schizophrenia. *American Journal of Psychiatry* 145: 11–18.

Address for correspondence

RW Buchanan
Department of Psychiatry
University of Maryland School of Medicine
Baltimore
MD 21228
USA

Neurological Evaluation Scale (NES)

1. Tandem walk	15. Rapid alternating movements
2. Romberg test	16. Finger-thumb opposition
3. Adventitious overflow	17. Mirror movements
4. Tremor	18. Extinction (face-hand test)
6. Cerebral dominance	20. Right/left confusion
7. Audio-visual integration	21. Synkinesis
8. Stereognosis	22. Convergence
9. Graphesthesia	23. Gaze impersistence
10. Fist-ring test	24. Finger to nose test
11. Fist-edge-palm test	25. Glabellar reflex
12. Ozeretski test	26. Snout reflex
13. Memory	27. Grasp reflex
14. Rhythm tapping test	28. Suck reflex

Assessments:
0 = Relatively normal
1 = Some disruption
2 = Major disruption

Abnormal Involuntary Movement Scale (AIMS)

Reference   Psychopharmacology Research Branch, NIMH. Abnormal Involuntary Movement Scale (AIMS). In: Guy W, ed ECDEU Assessment Manual for Psychopharmacology, revised DHEW Pub No (ADM) 76–338, Rockville, MD: National Institute of Mental Health, 1976, 534–37

Time taken 20 minutes (reviewer's estimate)
Rating by clinician

Main indications
Assessment of abnormal involuntary movement.

Commentary
The Abnormal Involuntary Movement Scale (AIMS) allows rating of seven body areas and global judgements of the severity of abnormal movements, incapacitation and also the patient's awareness of the abnormal movements. Formal instructions are given about the examination procedure, and brief definitions of each movement are incorporated in the scale. Inter-rater reliability varies from 0.5–0.8 for the seven body areas, with an overall agreement of 0.70. Test/retest reliability (which needs to be interpreted with caution, because the patient's clinical condition can obviously vary) is 0.7 on overall severity (Smith et al, 1979a, 1979b, 1990). Validity has been assessed against direct electronic counting of mouth movements, with a direct correlation against the total AIMS score of 0.72 (Chien et al, 1977). The AIMS has also been used to measure change (Galenberg et al, 1979).

Additional references
Smith J et al (1979a) An assessment of tardive dyskinesia in schizophrenic outpatients. *Psychopharmacology (Berlin)* **64**: 99–104.

Smith J et al (1979b) A systematic investigation of tardive dyskinesia in inpatients. *American Journal of Psychiatry* **136**: 918–22.

Chien C et al (1977) The measurement of persistent dyskinesia by piezoelectric recording and clinical rating scales. *Psychopharmacology Bulletin* **13**: 34–36.

Galenberg (1979) Choline and lethercen in the treatment of tardive dyskinesia. *American Journal of Psychiatry* **136**: 772–76.

Abnormal Involuntary Movement Scale (AIMS)

PATIENT NUMBER	DATA GROUP	EVALUATION DATE	PATIENT NAME

— — — —   — — — — — —   RATER NAME

aims   M   M   D   D   V   Y

INSTRUCTIONS:	Complete Examination Procedure (reverse side) before making ratings. MOVEMENT RATINGS: Rate highest severity observed.	Code:	1 = None 2 = Minimal, may be extreme normal 3 = Mild 4 = Moderate 5 = Severe

		(Circle One)
	1. Muscles of Facial Expression e.g., movements of forehead, eyebrows, periorbital area, cheeks; include frowning, blinking, smiling, grimacing	1 2 3 4 5
FACIAL AND ORAL MOVEMENTS:	2. Lips and Perioral Area e.g., puckering, pouting, smacking	1 2 3 4 5
	3. Jaw e.g., biting, clenching, chewing, mouth opening, lateral movement	1 2 3 4 5
	4. Tongue Rate only increase in movements both in and out of mouth, NOT inability to sustain movement.	1 2 3 4 5
EXTREMITY MOVEMENTS:	5. Upper (arms, wrists, hands, fingers) Include choreic movements (i.e., rapid. objectively purposeless, irregular, spontaneous), athetoid movements (i.e., slow, irregular, complex, serpentine). Do NOT include tremor (i.e., repetitive, regular, rhythmic).	1 2 3 4 5
	6. Lower (legs, knees, ankles, toes) e.g., lateral knee movement, foot tapping, heel dropping, foot squirming, inversion and eversion of foot	1 2 3 4 5
TRUNK MOVEMENTS:	7. Neck, shoulders, hips e.g., rocking, twisting, squirming, pelvic gyrations	1 2 3 4 5
GLOBAL JUDGMENTS:	8. Severity of abnormal movements	None, normal 1 Minimal 2 Mild 3 Moderate 4 Severe 5
	9. Incapacitation due to abnormal movements	None, normal 1 Minimal 2 Mild 3 Moderate 4 Severe 5
	10. Patient's awareness of abnormal movements Rate only patient's report	No awareness 1 Aware, no distress 2 Aware, mild distress 3 Aware, moderate distress 4 Aware, severe distress 5
DENTAL STATUS:	11. Current problems with teeth and/or dentures	No 1 Yes 2
	12. Does patient usually wear dentures?	No 1 Yes 2

EXAMINATION PROCEDURE

Either before or after completing the Examination Procedure, observe the patient unobtrusively, at rest (e.g.,in waiting room).

The chair to be used in this examination should be a hard, firm one without arms.

1.   *Ask patient to remove shoes and socks.*

2.   *Ask patient whether there is anything in his/her mouth (i.e., gum, candy, etc.) and if there is, to remove it.*

3.   *Ask patient about the current condition of his/her teeth. Ask patient if he/she wears dentures. Do teeth or dentures bother patient now?*

4.   *Ask patient whether he/she notices any movements in mouth, face, hands, or feet. If yes, ask to describe and to what extent they currently bother patient or interfere with his/her activities.*

5.   *Have patient sit in chair with hands on knees, legs slightly apart, and feet flat on floor. (Look at entire body for movements while in this position.)*

6.   *Ask patient to sit with hands hanging unsupported. If male, between legs, If female and wearing a dress, hanging over knees. (Observe hands and other body areas.)*

7.   *Ask patient to open mouth. (Observe tongue at rest in mouth.) Do this twice.*

8.   *Ask patient to protrude tongue. (Observe abnormalities of tongue movement.) Do this twice.*

9.   *Ask patient to tap thumb, with each finger, as rapidly as possible for 10 to 15 seconds; separately with right hand, then with left hand. (Observe facial and leg movements.)*

10. *Flex and extend patient's left and right arms (one at a time). (Note any rigidity.)*

11. *Ask patient to stand up. (Observe in profile. Observe all body areas again, hips included.)*

12. *Ask patient to extend both arms outstretched in front with palms down. (Observe trunk, legs, and mouth.)*

13. *Have patient walk a few paces, turn, and walk back to chair. (Observe hands and gait.) Do this twice.*

Reproduced with permission.

Chapter 5

Delirium

Three scales purport to measure the symptoms of delirium. Two are firmly based on DSM criteria for the diagnosis of delirium: the Delirium Rating Scale (DRS; page 230) and the Confusion Assessment Method (CAM; page 228). The Delirium Symptom Interview (DSI; page 227) and CAM are devised to be completed by non-specialists. This is clearly an advantage considering the proportion of patients in non-specialist settings who may suffer from delirium.

Readers should also be aware of another two rating scales for delirium: The Delirium Assessment Scale (O'Keefe S, 1994, Rating the severity of delirium – The Delirium Assessment Scale. *International Journal of Geriatric Psychiatry* 9: 551–6) and the Confusional State Evaluation (CSE) (Robertson B, Karlsson I. Styrud E, Gottfries C, 1997, Confusional state evaluation: an instrument for measuring severity of delirium in the elderly. *British Journal of Psychiatry* 170: 565–70).

For information on the Delirium Index (DI), please refer to Appendix 2.

Delirium Symptom Interview (DSI)

Reference Albert MS, Levkoff SE, Reilly C, Liptzin B, Pilgrim D, Cleary PD, Evans D, Rowe JW (1992) The Delirium Symptom Interview: an interview for the detection of delirium symptoms in hospitalized patients. *Journal of Geriatric Psychiatry and Neurology* 5: 14–21

Time taken 10–15 minutes
Rating by lay interviewer

Main indications

To rate the symptoms of delirium.

Commentary

The Delirium Symptom Interview (DSI) was developed by an interdisciplinary group of investigators. One of the stimuli was the lack of easily administered instruments for delirium, which was impeding studies on the subject. The importance of ratings on a daily basis (in view of rapid changes seen in delirium) and the need therefore for ratings to be made by non-clinicians were emphasized. Fifty patients on medical or surgical wards of an acute hospital were interviewed. Reliability for the various domains of the DSI range from 0.45 (sleep disturbance) to 0.80 (disturbance of consciousness), and ratings were made in the same interview. Reliability was 0.90 using a physicians' consensus. Sensitivity of the DSI in detecting delirium was 0.90, specificity 0.80, positive predictive value 0.87 and negative predictive value 0.84.

Address for correspondence

Marilyn S Albert
Department of Psychiatry and Neurology
Massachusetts General Hospital
Boston
MA
USA

Delirium Symptom Interview (DSI)

Symptom domains measured (from DSM III)
- Disorientation
- Sleep disturbance
- Perceptual disturbance
- Disturbance of consciousness
- Psychomotor activity
- General behaviour observations
- Fluctuating behaviour score

Domains assessed
Disorientation, disturbance of sleep, perceptual disturbance, disturbance of consciousness.

Observations
Disturbance of consciousness, incoherent speech, level of psychomotor activity, general behavioural observations, fluctuations in behaviour.

Score: or
1 = No
2 = Mild   1 = No
3 = Moderate   2 = Yes
4 = Severe   7 = Not applicable

A patient is defined as positive on the DSI if any one of the following is present: disorientation, disturbance of consciousness or perceptual disturbance.

Source: Albert MS, Levkoff SE, Reilly C, Liptzin B, Pilgrim D, Cleary P, Evans D, Rowe JW (1992) The Delirium Symptom Interview: an interview for the detection of delirium symptoms in hospitalized patients. *Journal of Geriatric Psychiatry and Neurology* 5: 14–20.

Confusion Assessment Method (CAM)

Reference   Inouye SK, van Dyck CH, Alessi CA, Balkin S, Siegal AP, Horwitz RI (1990) Clarifying confusion: the Confusion Assessment Method. *Annals of Internal Medicine* **113**: 941–8

Time taken 5 minutes
Rating by clinician

Main indications

For the non-psychiatric clinician to detect delirium. Some training required.

Commentary

The Confusion Assessment Method (CAM) instrument consists of nine operationalized criteria from DSM-III-R including the four cardinal features of acute onset and fluctuation, inattention, disorganized thinking and altered level of consciousness. Both the first and second feature, and either the third or fourth, are required. Face and content validity, concurrent validation, inter-rater reliability and convergent validity were all assessed. The results were validated against a psychiatric diagnosis and for cognitive tests. Sensitivity was 94% and 100% (in two study sites), with specificity 90% and 95% respectively. There was a good correlation with ratings on cognitive tests, and inter-rater reliability was around 0.81. Test/retest reliability was not carried out because of fluctuations in the clinical condition of the patients. Individual clinical features of the CAM include acute onset and fluctuating course, inattention and disorganized thinking, altered level of consciousness, disorientation, memory impairment, perceptional disturbance, abnormal psychomotor activity and altered sleeping cycle.

Address for correspondence

Sharon K Inouye
Yale–New Haven Hospital
20 York Street
Tomkins Basement 15
New Haven
CT 06504
USA

Confusion Assessment Method (CAM)

Acute onset
1. Is there evidence of an acute change in mental status from the patient's baseline?

Inattention*
2. A. Did the patient have difficulty focusing attention, for example, being easily distractible, or having difficulty keeping track of what was being said?

    Not present at any time during interview.
    Present at some time during interview, but in mild form.
    Present at some time during interview, in marked form.
    Uncertain.

    B. (If present or abnormal) Did this behavior fluctuate during the interview, that is, tend to come and go or increase and decrease in severity?

    Yes.
    No.
    Uncertain.
    Not applicable.

    C. (If present or abnormal) Please describe this behavior:

Disorganized thinking
3. Was the patient's thinking disorganized or incoherent, such as rambling or irrelevant conversation, unclear or illogical flow of ideas, or unpredictable switching from subject to subject?

Altered level of consciousness
4. Overall, how would you rate this patient's level of consciousness?

    Alert (normal).
    Vigilant (hyperalert, overly sensitive to environmental stimuli, startled very easily).
    Lethargic (drowsy, easily aroused).
    Stupor (difficult to arouse).
    Coma (unrousable).
    Uncertain.

*The questions listed under this topic are repeated for each topic where applicable.

Disorientation
5. Was the patient disoriented at any time during the interview, such as thinking that he or she was somewhere other than the hospital, using the wrong bed, or misjudging the time of day?

Memory impairment
6. Did the patient demonstrate any memory problems during the interview, such as inability to remember events in the hospital or difficulty remembering instructions?

Perceptual disturbances
7. Did the patient have any evidence of perceptual distrubances, for example, hallucinations, illusions, or misinterpretations (such as thinking something was moving when it was not)?

Psychomotor agitation
8. Part 1.
    At any time during the interview, did the patient have an unusually increased level of motor activity, such as restlessness, picking at bedclothes, tapping fingers, or making frequent sudden changes of position?

Psychomotor retardation
8. Part 2.
    At any time during the interview, did the patient have an unusually decreased level of motor activity, such as sluggishness, staring into space, staying in one position for a long time, or moving very slowly?

Altered sleep–wake cycle
9. Did the patient have evidence of disturbance of the sleep–wake cycle, such as excessive daytime sleepiness with insomnia at night?

Annals of Internal Medicine, **113**, 941–948, 1990. Copyright 1990, the American College of Physicians. Reprinted by permission.

Delirium Rating Scale (DRS)

Reference   Trzepacz PT, Baker RW, Greenhouse J (1988) A symptom rating scale for delirium. *Psychiatry Research* 23: 89–97

Time taken 5–10 minutes
Rating by clinician

Main indications

Assessment of symptoms of delirium.

Commentary

The Delirium Rating Scale (DRS) consists of ten items based on DSM-III criteria for delirium. Twenty patients with delirium were compared against nine with chronic schizophrenia, nine with dementia and nine medically ill subjects. Other ratings included the Mini-Mental State Examination (MMSE; page 34), the Trail Making Test and the Brief Psychiatric Rating Scale (BPRS; page 194).

Inter-rater reliability was 0.97. Ratings on the DRS were significantly higher for the delirium group compared with the other three groups. It is suggested that the test can be used in conjunction with the electroencephalogram and cognitive tests to measure delirium.

Address for correspondence

PT Trzepacz
Allegheny General Hospital
320 E North Avenue
Pittsburgh
PA 15213
USA

Delirium Rating Scale (DRS)

Item 1: Temporal onset of symptoms
0. No significant change from longstanding behavior, essentially a chronic or chronic-recurrent disorder.
1. Gradual onset of symptoms, occurring within a 6-month period.
2. Acute change in behavior or personality occurring over a month.
3. Abrupt change in behavior, usually occurring over a 1- to 3-day period.

Item 2: Perceptual disturbances
0. None evident by history or observation.
1. Feelings of depersonalization or derealization.
2. Visual illusions or misperceptions including macropsia, micropsia, e.g. may urinate in wastebasket or mistake bedclothes for something else.
3. Evidence that the patient is markedly confused about external reality, not discriminating between dreams and reality.

Item 3: Hallucination type
0. Hallucinations not present.
1. Auditory hallucinations only.
2. Visual hallucinations present by patient's history or inferred by observation, with or without auditory hallucinations.
3. Tactile, olfactory, or gustatory hallucinations present with or without visual or auditory hallucinations.

Item 4: Delusions
0. Not present.
1. Delusion are systematized, i.e. well-organized and persistent.
2. Delusions are new and not part of a preexisting primary psychiatric disorder.
3. Delusions are not well circumscribed; are transient, poorly organized, and mostly in response to misperceived environmental cues; e.g. are paranoid and involve persons who are in reality caregivers, loved ones, hospital staff, etc.

Item 5: Psychomotor behavior
0. No significant retardation or agitation.
1. Mild restlessness, tremulousness, or anxiety evident by observation and a change from patient's usual behavior.
2. Moderate agitation with pacing, removing i.v.'s etc.
3. Severe agitation, needs to be restrained, may be combative; or has significant withdrawal from the environment, but not due to major depression or schizophrenic catatonia.

Item 6: Cognitive status during formal testing
0. No cognitive deficits, or deficits which can be alternatively explained by lack of education or prior mental retardation.

1. Very mild cognitive deficits which might be attributed to inattention due to acute pain, fatigue, depression, or anxiety associated with having a medical illness.
2. Cognitive deficit largely in one major area tested, e.g. memory, but otherwise intact.
3. Significant cognitive deficits which are diffuse, i.e. affecting many different areas tested; must include periods of disorientation to time or place at least once each 24-hr period; registration and/or recall are abnormal; concentration is reduced.
4. Severe cognitive deficits, including motor or verbal perseverations, confabulations, disorientation to person, remote and recent memory deficits, and inability to cooperate with formal mental status testing.

Item 7: Physical disorder
0. None present or active
1. Presence of any physical disorder which might affect mental state.
2. Specific drug, infection, metabolic, central nervous system lesion, or other medical problem which can be temporally implicated in causing the altered behavior or mental status.

Item 8: Sleep-wake cycle disturbance
0. Not present, awake and alert during the day, and sleeps without significant disruption at night.
1. Occasional drowsiness during day and mild sleep continuity disturbances at night; may have nightmares but can readily distinguish from reality.
2. Frequent napping and unable to sleep at night, constituting a significant disruption of or a reversal of the usual sleep-wake cycle.
3. Drowsiness prominent, difficulty staying alert during interview, loss of self-control over alertness and somnolence.
4. Drifts into stuporous or comatose periods.

Item 9: Lability of mood
0. Not present; mood stable.
1. Affect/mood somewhat altered and changes over the course of hours; patient states that mood changes are not under self-control.
2. Significant mood changes which are inappropriate to situation, including fear, anger, or tearfulness; rapid shifts of emotion, even over several minutes.
3. Severe disinhibition of emotions, including temper outbursts, uncontrolled inappropriate laughter, or crying.

Item 10: Variability of symptoms
0. Symptoms stable and mostly present during daytime.
2. Symptoms worsen at night.
4. Fluctuating intensity of symptoms, such that they wax and wane during a 24-hr period.

Chapter 6

Caregiver assessments

This is an ever expanding field with much current interest in the views and experiences of carers. Psychological distress is best measured using the General Health Questionnaire (GHQ; page 246) – the gold standard in terms of the rating of psychological distress. Lists of the number of problems exist, and other scales cover activity, imtimacy and hassles in more detail. The gold standard remains Gilleard's Problem Checklist and Strain Scale (page 234). Other inventories include the Screen for Caregiver Burden (SCB; page 238), the Caregiving Hassles Scale (page 240), the Revised Memory and Behavior Problems Checklist (page 244), the TRIMS Behavioral Problem Checklist (BPC; page 248) and the Geriatric Evaluation by Relative's Rating Instrument (GERRI; page 250). More detailed information, looking at the mechanisms of strain, is dealt with by the Marital Intimacy Scale (page 242) and the Ways of Coping Checklist (page 236). The Caregiver Activity Survey (CAS; page 245) measures time spent, while the Zung Self-Rating Depression Scale (page 252) and GHQ are included as they are commonly used assessments of psychological disturbance and depression in relatives.

Problem Checklist and Strain Scale

Reference   Gilleard CJ (1984) *Living with dementia: community care of the elderly mental infirm.* Beckenham: Croom Helm

Time taken 20 minutes (reviewer's estimate)
Rating by interviewer

Main indications

Problem Checklist: assessment of problems experienced by carers of patients with dementia. Strain Scale: assessment of strain.

Commentary

The Problem Checklist was derived from three main studies on day patients, largely in the Edinburgh region of Scotland (Gilleard and Watt, 1982). The 34-item Problem Checklist is rated on a three-point scale: not present, occasionally occurring and frequently/continually occurring, with those items rated as occasionally or frequently further rated as no problem, a small problem or a great problem. The Strain Scale is derived from Machin (1980) and contains 12 items.

Additional references

Gilleard CJ, Watt G (1982) The impact of psychogeriatric day care on the primary supporter of the elderly mentally infirm. In Taylor R, Gilmore A, eds. *Current trends in British gerontology.* Aldershot: Gower Publishing, 139–47.

Machin E (1980) A survey of the behaviour of the elderly and their supporters at home. Unpublished MSc thesis, University of Birmingham.

Address for correspondence

CJ Gilleard
Director of Psychology
Department of Psychology
Springfield Hospital
61 Glenburnie Road
Tooting
London SW17 7DJ
UK

Problem Checklist and Strain Scale

Problem Checklist

1. Unable to dress without help
2. Demands attention
3. Unable to get in and out of a chair without help
4. Uses bad language
5. Unable to get in and out of bed without help
6. Disrupts personal and social life
7. Unable to wash without help
8. Physically aggressive
9. Needs help at mealtimes
10. Vulgar habits (e.g. spitting, table manners)
11. Incontinent – soiling
12. Creates personality clashes
13. Forgets things that have happened
14. Temper outbursts
15. Falling
16. Rude to visitors
17. Unable to manage stairs
18. Not safe if outside the house alone
19. Cannot be left alone for even one hour
20. Wanders about the house at night
21. Careless about own appearance
22. Unable to walk outside house
23. Unable to hold a sensible conversation
24. Noisy, shouting
25. Incontinent – wetting
26. Shows no concern for personal hygiene
27. Unsteady on feet
28. Always asking questions
29. Unable to take part in family conversations
30. Unable to read newspapers, magazines, etc.
31. Sits around doing nothing
32. Shows no interest in news about friends and relatives
33. Unable to watch and follow television (or radio)
34. Unable to occupy himself/herself doing useful things

Strain Scale

Dangers
1. Do you fear accidents or dangers concerning the elderly person (e.g. fire, gas, falling over, etc.)?

Embarrassment
2. Do you ever feel embarrassed by the elderly person in any way?

Sleep
3. Is your sleep ever interrupted by the elderly person?

Coping
4. How often do you feel it is difficult to cope with the situation you are in and in particular with the elderly person?

Depression
5. Do you ever get depressed about the situation?

Worry
6. How much do you worry about the elderly person?

Household routine
7. Has your household routine been upset in caring for the elderly relative?

Frustration
8. Do you feel frustrated with your situation?

Enjoyment of role
9. Do you get any pleasure from caring for the elderly person?

Holidays
10. Do the problems of caring prevent you from getting away on holiday?

Finance
11. Has your standard of living been affected in any way due to the necessity of caring for your elderly relative?

Health
12. Would you say that your health had suffered from looking after your relative?

Attention
13. Do you find the demand for companionship and attention from the elderly person gets too much for you?

Scoring system:
Problem checklist:
0 = Not present
1 = Occasionally occurring
2 = Frequently/continually occurring

Strain scale:
5 = A great deal of the time
4 = Sometimes
3 = Never

Scoring for item 9 is reversed

Reproduced with permission of Dr Christopher J Gilleard.

Ways of Coping Checklist

Reference Vitaliano PP, Russo J, Carr JE, Maiuro RD, Becker J (1985) The Ways of Coping Checklist: revision and psychometric properties. *Multivariate Behavioral Research* 20: 3–26

Time taken 20 minutes (reviewer's estimate)
Rating by self-report

Main indications

To assess coping strategies in carers of patients with Alzheimer's disease.

Commentary

The authors identified the need for a short version of the original Ways of Coping Checklist (Folkman and Lazarus, 1980), and developed the revised version on three groups of subjects: medical students, psychiatric outpatients and spouses of patients with Alzheimer's disease. The 68 items were reduced to 41 items. Validity was assessed by comparison with the SCL-90 (Derogatis, 1977), the Beck Depression Inventory (BDI; page 6) and the Hamilton Depression Scale (page 4). Internal consistency, reliability, intercorrelations and comparisons of the factor structure of the original and revised scales showed that the revision was more reliable than the original scale.

Additional references

Derogatis LR (1977) *The SCL-90-R: administration, scoring and procedures manual I.* Baltimore, MD: Clinical Psychometric Research Unit, Johns Hopkins University.

Derogatis LR (1983) *The SCL-90-R: administration, scoring and procedures manual II.* Baltimore, MD: Clinical Psychometric Research Unit, Johns Hopkins University.

Folkman S, Lazarus RS (1980) An analysis of coping in a middle-aged community sample. *Journal of Health and Social Behavior* 21: 219–39.

Address for correspondence

PP Vitaliano
Department of Psychiatry and Behavioral Sciences
University of Washington
Washington, DC
USA

Ways of Coping Checklist

Revised scale		Original item source
Problem-focused		
1.	Bargained or compromised to get something positive from the situation.	P
2.	Concentrated on something good that could come out of the whole thing.	P
3.	Tried not to burn my bridges behind me, but left things open somewhat.	W
4.	Changed or grew as a person in a good way.	G
5.	Made a plan of action and followed it.	P
6.	Accepted the next best thing to what I wanted.	W
7.	Came out of the experience better than when I went in.	G
8.	Tried not to act too hastily or follow my own hunch.	W
9.	Changed something so things would turn out all right.	P
10.	Just took things one step at a time.	P
11.	I know what had to be done, so I doubled my efforts and tried harder to make things work.	P
12.	Came up with a couple of different solutions to the problem.	P
13.	Accepted my strong feelings, but didn't let them interfere with other things too much.	W
14.	Changed something about myself so I could deal with the situation better.	G
15.	Stood my ground and fought for what I wanted.	P
Seeks social support		
1.	Talked to someone to find out about the situation.	M
2.	Accepted sympathy and understanding from someone.	S
3.	Got professional help and did what they recommended.	M
4.	Talked to someone who could do something about the problem.	P
5.	Asked someone I respected for advice and followed it.	M
6.	Talked to someone about how I was feeling.	S
Blamed self		
1.	Blamed yourself.	B
2.	Criticized or lectured yourself.	B
3.	Realized you brought the problem on yourself.	B
Wishful thinking		
1.	Hoped a miracle would happen.	W
2.	Wished I was a stronger person – more optimistic and forceful.	W
3.	Wished that I could change what had happened.	W
4.	Wished I could change the way that I felt.	W
5.	Daydreamed or imagined a better time or place than the one I was in.	W
6.	Had fantasies or wishes about how things might turn out.	W
7.	Thought about fantastic or unreal things (like perfect revenge or finding a million dollars) that made me feel better.	M
8.	Wished the situation would go away or somehow be finished.	W
Avoidance		
1.	Went on as if nothing had happened.	Min
2.	Felt bad that I couldn't avoid the problem.	W
3.	Kept my feelings to myself.	W
4.	Slept more than usual.	M
5.	Got mad at the people or things that caused the problem.	M
6.	Tried to forget the whole thing.	Min
7.	Tried to make myself feel better by eating, drinking, smoking, taking medications.	M
8.	Avoided being with people in general.	M
9.	Kept others from knowing how bad things were.	W
10.	Refused to believe it had happened.	M

Abbreviations for scales are:

P, Problem-focused; W, Wishful thinking; G, Growth; M, Mixed; Min, Minimized; B, Blamed self; S, Seeks social support

From *Multivariate Behavioral Research* (pp. 11–13), by PP Vitaliano, J Russo, JE Carr, RD Maiuro, J Becker, 1985, New Jersey, USA: Lawrence Erlbaum Associates. Copyright 1985 by Lawrence Erlbaum Associates. Reprinted with permission.

Screen for Caregiver Burden (SCB)

Reference   Vitaliano PP, Russo J, Young HM, Becker J, Maiuro RD (1991) The Screen for Caregiver Burden. *Gerontologist* 31: 76–83

Time taken 20 minutes (reviewer's estimate)
Rating by interview

Main indications
The assessment of perceived burden of caring for a person with Alzheimer's disease.

Commentary
The Screen for Caregiver Burden (SCB) is a 25-item scale providing scores for objective and subjective burden. The former refers to the number of caregiver experiences occurring independently of their distress and the latter evaluates overall distress. Internal consistency of the two scales was above 0.85 and test/retest reliability between 0.64 and 0.70. Construct validity was examined with an explanatory model of distress previously described by the authors (Vitaliano et al, 1987). Convergent and divergent validity were examined in relation to measures taken of the patient's clinical condition and measures of anxiety and depression in the carers. The scale was also shown to be sensitive to changes over time, and correlate with changes in the same measures of the patient's functioning and ratings of the carer's mood.

Additional reference
Vitaliano PP, Maiuro RD, Bolton PA et al (1987) A psychoepidemiologic approach to the study of disaster. *Journal of Community Psychology* 15: 99–122.

Address for correspondence
PP Vitaliano
Department of Psychiatry and Behavioral Sciences
University of Washington
Washington, DC
USA

Screen for Caregiver Burden (SCB)

1. My spouse continues to drive when he/she shouldn't.
2. I have little control over my spouse's illness.
3. I have little control over my spouse's behavior.
4. My spouse is constantly asking the same questions over and over.
5. I have to do too many jobs/chores (feeding, shopping, paying bills) that my spouse used to perform.
6. I am upset that I cannot communicate with my spouse.
7. I am totally responsible for keeping our household in order.
8. My spouse doesn't cooperate with the rest of our family.
9. I have had to seek public assistance to pay for my spouse's medical bills.
10. Seeking public assistance in demeaning and degrading.
11. My spouse doesn't recognize me all the time.
12. My spouse has struck me on various occasions.
13. My spouse has gotten lost in the grocery store.
14. My spouse has been wetting the bed.
15. My spouse throws fits and has threatened me.
16. I have to constantly clean up after my spouse eats.
17. I have to cover up for my spouse's mistakes.
18. I am fearful when spouse gets angry.
19. It is exhausting having to groom and dress my spouse every day.
20. I try so hard to help my spouse but he/she is ungrateful.
21. It is frustrating trying to find things that my spouse hides.
22. I worry that my spouse will leave the house and get lost.
23. My spouse has assaulted others in addition to me.
24. I feel so alone — as if I have the world on my shoulders.
25. I am embarrassed to take my spouse out for fear that he/she will do something.

Burden Interview

Reference   Zarit SH, Reever KE, Bach-Peterson J (1980) Relatives of the impaired elderly: correlates of feeling of burden. *The Gerontologist* 20: 649–55

Time taken 25 minutes (reviewer's estimate)
Rating by self-report during an assessment interview

Main indications

Assessment of the feelings of burden of caregivers in caring for an older person with dementia.

Commentary

Twenty-nine patients with senile dementia and their caregivers were interviewed, and the Burden Interview was compared with measures of cognitive function (Khan Mental Status Questionnaire; Khan et al, 1960), a measure of mental state (Jacobs et al, 1977), a measure of the Memory and Problems Checklist and activities of daily living as assessed by scales described by Lawton (1971). The amount of burden assessed was found to be less when more visits were made by carers to the patient with dementia, and severity of behavioural problems was not associated with higher levels of burden. The paper was one of the earlier studies to underscore the importance of providing support to caregivers in the community care of older people with dementia.

Additional references

Jacobs JW, Bernhard JR, Delgado A et al (1977) Screening for organic mental syndromes in the medically ill. *Annals of Internal Medicine* 86: 40–6.

Khan RL, Goldfarb AI, Pollack J et al (1960) A brief objective measure for the determination of mental status of the aged. *American Journal of Psychiatry* 117: 326–8.

Lawton MP (1971) The functional assessment of elderly people. *Journal of the American Geriatrics Society* 19: 465–80.

Address for correspondence

Steve Zarit
Gerontology Center
College of Health and Human Development
Pennsylvania State University
105 Henderson Building South
University Park
PA 16802-6500
USA

Burden Interview

1. I feel resentful of other relatives who could but who do not do things for my spouse.
2. I feel that my spouse makes requests which I perceive to be over and above what s/he needs.
3. Because of my involvement with my spouse, I don't have enough time for myself.
4. I feel stressed between trying to give to my spouse as well as to other family responsibilities, job, etc.
5. I feel embarrassed over my spouse's behavior.
6. I feel guilty about my interactions with my spouse.
7. I feel that I don't do as much for my spouse as I could or should.
8. I feel angry about my interactions with my spouse.
9. I feel that in the past, I haven't done as much for my spouse as I could have or should have.
10. I feel nervous or depressed about my interactions with my spouse.
11. I feel that my spouse currently affects my relationships with other family members and friends in a negative way.
12. I feel resentful about my interactions with my spouse.
13. I am afraid of what the future holds for my spouse.
14. I feel pleased about my interactions with my spouse.
15. It's painful to watch my spouse age.
16. I feel useful in my interactions with my spouse.
17. I feel my spouse is dependent.
18. I feel strained in my interactions with my spouse.
19. I feel that my health has suffered because of my involvement with my spouse.
20. I feel that I am contributing to the well-being of my spouse.
21. I feel that the present situation with my spouse doesn't allow me as much privacy as I'd like.
22. I feel that my social life has suffered because of my involvement with my spouse.
23. I wish that my spouse and I had a better relationship.
24. I feel that my spouse doesn't appreciate what I do for him/her as much as I would like.
25. I feel uncomfortable when I have friends over.
26. I feel that my spouse tries to manipulate me.
27. I feel that my spouse seems to expect me to take care of him/her as if I were the only one s/her could depend on.
28. I feel that I don't have enough money to support my spouse in addition to the rest of our expenses.
29. I feel that I would like to be able to provide more money to support my spouse than I am able to now.

Caregiving Hassles Scale

Reference   Kinney JM, Stephens MAP (1989) Caregiving Hassles Scale: assessing the daily hassles of caring for a family member with dementia. *Gerontologist* 29: 328–32

Time taken 25 minutes (reviewer's estimate)

Rating by caregivers

Main indications

To examine the daily burden of caring for a patient with Alzheimer's disease.

Commentary

The Caregiving Hassles Scale was developed specifically to assess minor events of the day-to-day experience of caregiving rather than longer-term events or wider caregiver responsibilities. The development of the scale was based on the work of Lazarus and Folkman (1984), which regards stress as a measure of minor irritation of daily living. Sixty caregivers of patients with Alzheimer's disease were interviewed with measures of construct validity. Test/retest reliability and internal consistency were also measured. Originally, 110 items were considered (Kinney and Stephens, 1987). Statistically this was reduced to 42 items, and each was coded according to its relevance to a number of constructs: basic activities of daily living, instrumental activities of daily living, patient's cognitive status and behaviour and the caregiver's support network. Test/retest reliability was 0.83 and internal consistency 0.91. There were significant correlations with other measures of the impact of caregivers: the Caregiver's Impact Scale (Poulshock and Deimling, 1984), the SCL-90-R (an inventory to measure psychological distress: Derogatis, 1983) and the London Psychogeriatric Rating Scale.

Additional references

Derogatis LR (1983) *The SCL-90-R: administration, scoring and procedures manual II.* Baltimore, MD: Clinical Psychometric Research Unit, Johns Hopkins University.

Kinney JM, Stephens MAP (1987) *The Caregiving Hassles Scale: administration, reliability and validity.* Kent, OH: Psychology Department, The State University.

Lazarus RS, Folkman S (1984) *Stress, appraisal and coping.* New York: Springer.

Poulshock SW, Deimling GT (1984) Families caring for elders: issues in the measurement of burden. *Journal of Gerontology* 39: 230–9.

Caregiving Hassles Scale

1.	BEH	Care-recipient criticizing complaining.
2.	COG	Care-recipient declining mentally.
3.	BADL	Assisting care-recipient with walking.
4.	IADL	Extra expenses due to caregiving.
5.	SN	Friends not showing understanding about caregiving.
6.	BEH	Care-recipient losing things.
7.	COG	Undesirable changes in care-recipient's personality.
8.	BADL	Assisting with care-recipient's toileting.
9.	IADL	Transporting care-recipient to doctor/other places.
10.	BEH	Conflicts between care-recipient and family.
11.	COG	Care-recipient not showing interest in things.
12.	BADL	Bathing care-recipient.
13.	SN	Family not showing understanding about caregiving.
14.	BEH	Care-recipient yelling/swearing.
15.	BEH	Care-recipient's not cooperating.
16.	COG	Care-recipient's forgetfulness.
17.	BADL	Assisting care-recipient with exercise/therapy.
18.	IADL	Doing care-recipient's laundry.
19.	BEH	Care-recipient leaving tasks uncompleted.
20.	COG	Care-recipient being confused/not making sense.
21.	BADL	Lifting or transferring care-recipient.
22.	SN	Not receiving caregiving help from friends.
23.	BEH	Care-recipient frowning/scowling.
24.	COG	Care-recipient living in past.
25.	BADL	Helping care-recipient eat.
26.	IADL	Picking up after care-recipient.
27.	BEH	Care-recipient verbally inconsiderate; not respecting others' feelings.
28.	BEH	Being in care-recipient's presence.
29.	COG	Care-recipient talking about/seeing things that aren't real.
30.	BADL	Dressing care-recipient.
31.	SN	Not receiving caregiving help from family.
32.	BEH	Care-recipient asking repetitive questions.
33.	COG	Care-recipient not recognizing familiar people.
34.	BADL	Giving medications to care-recipient.
35.	IADL	Preparing meals for care-recipient.
36.	BEH	Care-recipient wandering off.
37.	COG	Care-recipient's agitation.
38.	BADL	Assisting care-recipient with health aids (e.g. dentures, braces)
39.	IADL	Care-recipient requiring day supervision.
40.	SN	Leaving care-recipient with others at home.
41.	BEH	Care-recipient hiding things.
42.	IADL	Care-recipient requiring night supervision.

BADL = Hassle assisting with basic ADL.
IADL = Hassle assisting with instrumental ADL.
COG = Hassle with care-recipient's cognitive status.
BEH = Hassle with care-recipient's behavior.
SN = Hassle with caregiver's support network.

Marital Intimacy Scale

Reference   Morris LW, Morris RG, Britton PG (1988) The relationship between martial intimacy, perceived strain and depression in spouse caregivers of dementia sufferers. *British Journal of Medical Psychology* 61: 231–6

Time taken 20 minutes (reviewer's estimate)
Rating essentially self-report but with guidance from interviewer

Main indications

This scale aims to assess the relationship between martial intimacy and that of strain and depression in spouse carers of individuals suffering from dementia.

Commentary

The Marital Intimacy Scale was adapted by Morris and his colleagues from the Waring Intimacy Questionnaire (Waring and Reddon, 1983; Waring and Patten, 1984). Nine areas were assessed: conflict resolution, affection, cohesion, sexuality, identity, compatibility, autonomy, expressiveness and desirability. Morris et al (1988) administered the 24-item questionnaire twice: once to obtain a measure of present intimacy with statements being rated as they applied at the time, and again to assess past intimacy where the caregivers were asked to rate the statements as they applied before the partner became ill. Essentially the questionnaire consists of a number of statements, with the person circling one of five choices: strongly agree, agree, undecided, disagree, strongly disagree. Twenty spouse caregivers were interviewed. A measure of subjective burden was assessed using a screen scale devised for the study: a seven-point bipolar rating scale anchored at each end by statements "I feel more strain because of the way my partner is nowadays" (1) to "I feel severe strain because of the way my partner is nowadays" (7). The Beck Depression Inventory (BDI; page 6) and the Problem Checklist and Strain Scale (page 234) were also administered to the carers. Higher levels of perceived strain and depression were found in carers who experienced lower levels of marital intimacy, the decline in intimacy being estimated from the difference between the levels of past and present intimacy.

The scale has been used in studies of dementia to assess the relationship between marital intimacy and behavioural problems in dementia (Fearon et al, 1998).

Additional references

Fearon M, Donaldson C, Burns A, Tarrier N (1998) Intimacy as a determinant of expressed emotion in carers of people with Alzheimer's disease. *Psychological Medicine* 28: 1085–90.

Waring E, Reddon J (1983) Waring Intimacy Questionnaire. *Journal of Clinical Psychology* 39: 53–7.

Waring E, Patton D (1984) Marital intimacy in depression. *British Journal of Psychiatry* 145: 641–4.

Marital Intimacy Scale

Introduction to rating of present intimacy

Please say whether you strongly agree, agree, are undecided, disagree or strongly disagree with each of the following statements as they apply to you AT PRESENT. It is best not to spend too long thinking about your answers. Please circle the letter that corresponds to your answer.

Introduction to rating of past intimacy

Please think back to the time before you suspected that your partner was ill. Please say whether you strongly agreed, agreed, have been undecided, disagreed or strongly disagreed with each of the following statements AT THAT TIME. Please try to remember as accurately as you can but it is best not to spend too long on each question. Circle the letter that corresponds to each answer.

		Strongly agree	Agree	Unde-cided	Disagree	Strongly disagree
1.	The feelings I have for my partner are warm and affectionate.	A	B	C	D	E
2.	My partner and I find it difficult to agree when making important decisions.	A	B	C	D	E
3.	I am very committed to my partner.	A	B	C	D	E
4.	My partner makes unreasonable demands on my spare time.	A	B	C	D	E
5.	All my partner's habits are good and desirable ones.	A	B	C	D	E
6.	I enjoy pleasant conversations with my partner.	A	B	C	D	E
7.	I wish my partner was more loving and affectionate to me.	A	B	C	D	E
8.	My partner has helped me to feel that I am a worthwhile person.	A	B	C	D	E
9.	I am unable to tell my partner in words that I love him/her.	A	B	C	D	E
10.	On occasion, I have told a small lie to my partner.	A	B	C	D	E
11.	My partner is liked and accepted by my relatives.	A	B	C	D	E
12.	I look outside my marriage for things that make life worthwhile and interesting.	A	B	C	D	E
13.	When I am unhappy about some aspect of our relationship I am able to tell my partner about it.	A	B	C	D	E
14.	My marriage has "smothered" my personality.	A	B	C	D	E
15.	I sometimes have thoughts and ideas I would not like to tell my partner.	A	B	C	D	E
16.	I am happy with the physical relationship in my marriage.	A	B	C	D	E
17.	My partner does not understand the way I feel.	A	B	C	D	E
18.	My relationship with my partner is the most important and meaningful relationship I have.	A	B	C	D	E
19.	I wish my partner worked harder to make our relationship more satisfying for us both.	A	B	C	D	E
20.	I have never had an argument with my partner.	A	B	C	D	E
21.	My partner confides his/her innermost thoughts and beliefs to me.	A	B	C	D	E
22.	I have become angry, upset or irritable because of things that occur in my marriage.	A	B	C	D	E
23.	My partner and I enjoy several mutually satisfying outside interests together.	A	B	C	D	E
24.	I am unable to say to my partner all that I would like.	A	B	C	D	E
25.	I sometimes boast in front of my partner.	A	B	C	D	E
26.	My partner and I share views on what is right and proper conduct.	A	B	C	D	E
27.	My partner is critical of decisions I make.	A	B	C	D	E
28.	My marriage helps me to achieve the goals I have set myself in life.	A	B	C	D	E
29.	My marriage suffers from disagreement concerning matters of leisure and recreation.	A	B	C	D	E
30.	Once in a while, I lose my temper and get angry with my partner.	A	B	C	D	E

Thank you for answering these questions.

Reproduced with kind permission from R Morris.

Revised Memory and Behavior Problems Checklist

Reference   Teri L, Truax P, Logsdon R, Uomoto J, Zarit S, Vitaliano PP (1992) Assessment of behavioral problems in dementia: the Revised Memory and Behavior Problems Checklist. *Psychology and Aging* 7: 622–31

Time taken 15–20 minutes (reviewer's estimate)
Rating from caregiver reports

Main indications

Assessment of behavioural problems in patients with dementia.

Commentary

The Revised Memory and Behavior Problems Checklist is a 24-item checklist which provides one total score and three subscores for the following problems: memory related, depression and disruptive behaviours. It assesses both the frequency of behaviours and caregiver reactions. Some 64 items were gathered from the original Memory and Problems Checklist (Zarit and Zarit, 1983) plus additional items. Validity was assessed by the Mini-Mental State Examination (MMSE; page 34), the Hamilton Depression Scale (page 4),

the Center for Epidemiological Studies – Depression Scale (CES-D; page 14) and the Caregiver Hassles Scale (page 240), and it was found to be good. Internal consistency was 0.75 for the frequency estimates and 0.87 for caregiver reactions. Some 201 subjects and their carers were examined.

Additional reference

Zarit SH, Zarit JM (1983) Cognitive impairment. In Lewinsohn PM, Teri L, eds. *Clinical geropsychology*. Elmsford, NY: Pergamon Press, 38–81.

Address for correspondence

Linda Teri
Department of Psychiatry and Behavioral Sciences
University of Washington Medical Center
RP-10 Seattle
WA 98195
USA

Revised Memory and Behavior Problems Checklist

1. Asking the same question over and over.
2. Trouble remembering recent events (e.g. items in the newspaper or on TV).
3. Trouble remembering significant past events.
4. Losing or misplacing things.
5. Foregetting what day it is.
6. Starting, but not finishing, things.
7. Difficulty concentrating on a task.
8. Destroying property.
9. Doing things that embarrass you.
10. Waking you or other family members up at night.
11. Talking loudly and rapidly.
12. Appears anxious or worried.
13. Engaging in behavior that is potentially dangerous to self or others.
14. Threats to hurt oneself.
15. Threats to hurt others.
16. Aggressive to others verbally.
17. Appears sad or depressed.
18. Expressing feelings of hopelessness or sadness about the future (e.g. "Nothing worthwhile ever happens," "I never do anything right").
19. Crying and tearfulness.
20. Commenting about death of self or others (e.g. "Life isn't worth living," "I'd be better off dead").
21. Talking about feeling lonely.
22. Comments about feeling worthless or being a burden to others.
23. Comments about feeling like a failure or about not having any worthwhile accomplishments in life.
24. Arguing, irritability, and/or complaining.

Rate both frequency and reaction as follows:

Frequency:
0 = Never occurred
1 = Not in past week
2 = 1–2 times in past week
3 = 3–6 times in past week
4 = Daily or more often
9 = Do not know/not applicable

Reaction:
0 = Not at all
1 = A Little
2 = Moderately
3 = Very much
4 = Extremely
9 = Do not know/not applicable

Reproduced with kind permission from Dr L Teri.

Caregiver Activity Survey (CAS)

Reference Davis KL, Marin DB, Kane R, Patrick D, Peskind ER, Raskind MA, Puder KL (1997) The Caregiver Activity Survey (CAS): development and validation of a new measure for caregivers of persons with Alzheimer's disease. *International Journal of Geriatric Psychiatry* 12: 978–88

Time taken 5 minutes
Rating by self-report

Main indications
A measure of time spent with the carer and caregiver burden.

Commentary
The Caregiver Activity Survey (CAS) was developed to assess the amount of time caregivers were spending looking after patients with Alzheimer's disease. Forty-two patients with Alzheimer's disease and their carers were studied with measures of test/retest reliability over a 3-week period and validity assessed by comparison with the Alzheimer's Disease Assessment Scale – Cognitive Section (ADAS-CoG; page 42) and the Mini-Mental State Examination (MMSE; page 34). The final version of the CAS consisted of six items. There was high test/retest reliability, intra-class correlation was 0.88 and conversion validity was high in comparison with the three scales. In the final scale, the inclusion of a dimension reflecting caregiver burden was not successful.

Address for correspondence
KL Davis
Department of Psychiatry
Mount Sinai School of Medicine
New York
NY 10029-6574
USA

Caregiver Activity Survey (CAS)

Areas assessed:

I	– Communication	III	– Dressing
II	– Using transportation	IV	– Eating
		V	– Looking after self-appearance
		VI	– Supervision necessary

Scoring is by the amount of time spent in the last 24 hours doing those activities assessed

Reproduced from Davis KL, Marin DB, Kane R, Patrick D, Peskind ER, Raskind MA, Puder KL (1997) The Caregiver Activity Survey (CAS): development and validation of a new measure for caregivers of persons with Alzheimer's disease. *International Journal of Geriatric Psychiatry* 12: 978–88. Copyright John Wiley & Sons Limited. Reproduced with permission.

Caregiver Activity Survey (CAS)

General Health Questionnaire (GHQ)

Reference Goldberg DP, Williams P (1988) *A User's Guide to the General Health Questionnaire.* Windsor: NFER-NELSON

Time taken depends on version (e.g. 5 minutes for 12-item GHQ)
Rating by self-rating

Main indications

A self-administered screening test in detecting psychiatric disorders in community settings and non-psychiatric clinical settings.

Commentary

The General Health Questionnaire (GHQ) is the most widely used self-rating instrument for the detection of psychiatric disorder and psychological morbidity. It is not used primarily in older people, but it is included here as it is used as a measure of psychological distress and psychiatric morbidity in carers of patients. For details, the rater is referred to the *User's Guide to the General Health Questionnaire*, and the 12-item questionnaire (GHQ-12), which is reproduced here. Essentially, four versions are available: 12-, 28-, 30- and 60-item questionnaires.

Where scaled subscores are required, the GHQ-28 should be used. For more intensive examination, with literate subjects with plenty of time the GHQ-60 is the best, but the GHQ-12 still does a good job with regard to sensitivity and specificity (e.g. GHQ-12, 89% sensitivity, 80% specificity; GHQ-28, 84% and 82% respectively; GHQ-30, 74% and 82% respectively; and GHQ-60, 78% and 87% respectively). These sensitivity and specificity measurements are in relation to the ability of the questionnaire to discriminate between cases and non-cases.

Address for correspondence

DP Goldberg
Director of Research and Development
Institute of Psychiatry
De Crespigny Park
Denmark Hill
London SE5 8AF
UK

General Health Questionnaire (GHQ-12)

Sample only

Please read this carefully:
We should like to know if you have had any medical complaints, and how your health has been in general, over the past few weeks. Please answer ALL the questions simply by underlining the answer which you think most nearly applies to you. Remember that we want to know about present and recent complaints, not those you had in the past. It is important that you try to answer ALL the questions.

Thank you very much for your co-operation.

HAVE YOU RECENTLY:

1	– been able to concentrate on whatever you're doing?	Better than usual	Same as usual	Less than usual	Much less than usual
2	– lost much sleep over worry?	Not at all	No more than usual	Rather more than usual	Much more than usual
3	– felt that you are playing a useful part in things?	More so than usual	Same as usual	Less useful than usual	Much less useful
4	– felt capable of making decisions about things?	More so than usual	Same as usual	Less so than usual	Much less capable
5	– felt constantly under strain?	Not at all	No more than usual	Rather more than usual	Much more than usual
6	– felt you couldn't overcome your difficulties?	Not at all	No more than usual	Rather more than usual	Much more than usual
7	– been able to enjoy your normal day-to-day activities?	More so than usual	Same as usual	Less so than usual	Much less than usual
8	– been able to face up to your problems?	More so than usual	Same as usual	Less able than usual	Much less able
9	– been feeling unhappy and depressed?	Not at all	No more than usual	Rather more than usual	Much more than usual
10	– been losing confidence in yourself?	Not at all	No more than usual	Rather more than usual	Much more than usual
11	– been thinking of yourself as a worthless person?	Not at all	No more than usual	Rather more than usual	Much more than usual
12	– been feeling reasonably happy, all things considered?	More so than usual	About same as usual	Less so than usual	Much less than usual

TRIMS Behavioral Problem Checklist (BPC)

Reference   Niederehe G (1988) TRIMS Behavioral Problem Checklist (BPC). *Psychopharmacology Bulletin* 24: 771–8

Time taken 25 minutes (reviewer's estimate)
Rating by carers

Main indications

The Texas Research Institute of Mental Science (TRIMS) Behavioral Problem Checklist (BPC) was developed for the assessment of the range of behavioural problems of patients with dementia and their effect on carers.

Commentary

Six subgroups were described as part of the BPC scale: cognitive symptoms, self-care deficits, instrumental activities of daily living deficits, dysphoric mood, acting-out behaviour and inactivity/withdrawal. The scales were all intercorrelated. Cronbach's alpha showed excellent internal consistency (0.93), and symptoms correlated with the measures of activities of daily living and AOLS.

Additional references

Zarit SH, Reever KE, Bach-Peterson J (1980) Relatives of the impaired elderly: correlates of feelings of burden. *Gerontologist* 20: 649–55.

Address for correspondence

George Niederehe
Mental Disorders of the Aging Research Branch
National Institute of Mental Health
Room 11C-03
5600 Fishers Lane
Rockville
MD 20857
USA

TRIMS Behavioral Problem Checklist (BPC)

Cognitive symptoms
Self-care deficits
Instrumental activities of daily living deficits

Dysphoric mood
Acting-out behaviour
Inactivity/withdrawal

Frequency: *How often does your relative show the problem?*
0 = Never happens (If behavior never happens, go on to next question)
1 = Has happened but not in the past week
2 = 1 to 2 times in past week
3 = 3 to 6 times in past week
4 = Happens daily or more often

Duration: *When did the problem begin?*
0 = Never happens
1 = Recently (1–6 months ago)
2 = Within the past year (7–12 months ago)
3 = Within the previous year (13–24 months ago)
4 = Over 2 years ago (2+ years ago)

Reaction: *How much does this problem bother or upset you?*
0 = Not at all
1 = A little
2 = A moderate amount
3 = Quite a lot
4 = Very much, extremely

Reproduced from Niederehe G (1988) TRIMS Behavioral Problem Checklist (BPC). *Psychopharmacology Bulletin* **24**: 771–8.

Geriatric Evaluation by Relative's Rating Instrument (GERRI)

Reference   Schwartz GE (1988) Geriatric Evaluation by Relative's Rating Instrument (GERRI).
Psychopharmacology Bulletin 24: 713–16

Time taken 20 minutes (reviewer's estimate)
Rating by carer

Main indications

Assessment of a number of behaviours in elderly people.

Commentary

The Geriatric Evaluation by Relative's Rating Instrument (GERRI) consists of 49 short phrases covering behavioural disturbances and problems with cognitive function, social functioning and mood. Ratings are on a five-point frequency scale from "almost all the time" to "almost never". The scale assesses behaviour over the last 2 weeks and can be repeated at this time interval. High inter-rater reliability and high internal consistency have been demonstrated (Schwartz, 1983), and it has been validated against the London Psychogeriatric Rating Scale, the Mini-Mental State Examination (MMSE; page 34) and an activities of daily living index (Sheikh et al, 1979).

Additional references

Schwartz GE (1983) Development and validation of the Geriatric Evaluation by Relative's Rating Instrument (GERRI). *Psychological Reports* 53: 479–88.

Sheikh K, Smith D, Meade T et al (1979) Repeatability and validity of a modified activities of daily living (ADL) index in studies of chronic disability. *Internal Rehabilitation Medicine* 1: 51–8.

.

Address for correspondence

Gerri E Schwartz
Janssen Research Foundation
40 Kingsbridge Road
Piscataway
NJ 08855-3998
USA

Geriatric Evaluation by Relative's Rating Instrument (GERRI)

1.	Remembers name of spouse/children living with him/her.	C
2.	Shaves or puts on makeup, combs hair without help.	S
3.	Prepares coffee, tea, or simple meals for self when necessary.	S
4.	Remembers where small items, such as keys, jewelry, or wallets are placed.	C
5.	Reports he/she feels sad.	M
6.	Appears restless and fidgety.	M
7.	Pays bills with checks.	S
8.	Remembers familiar phone numbers.	C
9.	Grasps point of newspaper articles, news broadcasts, etc.	C
10.	Reports feeling of hopelessness about the future.	M
11.	Forgets names of common objects.	C
12.	Handles incoming calls.	S
13.	Gets lost — leaves house and does not know where he/she lives.	C
14.	Remembers point in conversation after interruption.	C
15.	Handles money shopping for simple grocery items or newspaper or cigarettes.	S
16.	Reports feeling worthless.	M
17.	Continues to work on some favorite hobby.	S
18.	Does not recognize familiar people.	C
19.	Repeats same point in conversation over and over.	C
20.	Appears tearful.	M
21.	Leaves clothes soiled.	S
22.	Physically dirty or sloppy in appearance.	S
23.	Mood changes from day to day, happy one day, sad the other.	M
24.	Forgets the day of the week.	C
25.	Goes out inappropriately dressed.	S

26.	Embarrassing behavior.	S
27.	Forgets what he/she is looking for in the house.	C
28.	Forgets appointments.	C
29.	Remembers names of close friends.	C
30.	Acts childish.	S
31.	Continues to watch or "follow" favorite TV or radio program.	C
32.	When asked questions, seems quarrelsome and irritable.	M
33.	Does not pursue every day activities.	S
34.	Overquick or "jumpy" reaction to sudden noises or sights.	M
35.	Has difficulty concentrating or paying attention.	C
36.	Does not socialize with friends.	S
37.	Has fluctuations in memory — good one day, bad the next.	C
38.	Remembers where clothes are placed.	C
39.	Wants to have things his/her own way.	S
40.	Irregular eating habits, misses meals or eats meals consecutively.	S
41.	Remembers to lock door when leaving the house.	C
42.	Initiates phone contacts with friends.	S
43.	Appears to be easily annoyed or angered.	M
44.	Remembers to take medication.	C
45.	Reports feeling optimistic about future.	M
46.	Appears to be cheerful.	M
47.	Forgets to turn off stove.	C
48.	Appears friendly and positive in conversations with family members.	S
49.	Behaves stubbornly, such as refuses to take medication.	S

C = Cognitive functioning
S = Social functioning
M = Mood

Score:
1 = Almost all the time
2 = Most of the time
3 = Often
4 = Sometimes
5 = Almost never
6 = Does not apply

Reproduced with permission of author and publisher from: Schwartz, G.E. "Development and validation of the Geriatric Evaluation by Relatives Rating Instrument (GERRI)." *Psychological Reports*, 1983, **53**, 479–488. © Psychological Reports 1983.

Zung Self-Rating Depression Scale

Reference   Zung WWK (1965) A Self-Rating Depression Scale. *Archives of General Psychiatry* 12: 63–70

Time taken 3 minutes
Rating by self-rating

Main indications
Self-rating of depression.

Commentary
The 20-item Zung Self-Rating Depression Scale has been used extensively for the assessment of mood in older people, and has excellent reliability and interal consistency. It has been validated both as a screening instrument and as one sensitive to change (Zung, 1983). Like the Beck Depression Inventory (BDI; page 6), it has been used to assess depression in carers of patients with dementia. The scale was originally assessed on 56 patients, and validity was shown by its ability to discriminate between those with depressive disorders and those with other psychiatric conditions.

Additional reference
Zung W (1983) Self-rating scales for psychopathology. In Crook T, Ferris S, Bartus R, eds. *Assessment in geriatric psychopharmacology*. New Canaan: Mark Powley Associates.

Zung Self-Rating Depression Scale

1. I feel down-hearted and blue.*
2. Morning is when I feel the best.
3. I have crying spells or feel like it.*
4. I have trouble sleeping at night.*
5. I eat as much as I used to.
6. I still enjoy sex.
7. I notice that I am losing weight.*
8. I have trouble with constipation.*
9. My heart beats faster than usual.*
10. I get tired for no reason.*

11. My mind is as clear as it used to be.
12. I find it easy to do the things I used to.
13. I am restless and can't keep still.*
14. I feel hopeful about the future.
15. I am more irritable than usual.*
16. I find it easy to make decisions.
17. I feel that I am useful and needed.
18. My life is pretty full.
19. I feel that others would be better off if I were dead.*
20. I still enjoy the things I used to do.

Rating:
1=A little of the time
2=Some of the time
3=Good part of the time
4=Most of the time

Each is graded on a 4-point scale (1–4), there being 10 positive and 10 negative items, so that a global score out of a maximum of 80 gives a measure of the severity of depression. Converted to a percentage, >50% is suggested to indicate depression.

*rated 1–4
Others rated 4–1

Reproduced (with the permission of the American Medical Association) from Zung WWK (1965) A Self-Rating Depression Scale. *Archives of General Psychiatry* **12**: 63–70.

Behavioural and Mood Disturbance Scale (BMDS) and Relatives' Stress Scale (RSS)

Reference Greene JG, Smith R, Gardiner M, Timbury GC (1982) Measuring behavioural disturbance of elderly demented patients in the community and its effect on relatives: a factor analytic study. *Age and Ageing* **11**: 121–6

Time taken 15–20 minutes (BMDS); 5–10 minutes (RSS) (reviewer's estimate)
Rating by interview

Main indications

Assessment of behaviour and mood of a patient by a relative.

Commentary

The Behavioural and Mood Disturbance Scale (BMDS) aims to enable relatives to make a standard assessment of mood and behaviour disturbance shown by older people with dementia living at home. The scale grew out of existing literature such as the PAMIE Scale (page 180), the Stockton Geriatric Rating Scale (page 182), the Clifton Assessment Procedures for the Elderly (CAPE; page 48) and the Psychogeriatric Dependency Rating Scales

(PGDRS; page 174). Thirty-eight day patients with dementia and their carers were interviewed. The items (as below) were rated, with a 0–4 severity scale. Three factors were extracted: apathetic/withdrawn behaviour, active/disturbed behaviour, and mood disturbance. Validation was by means of factor analysis, and a test/retest study achieved satisfactory results.

The Relatives' Stress Scale (RSS) has 15 items validated on the same population. Personal distress, degree of life upset and negative feelings to the patient were the three factors identified.

Additional reference

Greene JG, Timbury GC (1979) A geriatric psychiatry day hospital service: a five-year review. *Age and Ageing* 8: 49–53.

Behavioural and Mood Disturbance Scale (BMDS)

Does he/she . . . .

*1.	Play or talk with the children?	21.	Ever seem lost in a world of his/her own?
*2.	Watch and follow television?	22.	Ever get lost in the house?
*3.	Read newspapers, magazines etc.?	23.	Ever fail to recognize familiar people?
*4.	Keep his/herself busy doing useful things?	24.	Ever get mixed up about the day, year, etc.?
*5.	Help out with domestic chores?	25.	Get mixed up about where he/she is?
6.	Sit around doing nothing?	26.	Ever moan and complain?
*7.	Take part in family conversations?	27.	Ever talk out loud to him/herself?
8.	Ever talk nonsense?	28.	Ever mutter to him or herself?
*9.	Understand what is said to him/he?	29.	Ever get up unusually early in the morning?
*10.	Ever start and maintain a sensible conversation?	30.	Ever go on and on about certain things?
*11.	Respond sensibly when spoken to?	31.	Wander outside the house at night?
12.	Ever wander off the subject?	32.	Wander outside the house and get lost?
*13.	Show an interest in news about friends and relatives?	33.	Have to be prevented from wandering outside the house?
14.	Ever cry for no obvious reason?	34.	Ever accuse people of things?
15.	Ever become angry and threatening?	35.	Ever hoard useless things?
16.	Ever appear unhappy and depressed?	36.	Ever endanger him/herself?
17.	Ever appear restless and agitated?	37.	Ever pace up and down wringing his or her hands?
18.	Ever look frightened and anxious?	38.	Talk all the time?
19.	Ever become irritable and easily upset?	39.	Ever shout at the children?
20.	Mood ever change for no apparent reason?	40.	Attempt to help with the housework but prove more of a hindrance than help?

Score: 0 = Never.
   1 = Rarely, now and again.
   2 = Sometimes, in between.
   3 = Frequently, most of the time, quite a bit.
   4 = Always, all the time.
   * = Scoring reversed.

Identifying Pleasant Activities for Alzheimer's Disease Patients: The Pleasant Events Schedule – AD

Reference   Teri L, Logsdon RG (1991) Identifying pleasant activities for Alzheimer's disease patients: The Pleasant Events Schedule – AD. *Gerontologist* 31: 124–27

Time taken less than 30 minutes
Rating by caregiver

Main indications

To help caregivers identify appropriate and pleasant activities for patients with Alzheimer's disease.

Commentary

The Pleasant Events Schedule – AD was developed from two earlier schedules: Lewinshon and Talkington (1979) and one modified for the elderly by Teri and Lewinshon (1982). The amendments consist of the deleting of items not relevant to patients with Alzheimer's disease. The 53 items are each rated three times: the number of times the event occurred in the last month is rated on a 3-point scale (not at all, a few times, and often); each item is rated according to the availability or opportunities the patient has had to engage in the activity on the same 3-point scale; and a 2-point scale rates enjoyability (now enjoys and enjoyed in the past). The psychometric properties of the previous scales are documented (Cronbach's alpha 0.98).

Logston and Teri (1977) describe a short 20-item version validated on 42 patients with Alzheimer's disease. Items are rated with regard to their frequency and availability during the last month on a 3-point scale [not at all, a few times (1–6 times) and often (7 or more times)]. The rating is also made as to whether the patient enjoys the activity now and whether the activity was enjoyed in the past. An overall summary score of frequency of enjoyable activities is a cross product of current enjoyment with frequency, and is calculated for each item. Each item there-

fore receives a score of 0 (either does not enjoy or has not done in the past month), 1 (enjoys and has done a few times) and 2 (enjoys and has done often). The sum of these items' scores represents the frequency of pleasant activities during the last month and is called the ENJOY. Internal consistency and split half reliability of the scales were excellent. The 20-item version was obtained by excluding 33 items – three were judged by the author to be difficult to rate, eight were enjoyed by fewer than 30% of the subjects and so eliminated, and items with item total correlations below 0.35 were also eliminated (22).

Address for correspondence

Linda Teri
University of Washington
Department of Psychiatry and Behavioural Science
1959 NE Pacific St
Seattle
WA 98195
USA

Additional references

Lewinshon PM, Talkington J (1979) Studies on the measurement of unpleasant events and relations with depression. *Applied Psychological Measurement* 3: 83–101.

Logston R, Teri L (1977) The Pleasant Event Schedule – AD. *Gerontologist* 37: 40–5.

Teri L, Lewinshon PM (1982) Modification of pleasant and unpleasant events schedules for use with the elderly. *Journal of Consulting and Clinical Psychology* 50: 444–5.

Identifying Pleasant Activities for Alzheimer's Disease Patients: The Pleasant Events Schedule – AD

	Frequency			Availability			Enjoyability	
	Not at all	A few times	Often	Not at all	A few times	Often	Now enjoys	Enjoyed in the past

*1.   Being outside (sitting outside, being in the country)
2.   Meeting someone new or making new friends
3.   Planning trips or vacations, looking at travel brochures, traveling
*4.   Shopping, buying things (for self or others)
5.   Being at the beach
*6.   Reading or listening to stories, novels, plays, or poems
*7.   Listening to music (radio, stereo)
*8.   Watching T.V.
9.   Camping
10.   Thinking about something good in the future
11.   Completing a difficult task
*12.   Laughing
13.   Doing jigsaw puzzles, crosswords, and word games
*14.   Having meals with friends or family (at home or out, special occasions)
15.   Taking a shower or bath
16.   Being with animals or pets
17.   Listening to nonmusic radio programs (talk shows)
*18.   Making or eating snacks
*19.   Helping others, helping around the house, dusting, cleaning, setting the table, cooking
20.   Combing or brushing my hair
21.   Taking a nap
*22.   Being with my family (children, grandchildren. siblings, others)
23.   Watching animals or birds (in a zoo or in the yard)
*24.   Wearing certain clothes (such as new, informal, formal, or favorite clothes)
*25.   Listening to the sounds of nature (birdsong, wind, surf)
26.   Having friends come to visit
*27.   Getting/sending letters, cards, notes
28.   Watching the clouds, sky, or a storm
*29.   Going on outings (to the park, a picnic, a barbeque, etc.)
30.   Reading, watching, or listening to the news
31.   Watching people
*32.   Having coffee, tea, a soda, etc. with friends
*33.   Being complimented or told I have done something well
34.   Being told I am loved
35.   Having family members or friends tell me something that makes me proud of them
36.   Seeing or speaking with old friends (in person or on the telephone)
37.   Looking at the stars or moon
38.   Playing cards or games
39.   Doing handwork (crocheting, woodworking, crafts, knitting, painting, drawing, ceramics, clay work, other)
*40.   Exercising (walking, aerobics, swimming, dancing, other)
41.   Indoor gardening or related activities (tending plants)
42.   Outdoor gardening or related activities (mowing lawn, raking leaves, watering plants, doing yard work)
43.   Going to museums, art exhibits, or related cultural activities
44.   Looking at photo albums and photos
45.   Stamp collecting, or other collections
46.   Sorting out drawers or closets
*47.   Going for a ride in the car
48.   Going to church, attending religious ceremonies
49.   Singing
*50.   Grooming self (wearing makeup, having hair done)
51.   Going to the movies
*52.   Recalling and discussing past events
53.   Participating or watching sports (golf, baseball, football, etc.)

Chapter 7

Memory functioning

The scales here are self-explanatory, and measure symptoms of memory loss in older people.

Cognitive Failures Questionnaire (CFQ)

Reference   Broadbent DE, Cooper PF, FitzGerald P, Parkes KR (1982) Cognitive Failures Questionnaire (CFQ) and its correlates. *British Journal of Clinical Psychology* 21: 1–16

Time taken 10 minutes
Rating self-rating

Main indications

A measure of self-reported failures in perception, memory and motor function.

Commentary

The Cognitive Failures Questionnaire (CFQ) is only weakly correlated with indices of social desirability set or of neuroticism, but is significantly correlated with ratings of the respondent by his or her spouse. The score has been found to be reasonably stable over long periods; however, it does correlate with the number of current psychiatric symptoms. Responses relate to the last six months. Validity was assessed by correlations with the Short Inventory of Memory Experiences (Herrmann and Neisser, 1978) and a number of neuropsychological tests. The use of the CFQ in memory clinics may highlight areas of concern for the clinician.

Additional reference

Herrmann D, Neisser U (1978) An inventory of everyday memory experiences. In Gruneberg MM, Morris PE, Sykes RN, eds. *Practical aspects of memory*. London: Academic Press.

Cognitive Failures Questionnaire (CFQ)

The following questions are about minor mistakes which everyone makes from time to time, but some of which happen more than others. We want to know how often these things have happened to you in the last six months. Please circle the appropriate number.

		Very often	Quite often	Occasionally	Very rarely	Never
1	Do you read something and find you haven't been thinking about it and must read it again?	4	3	2	1	0
2	Do you find you forget why you went from one part of the house to the other?	4	3	2	1	0
3	Do you fail to notice signposts on the road?	4	3	2	1	0
4	Do you find you confuse right and left when giving directions?	4	3	2	1	0
5	Do you bump into people?	4	3	2	1	0
6	Do you find you forget whether you've turned off a light or a fire or locked the door?	4	3	2	1	0
7	Do you fail to listen to people's names when you are meeting them?	4	3	2	1	0
8	Do you say something and realize afterwards that it might be taken as insulting?	4	3	2	1	0
9	Do you fail to hear people speaking to you when you are doing something else?	4	3	2	1	0
10	Do you lose your temper and regret it?	4	3	2	1	0
11	Do you leave important letters unanswered for days?	4	3	2	1	0
12	Do you find you forget which way to turn on a road you know well but rarely use?	4	3	2	1	0
13	Do you fail to see what you want in a supermarket (although it's there)?	4	3	2	1	0
14	Do you find yourself suddenly wondering whether you've used a word correctly?	4	3	2	1	0
15	Do you have trouble making up your mind?	4	3	2	1	0
16	Do you find you forget appointments?	4	3	2	1	0
17	Do you forget where you put something like a newspaper or a book?	4	3	2	1	0
18	Do you find you accidentally throw away the thing you want and keep what you meant to throw away – as in the example of throwing away the matchbox and putting the used match in your pocket?	4	3	2	1	0
19	Do you daydream when you ought to be listening to something?	4	3	2	1	0
20	Do you find you forget people's names?	4	3	2	1	0
21	Do you start doing one thing at home and get distracted into doing something else (unintentionally)?	4	3	2	1	0
22	Do you find you can't quite remember something although it's on the tip of your tongue?	4	3	2	1	0
23	Do you find you forget what you came to the shops to buy?	4	3	2	1	0
24	Do you drop things?	4	3	2	1	0
25	Do you find you can't think of anything to say?	4	3	2	1	0

Reprinted with kind permission of the British Journal of Clinical Psychology.

Informant Questionnaire on Cognitive Decline in the Elderly (IQCODE)

References Jorm AF, Jacomb PA (1989) An Informant Questionnaire on Cognitive Decline in the Elderly (IQCODE): socio-demographic correlates, reliability, validity and some norms. *Psychological Medicine* 19: 1015–22.

Jorm AF, Scott R, Jacomb PA (1989) Assessment of cognitive decline in dementia by informant questionnaire. *International Journal of Geriatric Psychiatry* 4: 35–9

Time taken 10–15 minutes (reviewer's estimate)
Rating by interviewer

Main indications

The Informant Questionnaire on Cognitive Decline in the Elderly (IQCODE) is a questionnaire administered to an informant about changes in the everyday cognitive function of an elderly person and aims to assess cognitive decline independent of premorbid ability.

Commentary

These two companion papers outline the rationale behind the development of the IQCODE, emphasizing the three methods of assessing cognitive decline: comparison with estimated premorbid ability, self-reported questionnaires and a third informant's report (*n* = 362). Jorm analysed returns from a postal questionnaire, as well as a smaller and more direct validity exercise, on 31 volunteers from hostels and nursing homes in Canberra.

The internal consistency of the IQCODE was 0.93 and the validity measured against the Mini-Mental State Examination (MMSE; page 34) showed a correlation of 0.78.

Jorm and Jacomb (1989) provided some additional data showing test/retest reliability and a correlation of 0.75; patients with worse scores did move into institutional care at follow-up.

Further studies have shown that the IQCODE is as good as the MMSE in the diagnosis of dementia (Jorm et al, 1991, 1996). A 16-item version has been described and found to perform as well as the long version (Jorm, 1994). Validity has been affirmed by showing that ratings of moderate or severe decline have greater changes than quantitative tests over time (Jorm et al, 1996). The scale has also been successfully translated into French (Mulligan et al, 1996). A retrospective version is available (26 items) for analysis after a patient has died.

Additional references

Jorm AF, Scott R, Cullen JS, Mackinnon AJ (1991) Performance of the Informant Questionnaire on Cognitive Decline in the Elderly (IQCODE) as a screening test for dementia. *Psychological Medicine* 21: 785–90.

Jorm AF (1994) A short form of the Informal Questionnaire on Cognitive Decline in the Elderly (IQCODE): development and cross-validation. *Psychological Medicine* 24: 145–53.

Jorm AF, Broe GA, Creasey H et al (1996) Further data on the validity of the Informant Questionnaire on Cognitive Decline in the Elderly (IQCODE). *International Journal of Geriatric Psychiatry* 11: 131–9.

Mulligan R, Mackinnon A, Jorm AF (1996) A comparison of alternative methods of screening for dementia in clinical settings. *Archives of Neurology* 53: 532–6.

Address for correspondence

AF Jorm
NH & MRC Social Psychiatry Research Unit
The Australian National University
Canberra 0200
Australia

Informant Questionnaire on Cognitive Decline in the Elderly (IQCODE) (short form)

Now we want you to remember what your friend or relative was like 10 years ago and to compare it with what he/she is like now. 10 years ago was in 19__. Below are situations where this person has to use his/her memory or intelligence and we want you to indicate whether this has improved, stayed the same or got worse in that situation over the past 10 years. Note the importance of comparing his/her present performance with 10 years ago. So if 10 years ago this person always forgot where he/she had left things, and he/she still does, then this would be considered "Hasn't changed much". Please indicate the changes you have observed by circling the appropriate answer.

Compared with 10 years ago how is the person at:

	1	2	3	4	5
1. Remembering things about family and friends e.g. occupations, birthdays, addresses	Much improved	A bit improved	Not much change	A bit worse	Much worse
2. Remembering things that have happened recently	Much improved	A bit improved	Not much change	A bit worse	Much worse
3. Recalling conversations a few days later	Much improved	A bit improved	Not much change	A bit worse	Much worse
4. Remembering his/her address and telephone number	Much improved	A bit improved	Not much change	A bit worse	Much worse
5. Remembering what day and month it is	Much improved	A bit improved	Not much change	A bit worse	Much worse
6. Remembering where things are usually kept	Much improved	A bit improved	Not much change	A bit worse	Much worse
7. Remembering where to find things which have been put in a different place from usual	Much improved	A bit improved	Not much change	A bit worse	Much worse
8. Knowing how to work familiar machines around the house	Much improved	A bit improved	Not much change	A bit worse	Much worse
9. Learning to use a new gadget or machine around the house	Much improved	A bit improved	Not much change	A bit worse	Much worse
10. Learning new things in general	Much improved	A bit improved	Not much change	A bit worse	Much worse
11. Following a story in a book or on TV	Much improved	A bit improved	Not much change	A bit worse	Much worse
12. Making decisions on everyday matters	Much improved	A bit improved	Not much change	A bit worse	Much worse
13. Handling money for shopping	Much improved	A bit improved	Not much change	A bit worse	Much worse
14. Handling financial matters e.g. the pension, dealing with the bank	Much improved	A bit improved	Not much change	A bit worse	Much worse
15. Handling other every day arithmetic problems e.g. knowing how much food to buy, knowing how long between visits from family or friends	Much improved	A bit improved	Not much change	A bit worse	Much worse
16. Using his/intelligence to understand what's going on and to reason things through	Much improved	A bit improved	Not much change	A bit worse	Much worse

Sources: Jorm AF, Jacomb PA (1989) An Informant Questionnaire on Cognitive Decline in the Elderly (IQCODE): socio-demographic correlates, reliability, validity and some norms. *Psychological Medicine* **19**: 1015–22. Reproduced with kind permission from Cambridge University Press. Also Jorm AF, Scott R, Jacomb PA (1989) Assessment of cognitive decline in dementia by informant questionnaire. *International Journal of Geriatric Psychiatry* **4**: 35–9. Copyright John Wiley & Sons Limited. Reproduced with permission.

Metamemory in Adulthood (MIA) Questionnaire

Reference   Dixon RA, Hultsch DF, Hertzog C (1988) The Metamemory in Adulthood (MIA) Questionnaire. *Psychopharmacology Bulletin* 24: 671–88

Time taken 30 minutes (reviewer's estimate)
Rating self-rating

Main indications
Self-rating of memory function.

Commentary
The Metamemory in Adulthood (MIA) Questionnaire consists of 108 items divided into seven scales: strategy (knowledge and reported use of memory strategies), task (knowledge of basic memory process), capacity (beliefs regarding one's own memory), change (change in the ability to remember), anxiety (perceptions of the relationship between anxiety and memory performance), achievement (perception of one's own motivation to perform well in memory tasks) and locus (sense of control over memory skills). An eighth scale, activity (regularity of activities supportive of memory), has also been described, adding 12 items. A number of samples have been described in ages ranging from 18 to 84, and validation against personality, depression and other scales has been carried out (Hultsch et al, 1988). Internal consistency as assessed by Cronbach's alpha is high, and discriminant validity demonstrates that MIA constructs are not easily accounted for by other psychological indices such as depression or anxiety. While not meant as a device for measuring actual memory problems, it can measure knowledge, beliefs and affect about memory.

Additional reference
Hultsch DF, Hertzog C, Dixon RA et al (1988) Memory, self-knowledge and self-efficacy in the aged. In Howe ML, Brainerd CJ, eds. *Cognitive development in adulthood: progress in cognitive developmental research.* New York: Springer-Verlag, 65–92

Address for correspondence
Roger A Dixon
Department of Psychology
University of Victoria
Victoria BC
V8W 2Y2
Canada

Metamemory in Adulthood (MIA) Questionnaire

Main items:

Strategy	Anxiety
Task	Achievement
Capacity	Locus
Change	Activity

Reproduced from Dixon RA, Hultsch DF, Hertzog C (1988) The Metamemory in Adulthood (MIA) Questionnaire. *Psychopharmacology Bulletin* **24**: 671–88.

Memory Functioning Questionnaire (MFQ)

Reference Gilewski MJ, Zelinski EM (1988) Memory Functioning Questionnaire (MFQ). *Psychopharmacology Bulletin* 24: 665–70

Time taken 25 minutes (reviewer's estimate)
Rating self-rating

Main indications
Detection of memory complaints in elderly people.

Commentary
The Memory Functioning Questionnaire (MFQ) is a 64-item instrument with seven scales: general rating of memory, retrospective functioning, frequency of forgetting, frequency of forgetting when reading, remembering past events, seriousness of forgetting, and mnemonics usage. It is a revision of an earlier scale which had an additional 28 questions in nine scales (Zelinski et al, 1980). A principal components analysis of a larger scale in a population of some 800 adults revealed three factors: general frequency of forgetting, seriousness, and retrospective functioning/mnemonics. The parent question-naire has been shown to correlate significantly with formal tests of cognitive function (Zelinski et al, 1980).

Additional references
Zelinski EM, Gilewski MJ, Thompson LW (1980) Do laboratory tests relate to self-assessment of memory ability in the young and old? In Poon LW, Fozard JL, Cermak LS et al, eds. *New directions in memory and ageing: proceedings of the George A Talland Memorial Conference.* Hillsdaee, NJ: Erlbaum, 519–44.

Address for correspondence
Elizabeth M Zelinski
Leonard Davis School of Gerontology
University of Southern California
Los Angeles
CA 90089-0191
USA

Memory Functioning Questionnaire (MFQ)

Main items:
Memory rating
Retrospective functioning
Frequency of forgetting

Frequency of forgetting when reading
Remembering past events
Seriousness of forgetting
Mnemonics usage

Reproduced from Gilewski MJ, Zelinski EM (1988) Memory Functioning Questionnaire (MFQ). *Psychopharmacology Bulletin* **24**: 665–70.

Chapter 8

Other scales

These form a heterogeneous group of scales which do not easily fit elsewhere in the book. They comprise measures of the environment, assessments of quality of life and morale in older people, and an observational scale.

Multiphasic Environmental Assessment Procedure (MEAP)

Reference Moos RH, Lemke S (1992) *Multiphasic Environmental Assessment Procedure user's guide.* Palo Alto, CA: Center for Health Care Evaluation, Department of Veterans Affairs and Stanford University Medical Centers.

Time taken variable
Rating various

Main indications

The Multiphasic Environmental Assessment Procedure (MEAP) is a five-part procedure for making a comprehensive evaluation of the physical and social environments in group residential facilities for older people.

Commentary

The MEAP comprises five separate instruments corresponding to four conceptual domains as summarized below. A detailed analysis is beyond the scope of this book beyond the rater is referred to the User's Guide and appropriate references.

Overview of the Multiphasic Environmental Assessment Procedure (MEAP) instruments

Instrument	Aspect of environment assessed	Source
Resident and Staff Information Form (RESIF)	Suprapersonal factors, such as the average background and personal characteristics of people living or working the facility (6 subscales)	Records, interviews, and staff reports
Physical and Architectural Features Checklist (PAF)	Physical features, covering location, features inside and outside the facility, and space allowances (8 subscales)	Direct observation
Policy and Program Information Form (POLIF)	Facility policies, including types of rooms available, how the facility is organized, and what services are provided (9 subscales)	Facility administrator and staff reports
Sheltered Care Environment Scale (SCES)	Social milieu, including relationships, personal growth and system maintenance and change (7 subscales)	Resident and staff reports
Rating Scale	Physical environment and resident and staff functioning (4 subscales)	Direct observation

Moos RH, Lemke S, Multiphasic Environmental Assessment Procedure user's guide. Reprinted by permission of Sage Publications.

Philadelphia Geriatric Center Morale Scale

Reference Lawton MP (1975) Philadelphia Geriatric Center Morale Scale: a revision. *Journal of Gerontology* 30: 85–9

Time taken rating as one part of a 60-minute interview
Rating by interview

Main indications
Assessment of morale in elderly people.

Commentary
The original paper describes a principal components analysis of the scale on over 1000 elderly people. The work builds on the original description scale (Lawton, 1972) and a companion paper (Morris and Sherwood, 1975). Three consistently reproducible factors emerged: agitation, attitude towards own ageing and lonely dissatisfaction. Using 17 of the original items, internal consistency as determined by Cronbach's alpha statistics was 0.85, 0.81 and 0.85 respectively. The 17 items were designated as the revised Philadelphia Geriatric Center Morale Scale.

Additional references
Lawton MP (1972) The dimensions of morale. In Kent D, Kastenbaum R, Sherwood S, eds. *Research, planning and action for the elderly*. New York: Behavioral Publications.

Morris JN, Sherwood S (1975) A retesting and modification of the Philadelphia Geriatric Centre Morale Scale. *Journal of Gerontology* 15: 77–84.

Address for correspondence
M Powell Lawton
Philadelphia Geriatric Center
5301 Old York Road
Philadelphia
PA 19141
USA

Philadelphia Geriatric Center Morale Scale

	YES	NO
Agitation		
* Little things bother me more this year (no)	—	—
* I sometimes worry so much that I can't sleep (no)	—	—
I have a lot to be sad about (no)	—	—
* I am afraid of a lot of things (no)	—	—
* I get mad more than I used to (no)	—	—
Life is hard for me most of the time (no)	—	—
* I take things hard (no)	—	—
* I get upset easily (no)	—	—
Attitude toward own aging		
* Things keep getting worse as I get older (no)	—	—
* I have as much pep as I had last year (yes)	—	—
Little things bother me more this year (no)	—	—
* As you get older you are less useful (no)	—	—
* As I get older, things are better/worse than I thought they would be (better)	—	—
I sometimes feel that life isn't worth living (no)	—	—
* I am as happy now as when I was younger (yes)	—	—
Lonely dissatisfaction		
* How much do you feel lonely? (not much)	—	—
* I see enough of my friends and relatives (yes)	—	—
* I sometimes feel that life isn't worth living (no)	—	—
* Life is hard for much of the time (no)	—	—
* How satisfied are you with your life today? (satisfied)	—	—
* I Have a lot to be sad about (no)	—	—
People had it better in the old days (no)	—	—
A person has to live for today and not about tomorrow (yes)	—	—

High morale responses are indicated in parenthesis
(*) Items selected as best representative of the factor

Health of the Nation Outcome Scales for Older People (HoNOS 65+)

Reference   **Burns et al (in preparation)**

Time taken 5–10 minutes (by a professional who knows the patient and once all the information is collected); 30 minutes in semi-structured interview
Rating by trained interviewer

Main indications

Global rating of mental and physical functioning and social circumstances of older people.

Commentary

The UK government's directive on health, enshrined in the Health of the Nation document, was a stimulus to the development of simple scales to measure mental health outcomes. A Health of the Nation Outcome scale for younger people with mental health problems (Wing et al, 1998) was developed, and there was clearly a need to adapt it for use in older adults. The work was co-ordinated by the Royal College of Psychiatrists Research Unit, and a series of multiprofessional focus groups was held to adapt the scale. Inter-rate reliability studies gave satisfactory levels of cocordance in keeping with the general adult scale, and validity was assessed against the Mini-Mental State Examination (MMSE; page 34). The main amendments to the scale include specific ratings for agitation, restlessness and sleep disturbance, passive aspects of suicide ideation in the elderly, level of consciousness, and a clear steer as to where incontinence should be scored. Ratings of sensory deficits were also included. It is impor-tant to note that the HoNOS 65+ is not a rating of the aetiology of problems, merely a description of their presence. HoNOS 65+ was able to distinguish between patients with organic functional illness in all the items except physical disability, hallucinations, living condition and relationships. The HoNOS 65+ is still subject to further field trials and amendments.

Additional references

Burns et al (in preparation).

Curtis R, Beevor A (1995) Health of the Nation Outcome Scales. In Wing JK, ed. *Measurement of mental health: contributions from the College Research Unit. College Research Unit Publication No. 2.* London: Royal College of Psychiatrists Research Unit, 33–46.

Wing JK, Beevor AS, Curtis RH et al (1998) Health of the Nation Outcome Scales (HoNOS): research and development. *British Journal of Psychiatry* 172: 11–18.

Address for correspondence

Alistair Burns
Department of Psychiatry
Withington Hospital
West Didsbury
Manchester M20 8LR
UK

Health of the Nation Outcome Scales for Older People (HoNOS 65+)

1. Aggression	7. Depression
2. Self-harm	8. Other symptoms
3. Drug and alcohol use	9. Relationships
4. Cognitive problems	10. Activities of daily living
5. Physical illness and disability	11. Residential environment
6. Hallucinations and delusions	12. Day-time activities

Rating:

Each item rated on a 5-point individualized rating from 0 (no problem) – 4 (serious problem).

1–3	= Behaviour
4–5	= Impairment
6–8	= Symptoms
9–12	= Social

Cumulative Illness Rating Scale (CIRS)

Reference Conwell Y, Forbes NT, Cox C, Caine ED (1993) Validation of a measure of physical illness burden at autopsy: the Cumulative Illness Rating Scale. *Journal of the American Geriatrics Society* 41: 38–41

Time taken 20 minutes (reviewer's estimate)
Rating by trained examiners to complete medical examination and health history

Main indications

An objective measure of physical illness burden.

Commentary

The Cumulative Illness Rating Scale (CIRS) is useful in several scenarios – for example in predicting outcome in longitudinal studies of late-life affective illness, and as an outcome variable in studies of social factors or health behaviour on overall physical wellbeing. The CIRS is a measure of physical illness in which a cumulative score is derived from ratings of severity of impairment in each of 13 organ systems. Using information from physicians, interview and review of medical records, the CIRS was correlated with post-mortem ratings made independently at tissue autopsy on victims of suicide. Inter-rater reliability is about 0.83. CIRS ratings made by examination of tissue at autopsy were highly predictive of analogous ratings based on historical data, accounting for 75% of the variance in CIRS scores.

Additional reference

Linn MW, Linn BS, Gurel L (1967) Physical resistance in the aged. *Geriatrics* 22: 134–8.

Address for correspondence

Yeates Conwell
University of Rochester
300 Crittenden Blvd
Rochester
NY 14642
USA

Cumulative Illness Rating Scale (CIRS)

		Rating			
	Cardiovascular–Respiratory System		8.	Renal (kidneys only)	___
1.	Cardiac (heart only)	___	9.	Other GU (ureters, bladder, urethra, prostate, genitals)	___
2.	Vascular (blood, blood vessels and cells, marrow, spleen, lymphatics)	___		*Musculo-Skeletal-Integumentary System*	
3.	Respiratory (lungs, bronchi, trachea below larynx)	___	10.	MSI (muscles, bone, skin)	___
4.	EENT (eye, ear, nose, throat, larynx)	___		*Neuropsychiatric System*	
	Gastrointestinal System		11.	Neurologic (brain, spinal cord, nerves)	___
5.	Upper GI (esophagus, stomach, duodenum, biliary and pancreatic trees)	___	12.	Psychiatric (mental)	___
6.	Lower GI (intestines, hernias)	___		*General System*	
7.	Hepatic (liver only)	___	13.	Endocrine-Metabolic (includes diffuse infections, poisonings)	___
	Genitourinary System			Total	___

Rate as follows for each system:
0 = No impairment to organ/system
1 = Mild impairment
   No interference normal activity
   Treatment required
   Prognosis excellent
2 = Moderate impairment
   Interference with normal activity
   Treatment required
   Prognosis is good
3 = Severe impairment
   Disability
   Urgent treatment required
   Prognosis guarded
4 = Extrememly severe impairment
   Life threatening
   Treatment is emergent or of no avail
   Grave prognosis

Personality Inventory

Reference   Brooks DN, McKinlay W (1983) Personality and behavioural change after severe blunt head injury – a relative's view. *Journal of Neurology, Neurosurgery, and Psychiatry* 46: 336–44

Time taken 20 minutes (reviewer's estimate)

Rating on a visual analogue scale by relatives

Main indications

Assessment of personality changes after severe head injury; also used to assess personality in dementia.

Commentary

The original study using the Personality Inventory describes the scale ratings on 55 severely head-injured adults at 3, 6 and 12 months post-injury. No reliability or validity data were presented. Petry et al (1988) describe 30 control subjects pre- and post-retirement together with patients suffering from dementia of the Alzheimer type, and examined their changing score after the onset of dementia. No significant changes were found in the control group, but there were highly significant changes on 12 of the 18 items – patients became more passive, more coarse and less spontaneous. In this study, ratings were made on a –2 to +2, five-point rating scale with 0 indicating no change. Petry et al (1989) carried out a follow-up of the 30 original patients, describing four response pattern: change at onset with little subsequent change, ongoing change, no change and regression of previously disturbed behaviour. Cummings et al (1990) described personality changes in patients with dementia of the Alzheimer type and multi-infarct dementia, and found that while personality alterations were universal, patients with Alzheimer's disease had greater alterations in maturity and had less personal control compared with patients with vascular dementia, who had more apathy and remained more affectionate and easy-going. A few correlations were found between the severity of dementia and the magnitude of behavioural change.

Additional references

Cummings JL, Petry S, Dian L et al (1990) Organic personality disorder in dementia syndromes: an inventory approach. *Journal of Neuropsychiatry* 2: 261–7.

Petry S, Cummings JL, Hill MA et al (1988) Personality alterations in dementia of Alzheimer type. *Archives of Neurology* 45: 1187–90.

Petry S, Cummings JL, Hill MA et al (1989) Personality alterations in dementia of Alzheimer type: a three-year follow-up study. *Journal of Geriatric Psychiatry and Neurology* 2: 184–8.

Personality Inventory

	+2	+1	0	−1	−2	
Talkative	——	——	——	——	——	Quiet
Even-tempered	——	——	——	——	——	Quick-tempered
Relies on others	——	——	——	——	——	Does things himself
Affectionate	——	——	——	——	——	Cold
Fond of company	——	——	——	——	——	Dislikes company
Irritable	——	——	——	——	——	Easy-going
Unhappy	——	——	——	——	——	Happy
Excitable	——	——	——	——	——	Calm
Energetic	——	——	——	——	——	Lifeless
Down to earth	——	——	——	——	——	Out of touch
Rash	——	——	——	——	——	Cautious
Listless	——	——	——	——	——	Enthusiastic
Mature	——	——	——	——	——	Childish
Sensitive	——	——	——	——	——	Insensitive
Cruel	——	——	——	——	——	Kind
Generous	——	——	——	——	——	Mean
Unreasonable	——	——	——	——	——	Reasonable
Stable	——	——	——	——	——	Changeable

Journal of Neurology, Neurosurgery, and Psychiatry, 1983, **46**: 336–344, with permission from the BMJ Publishing Group.

Measurement of Morale in the Elderly

Reference   Pierce RC, Clarke MM (1973) Measurement of morale in the elderly. *International Journal of Aging and Human Development* 4: 83–101

Time taken 2–4 hours

Rating by clinical interviewer

Main indications

Designed to assess level of morale amongst older people with mental health problems.

Commentary

The Measurement of Morale in the Elderly scale was developed using original items and ones taken from previous studies (Thompson et al, 1960; Srole et al, 1962). There were eight identifiable factors for factor analysis: depression/satisfaction, will to live, equanimity (all referring to morale), positive or negative attitudes to ageing, social alienation (representing attitudes to ageing), physical health and sociability. The study was able to discriminate between two groups of ageing subjects; those with possible mental health problems and normal controls. A 1978 research version is also available, which has 35 items rated on a 4/5 point scale (agree strongly/never – disagree strongly/often).

Additional references

Srole L, Langner TS, Michael ST et al (1962) *Mental health in the metropolis: the midtown Manhattan study.* Vol. 1. New York: McGraw-Hill.

Thompson WE, Streib GF, Kosa J (1960) The effect of retirement on personal adjustment: a panel analysis. *Journal of Gerontology* 15: 165–9.

Address for correspondence

Robert C Pierce
99 Golden Hind Blvd
San Rafael
CA 94903
USA

1. How is your appetite? (Poor.)
2. How has you general health been this past year? (Extremely poor.)
3. Do you find you are less interested lately in things like your personal appearance and table manners and things like that? (No.)
4. Do you have as much energy as you did a year ago? (Less.)
5. Interviewer's rating of the subject's reaction to interview. (Any "abnormal" reaction.)
6. Interviewer's rating of the subject's affectivity. (Any "Abnormal" rating; e.g., tense, irritable, overly cheerful, tearful, etc.)
7. Interviewer's rating of the subject's cooperativeness. (Uncooperative.)
8. Do you often feel irritable and impatient? (No.)
9. Have you been worried during the past year for no reason? (No.)
10. Do you often feel moody and blue? (No.)
11. Have you felt lately that life is not worth living? (No.)
12. All in all, how much happiness would you say you find in life today? (Almost none.)
13. In general, how would you say you feel most of the time, in good spirits or in low spirits? (Usually low.)
14. On the whole, how satisfied would you say you are with your life today? (Not very satisfied.)
15. How often do you get the feeling that your life today is not very useful? (Hardly ever.)
16. How often do you find yourself feeling blue? (Hardly ever.)
17. How often do you get upset by the things that happen in your day-to-day life? (Hardly ever.)
18. These days I find myself giving up hope of trying to improve myself. (Disagree.)
19. Almost eveything these days is a racket. (Disagree.)
20. How much do you plan ahead the things that you will be doing the next week or week after? (Almost no plans.)
21. There's little use in writing to public officials because often they aren't interested in the problems of the average man. (Disagree.)
22. Nowadays a person has to live pretty much for today and let tomorow take care of itself. (Disagree.)
23. In spite of what some people say, the lot of the average man is getting worse, not better. (Disagree.)
24. It's hardly fair to bring children into the world with the way things look for the future. (Disagree.)
25. These days a person doesn't know who he can count on. (Disagree.)
26. Young people underestimate the capabilities of older people. (Disagree.)
27. When you are old there's not much use in going to a lot of trouble to look nice. (Disagree.)
28. I'd rather die than grow older. (Disagree.)
29. Old people can generally solve problems better because they have more experience. (Disagree.)
30. I'd like to live another 20 years. (Disagree.)
31. Life doesn't really being until 60. (Disagree.)
32. I feel sorry for old people. (Disagree.)
33. Sometimes I wish I were 25 or 30 again. (Disagree.)
34. Everybody takes advantage of older people. (Disagree.)
35. The main problem in old age is money. (Disagree.)
36. When you get old you begin to forget things. (Disagree.)
37. I have more friends now than I did when I was 50. (Disagree.)
38. Young people don't realize that old folks have problems. (Disagree.)
39. Lots of old people don't seem to care about keeping themselves neat and clean. (Disagree.)
40. When you're older you appreciate the world more. (Disagree.)
41. When you get old, more people go out of their way to be nice to you. (Disagree.)
42. When you're old you take longer to make up your mind. (Disagree.)
43. The only good things about being older is that you are near the end of your suffering. (Disagree.)
44. When you get old your thinking is not as good as it used to be. (Disagree.)
45. I can't think of any problems that older people have. (Disagree.)

Scale is continued overleaf

For each of the following items, please circle the number of the alternative that you feel applies best to you.

1. Do you ever fell moody?
    4 _____ Never
    3 _____ Once in a while
    2 _____ Fairly often
    1 _____ Often

2. I'd rather die than grow very old
    1 _____ Agree strongly
    2 _____ Agree moderately
    3 _____ Undecided
    4 _____ Disagree moderately
    5 _____ Disagree strongly

3. I'd like to live at least another twenty years
    1 _____ Disagree strongly
    2 _____ Disagree moderately
    3 _____ Undecided
    4 _____ Agree moderately
    5 _____ Agree strongly

4. I look forward to life in the next several years
    5 _____ Agree strongly
    4 _____ Agree moderately
    3 _____ Undecided
    2 _____ Disagree moderately
    1 _____ Disagree strongly

5. All in all, how much happiness would you say you find in life today?
    1 _____ Almost none
    2 _____ Some, but not much
    3 _____ A good deal

6. On the whole, how satisfied would you say you are with your way of life today?
    3 _____ Very satisfied
    2 _____ Fairly satisfied
    1 _____ Not very satisfied

7. Loud noises make me jump
    5 _____ Disagree strongly
    4 _____ Disagree moderately
    3 _____ Undecided
    2 _____ Agree moderately
    1 _____ Agree strongly

8. I've been feeling a lot of stress and strain recently
    5 _____ Agree strongly
    4 _____ Agree moderately
    3 _____ Undecided
    2 _____ Disagree moderately
    1 _____ Disagree strongly

9. In general, how would you say you feel most of the time, in good spirits or in low spirits?
    1 _____ Usually in low spirits
    2 _____ Sometimes in good, sometimes in low
    3 _____ Usually in good spirits

10. I've been feeling awfully jumpy lately
    5 _____ Disagree strongly
    4 _____ Disagree moderately
    3 _____ Undecided
    2 _____ Agree moderately
    1 _____ Agree strongly

11. Do you sometimes find yourself feeling impatient?
    1 _____ Often
    2 _____ Fairly often
    3 _____ Once in a while
    4 _____ Never

12. I think my life in the next few years will be better than ever
    5 _____ Agree strongly
    4 _____ Agree moderately
    3 _____ Undecided
    2 _____ Disagree moderately
    1 _____ Disagree strongly

13. I'd like to live to a ripe old age
    1 _____ Disagree strongly
    2 _____ Disagree moderately
    3 _____ Undecided
    4 _____ Agree moderately
    5 _____ Agree strongly

14. How often do you find yourself feeling blue?
    4 _____ Never
    3 _____ Once in a while
    2 _____ Fairly often
    1 _____ Often

15. I seem to get nervous very easily nowadays
    5 _____ Disagree strongly
    4 _____ Disagree moderately
    3 _____ Undecided
    2 _____ Agree moderately
    1 _____ Agree strongly

16. Do you get upset by the things that happen in your day-to-day life?
    1 _____ Often
    2 _____ Fairly often
    3 _____ Once in a while
    4 _____ Never

17. If things get any worse I think I'll kill myself
    1 _____ Agree strongly
    2 _____ Agree moderately
    3 _____ Undecided
    4 _____ Disagree moderately
    5 _____ Disagree strongly

18. I think I am a very calm person
    5 _____ Agree strongly
    4 _____ Agree moderately
    3 _____ Undecided
    2 _____ Disagree moderately
    1 _____ Disagree strongly

19. I hate it when things go wrong
    5 _____ Disagree strongly
    4 _____ Disagree moderately
    3 _____ Undecided
    2 _____ Agree moderately
    1 _____ Agree strongly

20. I'm generally pretty easygoing
    5 _____ Disagree strongly
    4 _____ Disagree moderately
    3 _____ Undecided
    2 _____ Agree moderately
    1 _____ Agree strongly

21. How often do you feel grouchy for no particular reason?
    4 _____ Never
    3 _____ Once in a while
    2 _____ Fairly often
    1 _____ Often

22. How often do you feel irritable?
    1 _____ Often
    2 _____ Fairly often

3 _____ Once in a while
4 _____ Never

23. How often do you get the feeling that your life today is not very useful?

4 _____ Never
3 _____ Once in a while
2 _____ Fairly often
1 _____ Often

24. Have you been worried during the past year for no reason?

1 _____ Often
2 _____ Fairly often
3 _____ Once in a while
4 _____ Never

25. Do you fly off the handle easy?

4 _____ Never
3 _____ Once in a while
2 _____ Fairly often
1 _____ Often

26. I'd like to take it easy, but circumstances won't allow me

5 _____ Disagree strongly
4 _____ Disagree moderately
3 _____ Undecided
2 _____ Agree moderately
1 _____ Agree strongly

27. I'm not as enthusiastic about things as I used to be

1 _____ Disagree strongly
2 _____ Disagree moderately
3 _____ Undecided
4 _____ Agree moderately
5 _____ Agree strongly

28. I'm contented with what I've done in life

5 _____ Agree strongly
4 _____ Agree moderately
3 _____ Undecided
2 _____ Disagree moderately
1 _____ Disagree strongly

29. I'm tired a lot

1 _____ Disagree strongly

2 _____ Disagree moderately
3 _____ Undecided
4 _____ Agree moderately
5 _____ Agree strongly

30. I feel discouraged

5 _____ Agree strongly
4 _____ Agree moderately
3 _____ Undecided
2 _____ Disagree moderately
1 _____ Disagree strongly

31. I've been having a hard time getting started lately

1 _____ Disagree strongly
2 _____ Disagree moderately
3 _____ Undecided
4 _____ Agree moderately
5 _____ Agree strongly

32. I'm generally satisfied with the way I am

5 _____ Agree strongly
4 _____ Agree moderately
3 _____ Undecided
2 _____ Disagree moderately
1 _____ Disagree strongly

33. Sometimes I just don't like myself

1 _____ Disagree strongly
2 _____ Disagree moderately
3 _____ Undecided
4 _____ Agree moderately
5 _____ Agree strongly

34. I have some bad qualities

5 _____ Agree strongly
4 _____ Agree moderately
3 _____ Undecided
2 _____ Disagree moderately
1 _____ Disagree strongly

35. Life has been pretty good to me

1 _____ Disagree strongly
2 _____ Disagree moderately
3 _____ Undecided
4 _____ Agree moderately
5 _____ Agree strongly

Scoring:

The individual taking the inventory should circle the number of the most appropriate alternative for each question.
To score the inventory, add the number of the alternative for the items composing the scales Satisfaction, Will-to-live, and Equanimity, as follows:

Satisfaction	Equanimity	Will-to-live
1	7	2
5	8	3
6	10	4
9	11	12
14	15	13
23	16	17
27	19	
28	20	
29	21	
30	22	
31	24	
32	25	
33	26	
34		
35		

Reproduced from Pierce RC, Clarke MM (1973) Measurement of morale in the elderly. *International Journal of Aging and Human Development* **4**: 83–101, published by Baywood Publishing Co.

Retrospective Postmortem Dementia Assessment (RCD-1)

Reference   Davis PB, White H, Price JL, McKeel D, Robins LN (1991) Retrospective Postmortem Dementia Assessment: validation of a new clinical interview to assist neuropathologic study. *Archives of Neurology* 48: 613–17

Time taken 40 minutes
Rating retrospective structured telephone interview

Main indications

Retrospective gathering of information about a patient after his or her death.

Commentary

The Retrospective Postmortem Dementia Assessment (RCD-1) is a screening interview for use after the death of a patient to enable retrospective information to be gathered so that a clinical diagnosis of the type of dementia can be achieved. It is particularly useful in studies looking at clinico-pathological correlations where one may not have had the opportunity to collect information prospectively. A number of different topics are included, including demographic data, family history, physical functioning, physical condition, drug and alcohol intake, hearing and vision, memory and orientation, neuropsychiatric features and particular signs such as aphasia.

Extracts from existing scales include the Blessed Dementia Scale (page 40) and the Clinical Dementia Rating (CDR; page 168). Agreement between RCD-1 interview and postmortem diagnosis was 91%, and between RCD-1 interview and medical records 100%.

Additional reference

Regier DA, Meyers JK, Kramer M et al (1984) The NIMH Epidemiologic Catchment Area Program. *Archives of General Psychiatry* 41: 934–40.

Address for correspondence

Paula Bonino
Senior Associate Geriatrician
Geriatric Care Services/Lutheran Affiliated Services
500 Wittenberg Way
Box 928
Mars
PA 16046–0928
USA

Retrospective Postmortem Dementia Assessment (RCD-1)

The assessment encompasses the following areas

Demographics
Family history – siblings, parents
Health status/physical functioning
Physical conditions

Medications
Hearing
Vision
Problems related to memory and orientation
Behaviour/changes in personality
Social support/functioning

EuroQol

Reference   The EuroQol Group (1990) EuroQol – a new facility for the measurement of health-related quality of life. *Health Policy* 16: 199–208

Time taken 10–15 minutes (reviewer's estimate)
Rating by self-assessment

Main indications

A non-disease specific instrument used to measure health-related quality of life.

Commentary

The EuroQol instrument is intended to complement other quality-of-life measures and to aid the collection of a common dataset for reference purposes. The instrument was devised by a small group of researchers and centres in five European countries. Studies were conducted in the UK, The Netherlands and in Sweden whereby the questionnaires were mailed to individuals selected at random on the general population. In each case Spearman's ρ was close to 1.0 and Kendal's coefficient of concordance w for the rank ordering of states across all three studies was high and significant ($w = 0.984$, $p<0.001$) – indicating broad agreement regarding the ranking of states. No specific studies have examined validity in the elderly.

Additional references

Bergner M, Bobitt RA et al (1976) The Sickness Impact Profile: conceptual formulation and methodology for the development of a health status measure. *International Journal of Health Services* 6: 393–415.

Hunt SM, McEwen J, McKenna SP (1986) *Measuring health status.* London: Croom Helm.

Patrick DL, Bush JW, Chen MM (1973) Toward an operational definition of health. *Journal of Health and Social Behaviour* 14: 6–23.

Rosser RM, Watts VC (1972) The measurement of hospital output. *International Journal of Epidemiology* 1: 361–8.

Address for correspondence

Alan Williams
Centre for Health Economics
University of York
York YO1 5DD
UK

EuroQol (Descriptive classification)

Mobility
1. No problems walking about
2. Unable to walk about without a stick, crutch or walking frame
3. Confined to bed

Self-care
1. No problems with self-care
2. Unable to dress self
3. Unable to feed self

Main activity
1. Able to perform main activity (e.g. work, study, housework)
2. Unable to perform main activity

Social relationships
1. Able to pursue family and leisure activities
2. Unable to pursue family and leisure activities

Pain
1. No pain or discomfort
2. Moderate pain or discomfort
3. Extreme pain or discomfort

Mood
1. Not anxious or depressed
2. Anxious or depressed

Quality of Life in Dementia

Reference   Blau TH (1977) Quality of life, social indicators, and criteria of change. *Professional Psychology* November, 464–73

Time taken 15 minutes (reviewer's estimate)
Rating self-rated

Main indications
Assessment of quality of life.

Commentary
The Quality of Life in Dementia rating scale was developed to assess quality of life, based on a theoretical model of trying to distinguish between the variety of approaches to quality of life: social, economic and psychological approaches and attempts to operationalize quality of life itself. The scale was developed to assess those features regarded as important by people undergoing psychotherapy. The main reason for its inclusion here is that it has been used (adapted slightly) to measure change in quality of life in patients with Alzheimer's disease undergoing clinical trials (Rogers et al, 1996).

Additional reference
Rogers S, Friedhoff L et al (1996) The efficacy and safety of donepezil in patients with Alzheimer's disease. *Dementia* 7: 293–303.

Quality of Life in Dementia

Evaluation

1. Working	5. Social contact
2. Leisure	6. Earning
3. Eating	7. Parenting
4. Sleeping	8. Loving
	9. Environment
	10. Self-acceptance

Score:
Rated on a line score of 0–50
  0 = Non-existent or no opportunity
10 = Minimal
30 = Adequate
50 = Best possible score

Lancashire Quality of Life Profile (Residential)

Reference   Oliver J, Mohamad H (1996) The quality of life of the chronic mentally ill: a comparison of public, private and voluntary residential provisions. *British Journal of Social Work* 22: 391–404

Time taken
Rating by trained interviewer

Main indications
Measurement of quality of life in older people in residential care.

Commentary
The Lancashire Quality of Life Profile is an extensive instrument assessing quality of life in a number of different populations. It has been adapted for use in residential care, and work currently underway (Huxley, Challis, Burns et al, Quality of Life in Residential and Nursing Home Care, University of Manchester) will provide further information specifically on its use for elderly people in these settings.

The Quality of Life Profile is divided into objective and subjective wellbeing. A number of well accepted measures have been incorporated into the scale: life domains (Lehman, 1983), social indicators (Campbell et al, 1976; Lehman, 1983), a quality-of-life uni-scale (Spitzer and Dobson, 1981), Cantrell's ladder (Cantrell, 1965), delighted–terrible scale (Lehman, 1983), affect balance scale (Bradburn, 1969), critical incidence and disability adaptation (Flannigan, 1982), self-esteem scale (Rosenberg, 1965) and happiness scale (Bradburn, 1969).

Additional references
Bradburn N (1969) *The structure of psychological wellbeing.* Chicago, IL: Aldheim Publishing.

Campbell A et al (1976) Subjective measures and wellbeing. *American Psychologist* 31: 117–24.

Cantrill H (1965) *The pattern of human concerns.* New Brunswick, NJ: Rutgers.

Flannigan J (1982) Measurement of quality of life: current state of the art. *Archives of Physical Medicine and Rehabilitation* 63: 56–9.

Lehman A (1983) The wellbeing of chronic mental patients. *Archives of General Psychiatry* 40: 4369–73.

Oliver J, Huxley P, Bridges K et al (1996) *Quality of life in mental health Services.* London: Routledge.

Rosenberg M (1965) *Society and the adolescent image.* Princeton, NJ: Princeton University Press.

Spitzer W, Dobson A (1981) Measuring the quality of life in cancer patients. *Journal of Chronic Diseases* 34: 585–97.

Address for correspondence
Peter Huxley
Department of Psychiatry
12th Floor, Maths Tower
University of Manchester
Oxford Road
Manchester M13
UK

Lancashire Quality of Life Profile

Items included are:
Leisure/participation
Family relations
Religion
Living situation
Social relations
Health
General wellbeing

Section I: General Wellbeing Today
Can you tell me how you feel about your life as a whole today?

Section 2: Leisure/Participation
10 questions regarding being outside, watching TV or listening to the radio. Rating of pleasure (5-point scale) associated with that.

Section 3: Family Relations
7 questions about family, children, grandchildren and contact with them.

Section 4: Religion
5 questions concerning importance of and practice of religion.

Section 5: Living Situation
10 questions regarding living arrangements, independence, privacy, food, opportunities for occupation.

Section 6:
5 questions about friends and contacts in and outside the home.

Section 7: Health
11 questions about depression, walking, hearing and vision.

Section 8: Cartmel's Ladder
Bottom = "Life is as bad as it could possibly be"
Top = "Life is as good as it could possibly be"
Measured in millimetres.

Section 9: General Wellbeing
Most questions rated as 1 (very dissatisfied) – 5 (very satisfied).
Ratings of confidence in interveiew responses (reliable/mixed/unreliable) made at the end of every section.

Reproduced from Oliver J, Mohamad H (1996) The quality of life of the chronic mentally ill: a comparison of public, private and voluntary residential provisions. *British Journal of Social Work* **22**: 391–404, by permission of Oxford University Press.

Quality of Interactions Schedule (QUIS)

Reference   Dean R, Proudfoot R, Lindesay J (1993) The Quality of Interactions Schedule (QUIS): development, reliability and use in the evaluation of two domus units. *International Journal of Geriatric Psychiatry* 8: 819–26

Time taken observation period can be varied
Rating by trained observer

Main indications

An observer-rated measure of interactions between residents and care staff.

Commentary

In some situations, direct observations of interactions between staff and residents are valuable in evaluating and planning services. Event-sampling strategies have been devised (Godlove et al, 1982) and shorter versions validated (Macdonald et al, 1985). The Quality of Interactions Schedule (QUIS) was developed to assess the number and quality of interactions as part of a prospective evaluation of two residential units for elderly people with mental illness. The number and quality of interaction are estimated on the basis of a series of ten 15-minute observation times across the working day, over a period of approximately two weeks. Interactions are coded in one of five categories: positive social, positive care, neutral, negative protective and negative restrictive, based on the work of Clark and Bowling (1989). Observation and coding consistently produce kappa reliability statistics of above 0.75, with a range of 0.60–0.91.

Additional references

Clark P, Bowling A (1989) Observational study of quality of life in nursing homes and a long stay ward for the elderly. *Ageing Soc* 9: 123–48.

Godlove C, Richard L, Rodwell G (1982) *Time for action. An observational study of elderly people in four different care environments. Social Services Monographs, Research in Practice.* Sheffield: Community Care, University of Sheffield, Joint Unit for Social Services Research.

Macdonald AJD, Craig TKJ, Warner LAR (1985) The development of short observation method for the study of activity and contacts of old people in residential settings. *Psychological Medicine* 15: 167–72.

Address for correspondence

James Lindesay
Leicester General Hospital
Gwendolen Road
Leicester LE5 4PW
UK

Quality of Interactions Schedule (QUIS): guidelines and examples for coding interactions

Positive social
Interaction principally involving "good, constructive, beneficial" conversation and companionship.

Positive care
Interactions during the appropriate delivery of physical care.

Neutral
Brief, indifferent interactions not meeting the definitions of the other categories.

Negative protective
Providing care, keeping safe or removing from danger, but in a restrictive manner, without explanation or reassurance.

Negative restrictive
Interactions that oppose or resist residents' freedom of action without good reason, or which ignore resident as a person.

Reproduced from Dean R, Proudfoot R, Lindesay J (1993) The Quality of Interactions Schedule (QUIS): development, reliability and use in the evaluation of two domus units. *International Journal of Geriatric Psychiatry* **8**: 819–26. Copyright John Wiley & Sons Limited. Reproduced with permission.

INSIGHT

Reference   Verhey FRJ, Rozendaal N, Ponds RWHM, Jolles J (1993) Dementia, awareness and depression. *International Journal of Geriatric Psychiatry* 8: 851–6

Time taken 5 minutes
Rating by interview

Main indications
Assessment of awareness of cognitive decline.

Commentary
Awareness of cognitive decline in dementia is an important area, and the terms "unawareness of deficit", "lack of insight" and "anosognosia" are usually used interdependently. Generally, insight tends to decrease with increasing severity of dementia (McGlynn and Schachter, 1989). The authors of the original paper on INSIGHT rated insight in 170 patients, the majority of whom had Alzheimer's disease. Standard guidelines were used to rate the awareness of cognitive decline, the final rating being made on a four-point scale. Level of awareness was significantly related to the severity of dementia but not depression.

Additional reference
McGlynn SM, Schachter DL (1989) Unawareness of deficits in neuropsychological syndromes. *Journal of Experimental Neuropsychology* 1: 143–205.

Address for correspondence
FRJ Verhey
Department of Psychiatry
University Hospital of Maastricht
PO Box 5800
6202 AZ Maastricht
The Netherlands

INSIGHT

Please tell me about the problems you are here for. Why did Dr . . . send you to this clinic?

When the patient has other complaints not directly related to dementia:

Do you have any other complaints?

When the patient has no spontaneous complaints about his cognitive functions:

How is your memory functioning? Do you think you have a poor memory?

When the patient denies deficits of memory or other cognitive functions:

So, there are no memory problems at all? Is everything going all right for you?

Complaints are then discussed and the same question adopted to ask the caregiver.

Scoring:
4 = Adequate
3 = Mildly disturbed
2 = Moderately disturbed
1 = Severely disturbed

Ischaemic Score

Reference Hackinski VC, Iliff LD, Zilka E et al (1975) Cerebral blood flow in dementia. *Archives of Neurology* 32: 632–7

Time taken 2 minutes (once all the information is gathered)
Rating by clinician

Main indications

Assessment of vascular contribution to the aetiology of dementia.

Commentary

On the basis of the Ischaemic Score, the concept of multi-infarct dementia was introduced based on the assumption that in many patients dementia was as a result of single or multiple large infarctions. The Ischaemic Score was validated using functional brain imaging to divide patients with dementia into those with vascular disease and those with primary degenerative dementia. The average age of the group was 63, and there seems to be a bimodal distribution of the scores in relation to the appearances on the scan, reflecting cerebral blood flow. A score of 4 or below was indicative of a primary degenerative dementia and 7 or above of vascular dementia. A number of authors have commented on the scale and adaptations have been suggested. The most obvious omission is the lack of evidence from brain imaging to show vascular changes in the brain. Hachinski (1983) confirmed that the scale is designed to identify strokes and so is considered by many to be more of an infarct than an ischaemic scale. Validity studies with amended versions of the scale have been published (e.g. Rosen et al, 1980; Loeb and Godolfo, 1983; Fischer et al, 1991). Grasel et al (1990) found the best discriminating factors to be fluctuation course, stepwise deterioration, abrupt onset, history of strokes, and the presence of focal neurological signs and symptoms.

Additional references

Fischer P et al (1991) Neuropathological validation of the Hachinski scale *Journal of Neural Transmission* 1: 57.

Grasel E et al (1990) What contribution can the Hachinski ischaemic scale make to the differential diagnosis between multi-infarct dementia and primary degenerative dementia? *Arch Gerontol Geriatr* 11: 63–75.

Hachinski C (1983) Multifocal dementia. *Neurologic Clinics* 1: 27–36.

Loeb C, Godolfo C (1983) Diagnostic evaluation of degenerative and vascular dementia. *Stroke* 14: 399–401.

Rosen WG et al (1980) Pathological verification of ischaemic score in dementias. *Annals of Neurology* 7: 486–8.

Ischaemic Score

Abrupt onset	2	Emotional incontinence	1
Stepwise deterioration	1	History of hypertension	1
Fluctuating course	2	History of strokes	2
Nocturnal confusion	1	Generalized atherosclerosis	1
Relative preservation of personality	1	Focal neurological symtoms	2
Depression	1	Focal neurological signs	2
Somatic complaints	1		

Quality of Life in Alzheimer's Disease: Patient and Caregiver Report (QOL-AD)

Reference   Logsdon RG, Gibbons LE, McCurry SM, Teri L (1998) Quality of life in Alzheimer's disease: patient and caregiver reports. *Journal of Mental Health and Aging* (in press).

Time taken 10 minutes each (reviewer's estimate)

Rating self and caregiver reports

Main indications

Assessment of quality of life in dementia.

Commentary

The Quality of Life in Alzheimer's Disease: Patient and Caregiver Report (QOL-AD) is a 13-item self and and caregiver measure of quality of life. 77 patients with Alzheimer's disease were assessed and ratings made of quality of life, Mini-Mental State Examination (MMSE; page 34), Activities of daily living, PSMS (page 129), depression (the Hamilton Depression Rating Scale; page 4), the Geriatric Depression Scale (page 2), and the Pleasant Events Schedule (page 254). The 13 items are rated on a 4-point scale, with 1 being poor and 4 being excellent, with a total score of between 13 and 52. To give a composite score which weights the patient rating more heavily than that of the caregiver, the patient's score is multiplied by 2, the caregiver score is multiplied by 2, the caregiver score added and the sum divided by 3. Internal consistency of the scale was good (Cronbach's alpha 0.88). Acceptable validity was found in comparison with the other instruments. Patient and caregiver quality of life were correlated, and moderate levels of cognitive impairment did not compromise reliability or validity.

Address for correspondence

Rebecca Logsdon
Psychosocial & Community Health
Box 357263
University of Washington
Seattle
WA 98195-7263
USA

Quality of Life in Alzheimer's Disease

Instructions for Interviewers

The QOL-AD is administered in interview format to individuals with dementia, following the instructions below.

Hand the form to the participant, so that he or she may look at it as you give the following instructions (instructions should closely follow the wording given in **bold type**):

I want to ask you some questions about your quality of life and how you rate different aspects of your life using one of four words; poor, fair, good, or excellent.

Point to each word (poor, fair, good, and excellent) on the form as you say it.

When you think about your life, there are different aspects, like your physical health, energy, family, money, and others. I'm going to ask you to rate each of these areas. We want to find out how you feel about your current situation in each area.

If you're not sure about what a question means, you can ask me about it. If you have difficulty rating any item, just give it your best guess.

It is usually apparent whether an individual understands the questions, and most individuals who are able to communicate and respond to simple questions can understand the measure. If the participant answers all questions the same, or says something that indicates a lack of understanding, the interviewer is encouraged to clarify the question. However, under no circumstances should the interviewer suggest a specific response. Each of the four possible responses should be presented, and the participant should pick one of the four.

If a participant is unable to choose a response to a particular item or items, this should be noted in the comments. If the participant is unable to comprehend and/or respond to two or more items, the testing may be discontinued, and this should be noted in the comments.

As you read the items listed below, ask the participant to circle her/his response. If the participant has difficulty circling the word, you may ask her/him to point to the word or say the word, and you may circle it for him or her. You should let the participant hold his or her own copy of the measure, and follow along as you read each item.

1. First of all, how do you feel about your physical health? Would you say it's. poor, fair, good, or excellent? Circle whichever word you think beat describes your physical health right now.
2. How do you feel about your energy level? Do you think it is poor, fair, good, or excellent? If the participant says that some days are better than others, ask him or her to rate how she/he has been feeling most of the time lately.

3. How has your mood been lately? Have your spirits been good, or have you been feeling down? Would you rate your mood as. poor, fair, good, or excellent?

4. How about your living situation? How do you feel about the place you have now? Would you say it's poor, fair, good, or excellent?

5. How about your memory? Would you say it is poor, fair, good, or excellent?

6. How about your family and your relationship with family members? Would you describe it as poor, fair, good, or excellent? If the respondent says they have no family, ask about brothers, sisters, children, nieces, nephews.

7. How do you feel about your marriage? How is your relationship with (spouse's name). Do you feel it's poor, fair, good, or excellent? Some participants will be single, widowed, or divorced. When this is the case. ask how they feel about the person with whom they have the closest relationship, whether it's a family member or friend. If there is a family caregiver, ask about their relationship with this person. If there is no one appropriate, or the participant is unsure, score the item as missing.

8. How would you describe your current relationship with your friends? 'Would you say it's poor, fair, good, or excellent? If the respondent answers that they have no friends, or all their friends have died, probe further. Do you have anyone you enjoy being with besides your family? Would you call that person a friend? It the respondent still says they have no friends, ask how do you feel about having no friends—poor, fair, good, or excellent?

9. How do you feel about yourself—when you think of your whole self and all the different things about you, would you say it's poor, fair, good, or excellent?

10. How do you feel about your ability to do things like chores around the house or other things you need to do? Would you say it's poor, fair, good, or excellent?

11. How about your ability to do things for fun, that you enjoy? Would you say it's poor, fair, good, or excellent?

12. How do you feel about your current situation with money, your financial situation? Do you feel it's poor, fair, good, or excellent? If the respondent hesitates, explain that you don't want to know what their situation is (as in amount of money), just how they feel about it

13. How would you describe your life as a whole. When you think about your life as a whole, everything together, how do you feel about your life? Would you say it's poor, fair, good, or excellent?

UWMC/ADPR/QOL
Aging and Dementia: Quality of Life in AD
Quality of Life: AD
(Participant Version)

ID Number
☐☐☐☐☐☐

Assessment Number
☐☐

Interview Date
☐☐ ☐☐ ☐☐
Month Day Year

Instructions: Interviewer administer according to standard instructions.
Circle participant responses.

1.	Physical health.	Poor	Fair	Good	Excellent
2.	Energy.	Poor	Fair	Good	Excellent
3.	Mood.	Poor	Fair	Good	Excellent
4.	Living situation.	Poor	Fair	Good	Excellent
5.	Memory.	Poor	Fair	Good	Excellent
6.	Family.	Poor	Fair	Good	Excellent
7.	Marriage.	Poor	Fair	Good	Excellent
8.	Friends.	Poor	Fair	Good	Excellent
9.	Self as a whole.	Poor	Fair	Good	Excellent
10.	Ability to do chores around the house	Poor	Fair	Good	Excellent
11.	Ability to do things for fun.	Poor	Fair	Good.	Excellent
12.	Money.	Poor	Fair	Good	Excellent
13.	Life as a whole.	Poor	Fair	Good	Excellent

Comments:

Scale is continued overleaf

UWMC/ADPR/QOL
Aging and Dementia: Quality of Life in AD
Quality of Life: AD
(Family Version)

ID Number

☐☐☐☐☐☐

Assessment Number

☐☐

Interview Date

☐☐   ☐☐   ☐☐
Month   Day   Year

Instructions: *Please rate your relative's current situation, as you see it.*
Circle your responses.

1.	Physical health.	Poor	Fair	Good	Excellent
2.	Energy.	Poor	Fair	Good	Excellent
3.	Mood.	Poor	Fair	Good	Excellent
4.	Living situation.	Poor	Fair	Good	Excellent
5.	Memory.	Poor	Fair	Good	Excellent
6.	Family.	Poor	Fair	Good	Excellent
7.	Marriage.	Poor	Fair	Good	Excellent
8.	Friends.	Poor	Fair	Good	Excellent
9.	Self as a whole.	Poor	Fair	Good	Excellent
10.	Ability to do chores around the house	Poor	Fair	Good	Excellent
11.	Ability to do things for fun.	Poor	Fair	Good	Excellent
12.	Money.	Poor	Fair	Good	Excellent
13.	Life as a whole.	Poor	Fair	Good	Excellent

Comments:

Reproduced with kind permission from Dr L Teri.

Appendix 1

What to use and when

Clinical or research issue	Suggested scales	Page No.
Depression		
Screening for depression:		
General practice	GDS	2
	BASDEC	10
	SELFCARE (D)	12
Medical/geriatric	GDS	2
Inpatients	BASDEC	10
Community surveys	CES-D	14
	GMSS	200
	Canberra Interview for the Elderly	201
	CAMDEX	208
In nursing/residential homes	GDS	2
	BASDEC	10
	SELFCARE (D)	12
With cognitive impairment	DSS	16
	NIMH Dementia Mood Assessment Scale (DMAS)	26
	Cornell Scale for Depression in Dementia	8
Rating severity of depression	Hamilton Depression Rating Scale	4
Symptom profile in depression	Hamilton Depression Rating Scale	4
Self-rating scales	GDS	2
	BDI	6
	Zung Self-Rating Depression Scale	252
Monitoring change	MADRS	7
	Hamilton Depression Rating Scale	4
Cognitive impairment		
Screening for cognitive impairment:		
General practice	MMSE	34
	MTS/AMTS	38
	Clock Drawing Test	44
	SKT	62

Clinical or research issue	Suggested scales	Page No.
	7 Minute Neurocognitive Screening Battery	70
Nursing/residential homes	MMSE	34
Medical/geriatric inpatients	MMSE	34
	Clock Drawing Test	44
In depressed patients	MMSE	34
	Clock Drawing Test	44
Community surveys	SIDAM	197
	GMSS	200
	Canberra Interview for the Elderly	201
	CAMDEX	208
Global ratings of psychiatric symptomatology	Psychogeriatric Assessment Scales	199
Dementia		
Detailed profile of cognitive deficits	ADAS-Cog	42
Global ratings	GDS	166
	CDR	168
Staging of disease	GDS	166
	CDR	168
Measuring therapeutic effects:		
Cognitive function	MMSE	34
	ADAS-Cog	42
Global changes	CIBIC and variants	170
	ADCS-CGIC	297
Noncognitive features of dementia:		
General measures	BEHAVE-AD	75
	NPI	78
	CUSPAD	79
	MOUSEPAD	82
	CERAD	88
Specific features:		
Personality change	Brooks and McKinlay scale	272
Agitation	BARS	108
	CMAI	110
	Pittsburgh Agitation Scale	112
Aggression	RAGE	92
	Overt Aggression Scale	94
	Ryden Aggression Scale	104
Behavioural disturbances in dementia	NRS	96
	COBRA	98
	PGDRS	174
	NOSGER	210
	DBRS	102
Global ratings of dementia severity	Dementia Behavior Disturbance Scale	111

Clinical or research issue	Suggested scales	Page No.
Activities of Daily Living:		
Specific for dementia	IADL	128
	IDDD	130
	FAQ	134
	DAFS	140
	CSADL	143
	DAD	295
	ADFACS	296
Generic scales	ADL index	142
	FDS	152
	Rapid Disability Rating Scale – 2 (RDRS-2)	150
Other disorders		
Global measures of psychiatric symptomatology	BPRS	194
	RAGS	196
	GAPS	198
	Psychogeriatric Assessment Scales	199
	GMSS	200
	SPAS	202
Parkinsonian signs/side-effects of drugs	Webster Scale	217
	TDRS	219
	AIMS	221
Caregiver burden	Problem Checklist and Strain Scale	234
	SCB	238
	Revised Memory and Behavior Problems Checklist	244
	CAS	245
Caregiver stress	BDI	6
	Problem Checklist and Strain Scale	234
	Ways of Coping Checklist	236
	Caregiving Hassles Scale	240
	GHQ	246
	Zung Self-Rating Depression Scale	252
Quality of life measures	QOL-AD	288
Memory complaints	CFQ	258
Delirium	Dementia Rating Scale	176
	DSI	227
	CAM	228
	DRS	230
	DI	298
Scales to consider when starting a memory clinic	MMSE	34
	Blessed	40
	ADAS-Cog	42
	ADAS	42
	BEHAVE-AD	75
	NPI	78
	CFQ	258
	Ischaemic Score	287

Appendix 2

Additional scales

The Disability Assessment for Dementia (DAD)

Reference Gelinas I, Gauthier L, McIntyre M, Gauthier S (1999) Development of a functional measure for persons with Alzheimer's Disease: The Disability Assessment for Dementia. *American Journal of Occupational Therapy*, in press

Time taken 20 minutes
Rating By trained observer

Main Indication
Rating of ADL in dementia

Commentary
The Disability for Assessment for Dementia Scale (DAD) is a new functional scale specifically developed for patients with Alzheimer's Disease, and incorporates activities combining basic and instrumental activities of daily living. The scale is rated by an informant, and has an inter-rater reliability of 0.95, test re-test reliability of 0.96, and internal consistency of 0.96.

The rates are measured in a number of different areas: initiation, planning and organisation, and effective performance. Examples of basic ADL activity include eating (deciding that he/she needs to eat, choosing appropriate utensils and seasonings when eating, and eating his/her meals at a normal pace with appropriate manners), initiation, planning and organisation and effective performance respectively.

An example of instrumental ADL assessed in the DAD is leisure and housework: showing an interest in leisure activities/taking an interest in household chores that he/she used to perform in the past (initiation); planning and organising household chores adequately that he/she performed in the past (planning and organisation); satisfactory completion of household chores performed in the past; and staying safely at home by him/herself when necessary (effective performance).

Additional references
Gauthier S, Bodick KN, Erzigkiet E et al (1997) Activities of daily living as an outcome measure in clinical trials of dementia drugs. *Alzheimer's Disease and Associated Disorders* 11 (Suppl 4): 6–7.

Gelinas I (1995) *Disability Assessment in Dementia of the Alzheimer Type*. Doctoral Thesis, Montreal: School of Physical and Occupational Therapy, McGill University.

Gelinas I, Auer S (1996) Functioning in Alzheimer's Disease. In: Gauthier S, (ed.), *Clinical Diagnosis and Management of Alzheimer's Disease*. London: Martin Dunitz Ltd, pp. 191–202.

Gelinas I, Gauthier S, Cyrus P et al (1998) The efficacy of metrifonate in enhancing the ability of Alzheimer's Disease patients to perform basic and instrumental activities of daily living. *Neurology* 50 (Suppl 4) a90–a91.

Address for Correspondence
Serge Gauthier
The McGill Center for Studies in Aging
Douglas Hospital
6825 LaSalle Boulevard
Verdun
Quebec H4H 1R3
Canada

The Alzheimer's Disease Functional Assessment and Change Scale (ADFACS)

Reference   Galasko D, Bennett D, Sano M et al (1997) An inventory to assess activities of daily living for clinical trials in Alzheimer's Disease. The Alzheimer's Disease co-operative study. *Alzheimer's Disease and Associated Disorders* 11 (Suppl 2): S33–9.

Time taken 20 minutes (reviewer's estimate)
Rating Informant-based

Main Indications

Assessment of ADL in patients with Alzheimer's Disease, with particular reference to outcomes in clinical trials

Commentary

The Alzheimer's Disease Functional Assessment and Change Scale has been used in drug trials, and consists of ten items for instrumental activities of daily living: ability to use the telephone, performing household tasks, using household appliances, handling money, shopping, preparing food, ability to get around both inside and outside the home, pursuing hobbies and leisure activities, handling personal mail and grasping situations or explanations.

These are rated on a five-point scale:

1 no impairment
2 mild impairment
3 moderate impairment
4 severe impairment
5 not assessable

Basic activities of daily living are assessed on a 6-point scale (an additional rating, very severe impairment, is included) – toiletting, feeding, dressing, personal hygiene and grooming, physical ambulation and bathing.

The scale was developed from 45 ADL items, with the chosen items having been shown to be sensitive to change over 12 months, to correlate with the MMSE (page 34) and to have good test re-test reliability (Galasko et al 1997).

Validity and Reliability of the Alzheimer's Disease Co-operative Study – Clinical, Global Impression of Change (ADCS-CGIC)

Reference   Schneider L, Olin J, Doody R et al (1997) Validity and reliability of the Alzheimer's Disease co-operative study – clinical global impression of change. *Alzheimer's Disease and Associated Disorders* 11 (suppl 2): S22–33.

Time taken about 40 minutes
Rating by trained rater, with at least one year's experience in clinical trials

Main Indication
Rating of global changes in Alzheimer's Disease

Commentary
The ADCS-CGIC consists of three parts: a baseline interview with the patient and informant, a follow-up interview and a rating review by the clinician. Raters are required to have one year's experience of making global ratings in clinical trials. The rating is made on a seven point scale:

1 marked improvement
2 moderate improvement
3 minimal improvement
4 no change
5 minimal worsening
6 moderate worsening
7 marked worsening

Validity and reliability data presented for the ADCS-CGIC are excellent, and satisfactory correlations are found between the instrument and The MMSE (page 34), CDR (page 168), Global Deterioration Scale (page 166) and FAST (page 164).

Instructions for Administration of the Alzheimer's Disease Cooperative Study-Clinical Global Impression of Change (ADCS-CGIC)

The ADCS-GCIC consists of two parts: Part I, baseline evaluation (includes information from both subjects and informant); Part II, ADCS-GCIC forms for both subject and informant.

The overall intent of the ADCS-CGIC is to provide a reliable means to assess global change from baseline in a clinical trial. It provides a semistructured format to enable clinicians to gather necessary clinical information from both the patient and informant to make a global impression of clinical change.

Part I is used to record baseline information to serve as a reference for future ratings. Part II is composed of two sections, a subject interview form and an informant interview form. These forms are used to record information from separate interviews with both subject and informant from which an impression of change score is made.

Method of Administration
Baseline Evaluation:
At baseline, the clinician interviews the patient and caregiver, recording onto Part I notes about baseline status for later reference. At baseline only, clinical information about the subject from any source can be used. The clinician indicates on a checklist the sources of information compiled during the baseline evaluation.

Parts I and II share a similar format for recording relevant clinical information. The column headed "Areas" identifies various areas that a clinician might consider while evaluating a patient for potential clinical change, including what might be expected to be assessed in performing an ordinary but brief comprehensive office interview to determine a subject's baseline status and eligibility for a clinical trial. The "Probes" column provides sample items that a clinician might find useful in assessing an area, and these are intended as guides for collecting relevant information. The last column provides space for notes. For the baseline form, there are separeate spaces for notes taken from the informant and patient interviews.

There is no specified amount of time to complete the baseline form.

Follow-up visits:
Part II is administered at each follow-up visit. At each follow-up visit, the order of interviews should be the same for all participants, with all subjects being interviewed first or, alternatively, all informants being interviewed first.

After completing the interviews, the clinician records the clinical impression of change on a 7-point Likert-type scale (from marked improvement to marked worsening). The ADCS-CGIC is a rating of change and not of severity. The clinician may refer to the baseline data in Part I.

The clinician, alone, must make decisions about change, without consulting other staff. The clinician should avoid asking opinions of the interviewee, which may contaminate the ratings, such as opinions regarding change in symptoms or side effects. At the beginning of the interview, the clinician may wish to caution the informant to refrain from mentioning this information.

The time allotted for the subsequent ratings of change is 20 min each per subject or informant interview. This time was chosen on the basis of the mean time reported by clinicians who often assess clinical charge.

Source: Schneider L, Olin J, Doody R et al (1997) Validity and reliabilityt f thee Alzheimer's Disease co-operative study-clinical global impression of change. *Alzheimer's Disease and Associated Disorders* **11** (suppl 2): 322–33. Reproduced with permission from Lippincott–Raven Publishers.

The Delirium Index (DI)

Reference   McCusker J, Cole M, Bellavance F, Primeau F (1998) Reliability and validity of a new measure of severity of delirium. *International Psychogeriatrics* 10: 421–33.

Time taken 5–10 minutes
Rating by trained observer

Main indication

To rate the severity of delirium

Commentary

The Delirium Index (DI) was designed from the Confusion Assessment Method (CAM; see page 228) and DSMIIIR Criteria for Delirium.

The final instrument is a 7 symptom rating scale, each scored on a 3 point measure, increased from an original 2 point scale, with a view to increasing sensitivity.

The scale was assessed in 3 studies looking at inter-rater reliability, and construct and criterion validity. Inter-rater reliability between a research assistant and psychiatrist ranged between 0.77 and 0.93. Criterion validity was assessed against the Delirium Rating Scale (Trzepacz et al 1998, page 230) and correlation with that instrument was high. Correlations with the Mini-Mental State Examination (page 34) and the Barthel Index (page 132) were 0.7 and 0.6 respectively. The DI is a measure of the severity of delirium, allowing standardised measurements of changes over time to be undertaken.

Address for Correspondence

Dr Jane McCusker
Department of Clinical Epidemiology and Community Studies
St Mary's Hospital Center, Room 2508
3830 Lacombe Avenue
Montreal
Quebec H3T 1M5
Canada

The Delirium Index (DI)

The DI is an instrument for the measurement of severity of symptoms of delirium that is based solely upon observation of the individual patient, without additional information from family members, nursing staff, or the patient medical chart. The DI was designed to be used in conjunction with the MMSE: At least the first five questions of the MMSE comprise the basis of observation. Additional questions may be necessary for scoring certain symptoms as noted.

1. Attention
  0 Attentive
  1 Generally attentive but makes at least one error in spelling "World" backwards.
  2 Questions can generally be answered but subject is distractible and at times has difficulty in keeping track of questions. May have some difficulty in shifting attention to new questions or questions may have to be repeated several times.
  3 Either unresponsive or totally unable to keep track of or answer questions. Has great difficulty in focusing attention and is often distracted by irrelevant stimuli.
  9 Cannot assess.

2. Disorganized Thinking
  0 Responses are logical, coherent, and relevant.
  1 Responses are vague or unclear.
  2 Thought is occasionally illogical, incoherent, or irrelevant.
  3 Either unresponsive or thought is fragmented, illogical, incoherent, and irrelevant.
  9 Cannot assess.

3. Level of Consciousness
  0 Normal.
  1 Hypervigilant or hypovigilant (glassy eyed, decreased reaction to questions).
  2 Drowsy/sleepy. Responds only to simple, loud questions.
  3 Unresponsive or comatose.

4 Disorientation (Additional questions on age, birthdate, and birthplace may be used.)
  0 Knows today's date (± 1 day) and the name of the hospital.
  1 Either does not know today's date (±1 day) or does not know the name of the hospital.
  2 Either does not know the month or year or does not know that he is in hospital.
  3 Either unresponsive or or does not know name or birthdate.
  9 Cannot assess.

5 Memory (Additional questions may be asked on how long patient has been in hospital, circumstances of admission.)
  0 Recalls 3 words and details of hospitalization.
  1 Either cannot recall 1 of the words or has difficulty recalling details of the hospitalization.
  2 Either cannot recall 2 of the 3 words or recalls very few details of the hospitalization.
  3 Either unresponsive or cannot recall any of the 3 words or cannot recall any details of the hospitalization.
  9 Cannot assess.

6 Perceptual Disturbance (Patient is asked whether he has had any unusual experiences and has seen or heard things that other people do not see or hear. If yes, he is asked whether these occur during the daytime or at night and how frequently. Patient is also observed for any evidence of disordered perception.)
  0 Either unresponsive or no perceptual disturbance observed or cannot assess.
  1 Misinterprets stimuli (for example, interpreting a door closing as a gunshot).
  2 Occasional nonthreatening hallucinations.
  3 Frequent, threatening hallucinations.

7. Motor Activity
  0 Normal.
  1 Responds well to questions but either moves frequently or is lethargic/sluggish.
  2 Moves continuously (and may be restrained) or very slow with little spontaneous movement.
  3 Agitated, difficult to control (restraints are required) or no voluntary movement.

Scoring
1 Total score is sum of 7 item scores.
2 If questions 1, 2 4 or 5 are checked "9" (e.g., patient refuses to answer questions), replace 9 by the score of Item 3.

Source: McCusker J, Cole M, Bellavance F, Primeau F (1998) Reliability and validity of a new measure of severity of delirium. *International Psychogeriatrics* **10**(4): 421–33. © 1998 Springer Publishing Company, Inc., New York 10012, used by permission.

Scales index

Oxford Revision Guides

AS & A Level

PE

Through Diagrams

David Morton
Nicholas Baugniet
Gillian Jones
rs

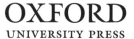

OXFORD
UNIVERSITY PRESS

Great Clarendon Street, Oxford OX2 6DP

Oxford University Press is a department of the
University of Oxford. It furthers the University's objective
of excellence in research, scholarship, and education by
publishing worldwide in

Oxford New York

Auckland   Cape Town   Dar es Salaam   Hong Kong   Karachi
Kuala Lumpur   Madrid   Melbourne   Mexico City   Nairobi
New Delhi   Shanghai   Taipei   Toronto

With offices in

Argentina   Austria   Brazil   Chile   Czech Republic   France   Greece
Guatemala   Hungary   Italy   Japan   Poland   Portugal   Singapore
South Korea   Switzerland   Thailand   Turkey   Ukraine   Vietnam

Oxford is a registered trade mark of Oxford University Press
in the UK and in certain other countries

A catalogue record for this book is available from the British Library.

ISBN: 978-0-19-918092-9

10 9 8 7 6 5 4 3 2 1

Printed in Great Britain by Bell and Bain Ltd, Glasgow

Paper used in the production of this book is a natural, recyclable product
made from wood grown in sustainable forests. The manufacturing process
conforms to the environmental regulations of the country of origin.

Where to find the information you need

AQA

Physiological and Psychological Factors which Improve Performance *2–24, 25–42, 43–46, 49–50, 110–115*

Socio-Cultural and Historical Effects on Participation in Physical Activity and their Influence on Performance *43-50*

Analysis and Improvement of Performance *51–70, 71–90, 91–97, 99–104, 123*

Physiological, Biomechanical and Psychological Factors which Optimise Performance *51–70, 71–90, 61–62, 94–97, 99–100*

Factors Affecting the Nature and Development of Elite Performance and Synoptic Assessment *91–97, 99–102*

OCR

An introduction to Physical Education *2–24, 26–42, 43–50, 51, 52–53, 69, 97*

Principles and concepts across different areas of Physical Education *51–70, 71–90, 91–96, 101–104, 105, 124, 125–130*

The improvement of effective performance and the critical evaluation of practical activities in Physical Education *97–100*

EDEXCEL

Participation in Sport and Recreation *2–24, 51, 52–53, 69, 105–108, 110–116, 125–130*

Preparation for Optimum Sports Performance *51–70, 71–90, 94–95, 101–104, 125–130*

Contents

Joints and movement types

> Joints are where bones meet. There are three types...

Fixed or immovable joints

Technical name: synarthrosis

The bones at an immovable joint are not able to move. They interlock or overlap, and are held together by tough fibre.

Example: the joints between plates (sutures) in the skull (cranium).

Freely movable joints

Technical name: diarthrosis

The bones at freely movable joints can move quite freely. These joints are also called synovial joints. A synovial, or freely movable, joint allows movement to occur, but may be restricted by the articular surfaces. There is a fluid-filled cavity which contains the ligaments and tendons that pass through the joint, as well as the cartilage. A synovial membrane encloses the synovial fluid which acts as a lubricant for the joint.

Examples: shoulder, hip, knee, elbow.

Slightly movable joints

Technical name: amphiarthrosis

The bones at a slightly movable joint can only move a little. They are held together by straps called ligaments and joined by pads of gristly cartilage.

Example: the joints between most vertebrae (backbone).

Cartilage

> protects bones and stops them knocking together.
> forms a cushion between bones at slightly movable joints (e.g. between vertebrae).
> forms a smooth, slippery coat on the ends of bones.
> acts as a shock absorber so the bones don't jar when you run and jump.

Ligaments

> are strong cords or straps that hold bones together.
> hold a joint in place.
> are slightly elastic – just enough to allow the bones to move the way they should.

Freely movable joints and their movements

There are six types...

1 Ball and sockets

The round end of one bone fits into a hollow in the other, and can turn in many directions.

Examples:
Shoulder (scapula-humerus): flexion, extension, abduction, adduction
Hip (acetabulum-femur): rotation, circumduction

2 Hinge

The joint can swing open until it is straight, like a door hinge.

Examples:
Elbow: flexion and extension only (humerus-ulna)
Fingers/toes: phalanges
Shin bone/ankle: talus

3 Pivot

A ring on one bone fits over a peg on the other, allowing rotation.

Examples:
Neck joint between the atlas and axis: rotation only
Elbow: rotation only (head of radius/head or ulna): supination/pronation

Movement types

Different joints allow different kinds of movement. There are 12 kinds of movement in the human body. Try doing them.

1 Flexion – bending

2 Extension – straightening

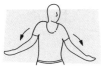

3 Plantar flexion – pointing the toes

4 Dorsi flexion – bringing the toes towards the tibia (leg)

5 Adduction – movement towards the body's midline

6 Abduction – movement from the body's midline

7 Circumduction – a combination of flexion, extension, adduction and abduction

8 Rotation – movement around the long axis of the bone (internal towards body axis; external away from body axis)

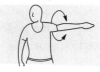

9 Pronation – turning the palm of the hand down

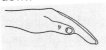

10 Supination – turning the palm up

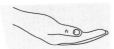

11 Inversion – turning the sole of the foot inwards

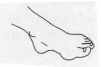

12 Eversion – turning the sole of the foot outwards

4 Condyloid

A bump on one bone sits in the hollow formed by another bone or bones. Movement is back and forward and from side to side. Ligaments prevent rotation.

Examples:
Wrist: flexion
Forearm bones – Carpals: extension
Femur and Tibia (structurally): adduction + adduction = circumduction (Condyloid but acts like a hinge)

5 Saddle

Part of one bone is saddle shaped; the other bone glides on it. Movement is back and forward and from side to side.

Examples:
Thumb – apposition of thumb

6 Gliding

Flat surfaces can glide over each other, giving a limited movement in all directions.

Examples:
Carpals and metacarpals
Femur – Patella
Tarsals and metatarsals
Vertebrae – Ribs

The mechanics of movement

> *Newtonian principles that govern all movements.*

Levers

The joints of our skeleton not only allow movement, they also act as levers. The joint itself is used as the turning point, the fulcrum, to 'take the strain' of pulling one bone nearer, or away from, another bone.

The human body is a system of levers and pulleys that enable us to move. The levers rotate around a series of joints, with the force being provided by muscles attached to bones (acting as pulleys). The resistance comes in the form of body weight and any implement used for sport (e.g. a bat or racquet).

Levers have two functions:

1 To apply force (strength) to an object – the longer the lever distance from the force to fulcrum the greater the force generated.

2 To move the resistance a greater distance or through a greater range of movement. The closer the effort is to the fulcrum, the greater the distance moved.

Joints work most efficiently at around a 90° angle of pull. At low angles and at high angles (120°+) greater strength (effort) is required to maintain the efficiency of the action. Think of any sporting activity: which part of the swing requires the most effort?

Orders of levers

1st order lever
This is a lever where the fulcrum occurs between the effort and resistance.

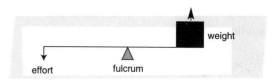

2nd order lever
This lever occurs where the load is between the effort and the fulcrum.

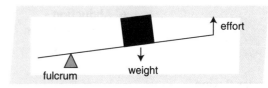

3rd order lever
This lever occurs where the effort lies between the fulcrum and resistance. This is very common in human movement.

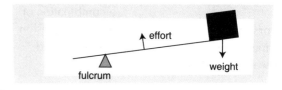

Motion

Force is used to move objects, to stop moving objects and to resist movement in stationary objects. Newton's Laws of Motion rely on an understanding of force.

> Force can be applied with varying sizes and is measured in Newtons (N). This depends on the mass of the body and the effect of gravity.
> Force can be applied in varying directions – the direction of the force dictates the direction of motion of an object if applied to its centre of gravity. This is also known as **linear motion**.
> When force is applied off-centre, it produces movement that is known as angular motion.

Newton's 1st Law

'A body will continue in its state of rest or motion unless another force acts on it.'

All objects have an inertia which must be overcome to change its state of motion (alter its velocity). For example, the 'jack' in bowls will only come to rest when friction force from the grass or mat has overcome its inertia of movement.

Newton's 2nd Law

'The rate of change of velocity (acceleration) of an object is directly proportional to the force acting on it.'

In sport we can propel objects further by imparting greater momentum to that object.

momentum = mass × velocity

For example, a golf ball will travel further if you hit it with the same force but with a heavier club.

Newton's 3rd Law

'Every action has an equal and opposite reaction.'

When one object produces force against another object, it exerts an equal force back in the opposite direction. For example, when a sprinter pushes against the blocks at the start of a race, they push back with equal force, propelling the runner forward.

Centre of gravity, rotation and balance

> *Maintaining balance and initiating rotation.*

Centre of gravity

This is the point in any object where all of its mass (weight) is said to be concentrated.

In an object – known as 'a uniform body' – the **centre of gravity** will be at its geometric centre.

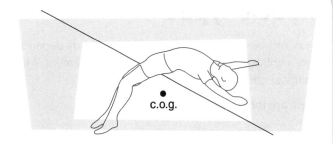

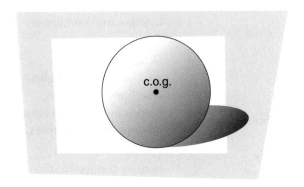

In the human body, the centre of gravity is constantly changing with movement. This is because the centre of gravity is determined by the distribution of mass and the density of the body.

The centre of gravity remains inside the physical body most of the time. However, in some activities the performer deliberately moves the centre of gravity outside the body to improve technique: for example, the high jumper arching over the bar.

Rotation

Rotation, or the turning of a body, occurs when force is applied to that body though not through the centre

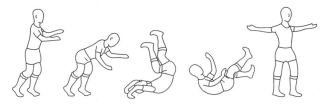

of gravity. When this force occurs, angular motion and rotation can occur around the centre of gravity.

A forward roll is initiated when the centre of gravity moves outside the area of support by a force that does not act through the centre of gravity. The force from the leg muscles pushing onto the ground and the ground returning that force to the feet enables you to shift your centre of gravity. This rotation continues into the forward roll.

Balance

A state of balance is achieved when the centre of gravity is over the area of support for the body. It allows you to hold a position without wobbling or falling over.

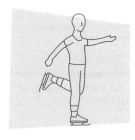

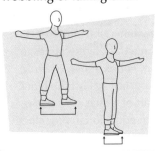

The larger the area of support the easier it is to maintain balance. Standing upright, legs astride is more balanced than on legs close together, or on one leg.

The stability of the balance is affected by the height of the centre of gravity. Lowering the height of the centre of gravity makes a balance much more stable. Headstands are easier to maintain with bent legs initially, than with legs stretched straight. Crouching low makes you harder to knock over in contact sports.

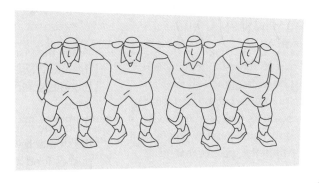

Muscles and muscle function (1)

> *The means of converting chemical energy into mechanical energy.*

Muscle types

Every movement that takes place in your body depends on muscles. They contract and lengthen to produce movement. Muscles convert chemical energy into mechanical energy.

There are three types of muscle:

1 Cardiac

> Called **myocardium** (or cardiac striped) **muscle.**

> Found only in the heart, where linked fibres act in unison.

> Acts as a single sheet of muscle because between the single cells is a very thin disc which has very low resistance to neural impulse (intercalated discs).

> Involuntary and has its own blood supply.

> The heart generates its own impulse to beat, so is called **myogenic.**

> Obeys the 'all-or-nothing law'.

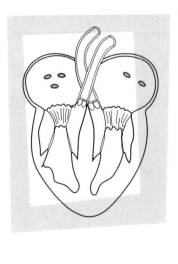

2 Visceral

> Involuntary muscles, because they work without you thinking about it. Controlled by involuntary parts of the nervous system.

> Associated with viscera (internal organs such as arteries, stomach, bowel).

> Composed of minute, spindle-shaped cells whose fibres are so fine they appear smooth.

> Often form circular or longitudinal coats.

> Each muscle fibre does *not* have a separate nerve to control it but the entire sheet is served by a nerve **plexus.**

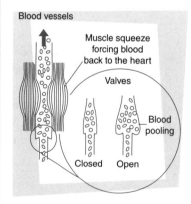

When the visceral muscle in the artery walls contracts, blood is squirted along the artery.

When the visceral muscle in the stomach wall contracts, it pushes food along.

3 Skeletal

> Attached to the skeleton, directly or indirectly.

> Controlled by voluntary parts of the nervous system.

> Composed of large, grooved cells bound together into bundles or sheets.

> Skeletal muscles are attached at their **origins** and **insertions** by a white, fibrous tissue which forms **tendons** or **aponeuroses.**

> The fascia is a tough, fibrous, connective tissue which surrounds muscle bundles.

> During movement the origins remain fixed whilst the insertions move.

> Each muscle fibre is served by a nerve fibre that is attached to the muscle via a 'motor end plate'. Skeletal muscles obey the 'all-or-nothing law'.

> The contraction of the whole muscle is proportional to the number of fibres stimulated.

> Muscle tone is maintained by a small number of fibres being stimulated constantly.

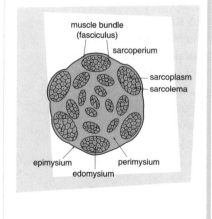

Muscle arrangements

Muscles are normally arranged in pairs so that when one is contracting the other is relaxing. As an example, when the biceps contracts, the triceps muscle relaxes – and the lower arm is raised. Then when the triceps contracts, the biceps must relax or the lower arm will not be lowered.

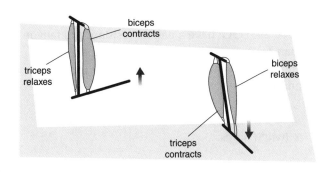

> Muscles that cause the joints to bend are known as **flexors**.
> Muscles that cause the joints to straighten are called **extensors**.
> The muscle that shortens to move the joint is the **prime mover** or **agonist**, whilst the muscle that relaxes is called the **antagonist**.
> Muscles which act as agonist for one movement, act as antagonist muscle for the opposite movement.
> Additionally, muscles which stabilise the origin, so only the insertion moves, are called **fixators** and **synergists**. Fixator muscles hold joints in position so the origin and insertion are on opposite sides of a stabilised joint. Synergist muscles hold the body in position to enable agonists to work.

Muscular contraction

There are four forms of muscle contraction:

1 Isometric (equal length) or static muscle contraction

There is generally no movement resulting from this contraction.

Examples: pushing against a fixed object (e.g. a wall); pushing one hand against the other; arm wrestling.

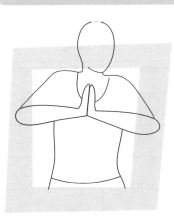

Force of muscle contraction = force expressed by resistance

2 Isotonic – concentric muscle contraction

Equal control. The muscles contract at a speed controlled by the individual. This produces positive movement (shortening of length), which closely mimics the sporting situation to which the training is applied.

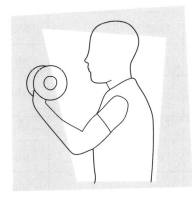

3 Isokinetic – concentric muscle contraction

Equal speed. The point at which the force acts or moves at a constant speed. Specialist machines are required.

4 Polymetrics – eccentric muscle contractions

It has been found that if maximum effort is put into an exercise whilst a muscle is lengthening, then the muscle exerts a much bigger force. This is eccentric or negative exercise.

Examples: bounding exercises; running downhill.

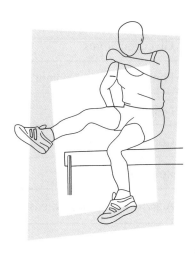

Muscles and muscle function (2)

> *What separates sprinters from marathon runners?*

Types of muscle fibre

By themselves muscle fibres are not very strong, but when lots of them are wrapped together in bundles they make a powerful mass of muscles.

There are two main types of muscle fibre.

Type 1: Slow twitch fibres

> Slow twitch fibres contract at a rate of about 20% slower than fast twitch fibres.

> They are smaller than fast twitch fibres and have smaller motor neurones, thus they generate force comparatively slowly.

> Slow twitch fibres do not fatigue as easily as fast twitch fibres, which makes them perfect for most low-level activities.

Type 2: Fast twitch fibres

Can be further sub-divided:

1 Type 2a: Fast Twitch High Oxidative Glycolytic (FOG) – used for longer sprint events.

2 Type 2b: Fast Twitch Glycolytic (FTG) – used for short sprint events.

Type 2a (FOG) have a greater resistance to fatigue than Type 2b (FTG). This is entirely due to endurance training which encourages muscular adaptation.

All muscles have a mixture of fast and slow twitch fibres.

Fibre-type characteristics

Characteristic	Type 1: slow twitch	Type 2: fast twitch	
Size		*FOG (2a) small*	*FTG (2b) large*
Myoglobin Content	High	High	Low
Capillary Density	High	Midway/High	Low
Mitochondrial Density	High	Midway	Low
Activity during low intensity exercise	High	Midway	Low
Glycogen Stores	Low	High	High
Phosphocreatine Content	Low	Midway	High
Fatigue Level	Low	Midway	High
Contractile Time	Slow	Midway	High
Relaxation Time	Slow	Midway	High
Activity during high intensity exercise	Slow	High	High

An individual muscle is composed of hundreds of **muscle fibres**.

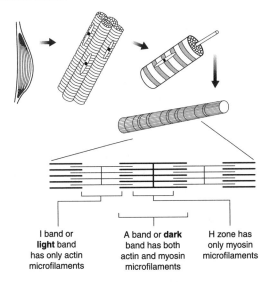

I band or **light** band has only actin microfilaments

A band or **dark** band has both actin and myosin microfilaments

H zone has only myosin microfilaments

Each muscle fibre is composed of many myofibrils.

A myofibril has a distinctive banding pattern due to **microfilaments**.

Sarcomere is the functional basic unit of a myofibril. Thousands of sarcomeres form a long chain in each myofibril.

The Z membrane indicates the boundaries between sarcomeres. The longitudinal protein filaments cause the striated appearance of muscle.

Thick Myosin Filaments (A + H Band)
Thin Action Filaments (A + I Band)

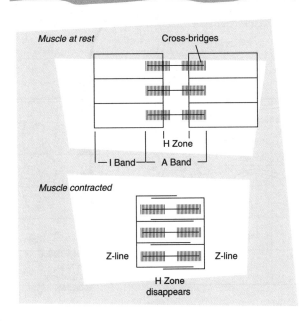

Muscle at rest — Cross-bridges

I Band — A Band — H Zone

Muscle contracted

Z-line — Z-line

H Zone disappears

Huxley's sliding filament theory

In the sarcomere the alternating bands of light and dark areas are caused because of the different thicknesses of actin and myosin. They give clues as to how Huxley's theory works:

> Areas of thicker myosin (A Band, H Zone) form the middle of the sarcomere.

> Areas of thinner actin (also troponin and tropomyosin) (I Band) form the outer parts of the sarcomere and attach to Z discs.

When an impulse arrives at the muscle cell, this triggers the release of calcium ions from 'T' vesicles (sacs within the cytoplasm of cells). The calcium ions bind to troponin and cause the binding sites on actin to be exposed.

Adenosine triphosphate (ATP) – main supplier of metabolic energy in living cells – is broken down and energy is released. This energy is used to power the myosin heads attachment to actin sites.

These cross-bridges (actin-myosin) attach, detach and re-attach further along the actin filament – pulling the actin past the myosin. This has the effect of shortening the length of the sarcomere, as the Z discs are pulled closer together – shortening the muscle.

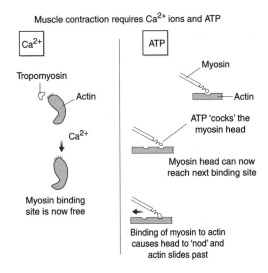

Muscle contraction requires Ca^{2+} ions and ATP

This process has been likened to the action of a person climbing a rope. The arms and legs represent the cross bridges. Movement occurs because the limbs reach and grasp then pull, break contact then reach and grasp then pull and so on; the cross bridges do the same.

Controlling muscular action

> *How the body applies just enough strength to do a job.*

A motor unit producing movement

A neurone (or neuron) forms the basic cellular unit of the nervous system. It is capable of carrying nerve impulses to muscles. A motor neurone controls large numbers of individual fibres – together they form a **motor unit**.

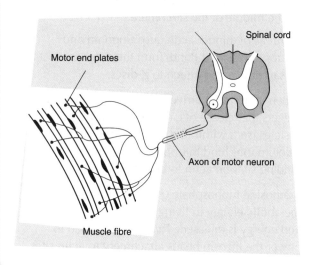

The axon branches as it reaches the muscle. The branches connect with a structure called the **motor end plate**.

Messages sent along motor neurones are electrochemical in nature. The generation of the messages relies upon an 'action potential' occurring in the axon. This occurs where the axon becomes 'leaky' and K^+ (potassium) ions diffuse out and N^+ (nitrogen) ions diffuse in.

To increase the speed of transfer, 'saltatory conduction' is used. This involves ion exchange occurring only at nodes on the axon known as 'nodes of Ranvier'[1].

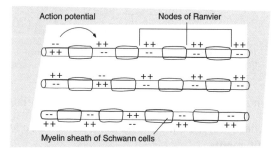

[1]named after Louis-Antoine Ranvier (1835-1922); the Schwann cells are named after Theodor Schwann (1810-1882)

The function of motor end plates

Motor end plates transfer the electrical impulse from motor neurones to muscle fibres.

> There is a delay of approximately 0.5 ms (microseconds) in order for the release of Acetylcholine (the carrier of the signal) from the synaptic knob.

> An area of depolarisation travels down the muscle cell which initiates the release of Ca^{2+} (calcium ions) from the 'T' vesicles (see page 9).

> This, in turn, causes the sliding filaments to begin their action.

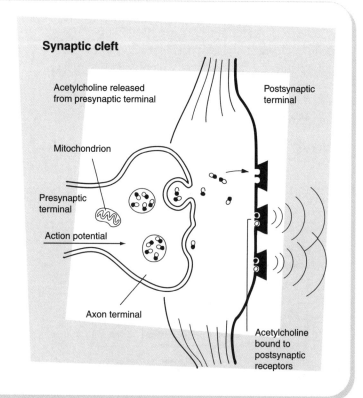

Motor neurone firing patterns

Neurones are of different types depending on their position in the nervous system. Motor neurones have short dendrons and long axons. Nerve impulses that are carried along the neurone are fired in various patterns.

Here are some of those firing patterns.

Muscle twitch

Stimuli received by neurone pools are transmitted to different motor units, which may not act in unison. The stimulus must be sufficiently strong to activate one motor unit in order to produce any contraction. **ALL** of the muscle fibres in that motor unit will contract maximally for a fraction of a second ('all-or-nothing law').

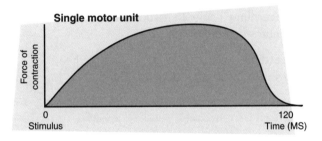

Graduation of contraction

Muscles contract for longer than a fraction of a second when a stimulus occurs that activates many motor neurones (different motor units will be involved, not necessarily in succession). This allows muscles to exert forces of graded strength. This skill is learned over time and through varied practice.

Wave summation

The strength of a muscle contraction can be increased in another way. If a second impulse is received by a neurone pool very quickly, there will not be time for relaxation before the next contraction starts. This increase in rate of stimulation to produce stronger contractions is **wave summation**.

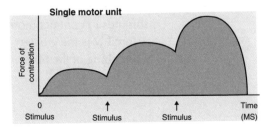

Absolute contraction

If stimuli arrive so fast there is no time for any relaxation, a state of 'absolute contraction' occurs.

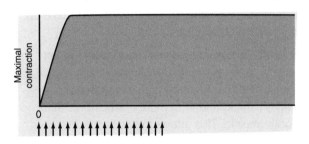

Spatial summation

This is the term given to the phenomenon of different motor units being stimulated across the whole muscle to produce contraction. Spatial summation allows the use of stores of ATP (adenosine triphosphate) to be shared around the whole muscle, thus reducing fatigue.

The *staggered* nature of the working of the motor units is an important factor in maintaining sustained contraction. Some motor units will be relaxing (and recovering) whilst others are contracting, which allows long periods of contraction.

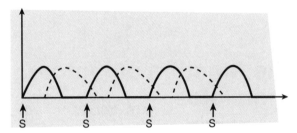

(Note: all muscle action requires the development of isometric tension in order to overcome inertia and to initiate movement.)

Co-ordinated contraction relies on the factors above and sensory feedback which adjusts contraction. These are produced by specialist proprioceptors and nerves, e.g.

Golgi -Tendon Apparatus + Muscle Spindles

The information received plays a role in decision making.

Reciprocal innervation is the constant adjustment of tension in antagonistic muscle groups based on sensory information from each muscle group. The **cerebellum** (brain) acts as a 'sorting office' for information which is then relayed to muscles to produce fine movement control.

The heart – structure

> *The never-tiring, non-stop muscle – the wellspring of the body.*

The body's pump

The heart is a muscular pump that beats nearly 4 million times a year. It pumps blood around the miles of arteries, veins and capillaries that make up the circulatory system.

The aorta carries oxygenated blood from the left ventricle to the systemic circulation. It is a typical elastic (conducting) artery with a wall that is relatively thick, and with more elastic fibres than smooth muscle. This allows the aorta to accommodate the surges of blood associated with the alternative contraction and relaxation of the heart.

The **pressure** generated by the left ventricle is greater than that generated by the right ventricle as the systemic circuit is more extensive than the pulmonary circuit.

The pressure generated by the atria is less than that generated by the ventricles since the distance from atria to ventricles is less than that from ventricles to circulatory system.

The same **volume** of blood passes through each side of the heart, so circulating volumes are also equal in the pulmonary and systemic circuits.

> When resting, the heart beats around 70 times a minute.
> It beats 100,000 times in a day.
> 7500 litres of blood pass through the heart each day – enough to fill a small road tanker.

Structures

Pericardium – the closed sac that surrounds the heart. It is fluid filled to reduce the effects of friction and to protect the heart.

Myocardium – cardiac muscle – composed of muscle cells with a single nucleus, but many mitochondria.

Endocardium – smooth tissues inside the heart chambers to aid blood flow.

Epicardium – outer layer of tissue of the heart. Links with inner layer of pericardium.

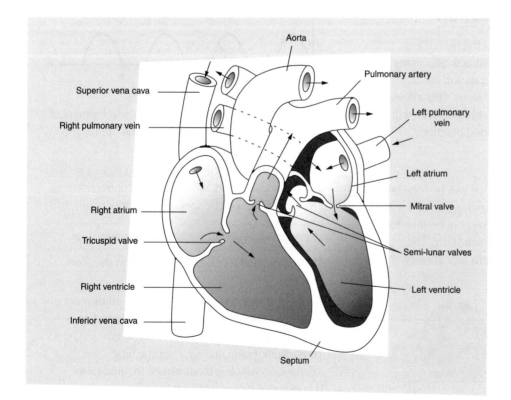

Starling's Law of the heart

Cardiac output is dependent on venous return (i.e. the amount of blood returned to the right side of the heart). During exercise venous return increases, thus cardiac output increases. This is because the myocardium is stretched and then contracts with greater force due to the increased stretch. The stimulus to contract more forcibly is the greater stretching of the fibres.

Heartbeat

Blood is supplied to the heart muscle itself via coronary arteries that branch from the aorta. Deoxygenated blood from the heart muscles is fed directly back to the right atrium via coronary veins and coronary sinus.

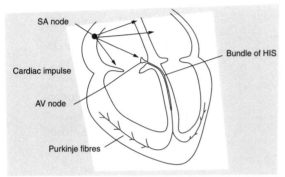

The heartbeat is initiated by electrical impulses which originate from the heart's 'pacemaker', the **sino-atrial node** (particularly excitable tissue in the wall of the right atrium; labelled as SA node). The impulse travels down the myocardium of the atrium until it reaches the **atrio-ventricular node** (AV node). A short delay occurs to allow atrial systole – see page 14 – to complete. The impulse then enters specialist tissues called **'Bundles of HIS'** which branch through the septum as **Purkinje fibres**[1]. These connect to myocardium fibres which cause the ventricles to contract (ventricular systole).

This process can be seen by tracing the electrical signals in the heart using an ECG (electrocardiogram).

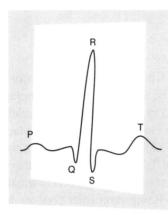

P = a wave of electrical energy just before the atria contract – impulse travelling from SA node to AV node.

Q, R, S = a wave of electrical energy just before the ventricles contract – impulse travelling from AV node along bundles of HIS and Purkinje fibres.

T = repolarisation of ventricle walls before relaxation (diastole).

1 **Intrinsic heart** rate is about 78 beats per minute.
2 **External (extrinsic)** factors may modify the basic heart rate:
> **vagus nerve** decreases heart rate
> **accelerator nerve** increases heart rate
> **adrenaline** and **thyroxine** increase heart rate.

1 Named after Jan Evangelista Purkinje (1787-1869)

Stroke volume (SV) – the amount of blood ejected from the heart when the ventricles contract[1].

(All figures approximate)

Untrained at rest	70 ml	Untrained maximal exercise	113 ml
Trained at rest	100 ml	Trained maximal exercise	179 ml

Heart rate (HR) – number of ventricular contractions in one minute

Untrained at rest	70 beats/minute	Untrained maximal exercise	195 beats/minute
Trained at rest	50 beats/minute	Trained maximal exercise	195 beats/minute

Cardiac output (Q) – the amount of blood ejected from the heart in one minute

Untrained at rest	5,000 ml (5 litres)	Untrained maximal exercise	22,000 ml (22 litres)
Trained at rest	5,000 ml (5 litres)	Trained maximal exercise	35,000 ml (35 litres)

Q = SV x HR

1 Stroke volume is increased due to (training) exercise as both the size of the heart and the muscle wall thickness increase. The larger and more powerful the heart, the fewer times it needs to beat in order to circulate the same amount of blood. Reduced heart rate at rest is known as 'bradycardia'.

The heart – cardiac cycle

> *How the heart works.*

Cardiac cycle

Two phases in the cycle:
> Relaxation – diastole 0.5 secs
> Contraction – systole 0.3 secs

The cycle starts

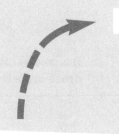

Systole

The SA node initiates an impulse causing a wave of contraction across the atrial myocardium, forcing the remaining blood out of the atria into the ventricles. Semi-lunar valves remain closed, but atrio-ventricular valves close after the passage of blood. This causes one of the heart sounds. The 'lub' of 'lub dub'. The impulse then reaches the AV node which then spreads a second contraction through the ventricle walls. Rising ventricular pressure forces open the semi-lunar valves to the lungs and systemic arteries.

Once the blood has left the heart and the contraction ceases the semi-lunar valves snap shut causing the 'dub' sound in the heart.

Diastole

Right and left atria fill with blood and the atrioventricular valves are closed (mitral & tricuspid).

Rising atrial pressure forces open the atrioventricular valves and the ventricles begin to fill. The semi-lunar valves to the aorta and pulmonary arteries are closed.

Heart rate regulation

This occurs via the sympathetic and parasympathetic nervous systems. These originate in the cardiac centre of the medulla oblongata (brain stem) – they work antagonistically. The effect of exercise is to speed up the heart rate (HR). This is achieved by the sympathetic nerves transmitting impulses to the SA node and the release of **norepinephrine,** a transmitter substance.

Baroreceptors located in the carotid artery and aorta respond to increased blood pressure by sending messages back to the cardiac centre. This, in turn, sends out impulses via the vagus nerve (parasympathetic nerves) to the SA node to slow down the heart rate.

THIS IS NEGATIVE FEEDBACK CONTROL.

Other factors affecting heart rate include:
> raised temperature
> hormonal release (e.g. adrenaline – this substance redirects blood flow and increases glycolysis)
> excess potassium can slow down HR
> age – HR drops with age one beat per year
> gender – females tend to have higher heart rates than males.

Heart rate is dependent upon a balance between sympathetic nerves (SNS) and parasympathetic nerves (PNS), which adjust to changing conditions.

Information received from peripheral sensors – e.g. baroreceptors (blood pressure); chemoreceptors (chemical sensors) and proprioceptors (in joints and tissues) – in the cardiac centre of the medulla oblongata is interpreted and redirected via SNS and PNS to the SA node.

Heart rate and exercise

1 Resting heart rate 60–70 beats/minute.
2 Pre-exercise anticipatory rise (adrenaline release).
3 Exercise begins – blood pressure increases, CO_2 content increases.
4 Steep rise in heart rate as exercise increases in intensity.
5 A plateau occurs near to age-predicted maximum heart rate despite an increase in exercise intensity.
6 Exercise ends and the heart rate immediately begins to rapidly fall, blood pressure decreases, CO_2 content decreases, venous return reduces.
7 Longer recovery period close to resting levels to help clear the by-products of tissue respiration.
8 Return to normal.

The body's transport system – blood

> *The fluid of life.*

Blood is the body's internal transport system. The blood vessels carry the raw materials along the network of arteries, veins and capillaries to all the consumers of the body – from major organs to each and every individual living cell.

Function: transport

> Food from alimentary canal
> Oxygen from lungs to tissues
> Waste from tissues to the excretory surface
> Hormones from the endocrine system
> White corpuscles to fight infection
> Heat.

Function: protection

> Salts to provide a buffering action to protect cells
> White corpuscles to fight disease
> Clotting properties
> White corpuscles to help wounds heal.

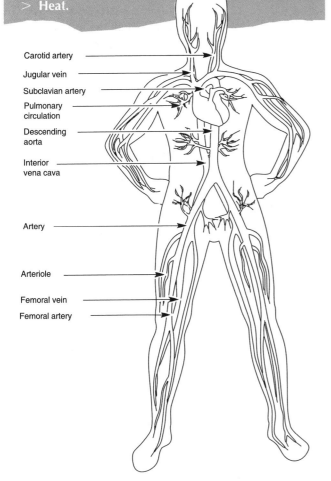

Carotid artery
Jugular vein
Subclavian artery
Pulmonary circulation
Descending aorta
Interior vena cava
Artery
Arteriole
Femoral vein
Femoral artery

What is blood?

If blood is spun for a few minutes in a high-speed centrifuge it separates into two layers:

1 Plasma (55%)

Straw-coloured fluid. At least 90% water, dissolved in which are salts, glucose, fatty acids, waste products, enzymes and hormones.

2 Cells (corpuscles) (45%)

Eosinophils

Neutrophils

Basophils

Lymphocytes

Red cells

Platelets (Thrombocytes)

Monocytes

> **red cells,** or **erythrocytes** – most numerous; red colour due to presence of haemoglobin (oxygen-carrying protein); relatively short lived. Carry oxygen (O_2), carbon dioxide (CO_2) and carbon monoxide (CO) around the body. Typical lifespan of a red cell is 19–20 days.

> **white cells,** or **leucocytes** – help to fight disease and injury in the body. There are various types: neutrophils (most abundant; very short lived; migrate from blood to tissues; replaced at the rate of 100000 million every day); monocytes (largest type; spend a short time in circulatory system before moving into the tissues); lymphocytes (30%; produced in bone marrow but continue to develop in lymph nodes, thymus gland and spleen; produce antibodies).

> **platelets,** or **thrombocytes** – fragments of cells which are involved in blood clotting.

> **basophils** – secrete large amounts of histamine (which increases swelling) and heparin (which helps to keep a balance between blood clotting and not clotting).

> **eosinophils** – help control the allergic response (e.g. secrete enzymes which activate histamine); numbers increase during an allergic reaction and in response to some parasitic infections.

The body's transport system – blood vessels

> *The motorways of the body.*

2 Arterioles

These have the same structure as arteries but are much narrower.

Function: to control blood flow into capillaries (due to vasomotor control).

1 Arteries

An artery is surrounded by 'smooth' muscle which controls the size of the lumen through which the blood flows. It carries oxygenated blood under pressure. This flows in spurts as the heart beats.

Thick elastic walls have three layers:

> **interna** – forms the inner lining of the vessel with endothelium

> **media** – formed of smooth muscle and elastin

> **externa** – formed of collagen and elastin to allow the walls to be elastic and cope with changes in blood volume.

3 Capillaries

Smallest blood vessels in the body – they pass through most muscle and other tissues.

Capillary bed – total capillary structure within a muscle or organ. The number of capillaries can be increased by training, thus O_2 and other nutrients can be delivered efficiently. Total cross-section of capillary bed is much greater than a single artery, so the speed of blood flow is dramatically reduced.

This allows greater efficiency in diffusion of O_2 into muscle tissue and diffusion of CO_2 out across the single cell layer of endothelium tissue. Once CO_2 and other waste products have been collected, the blood leaves the capillary bed and enters venules.

6 Vena cava

The final veins before blood gets back to the heart.

5 Veins

Blood vessels carrying deoxygenated blood from capillaries back to the heart. They have a muscular coat, which affects the tone of the veins due to venomotor control. This allows changes in capacity of blood flow.

4 Venules

These begin the journey of deoxygenated blood back to the heart. The blood pressure is low, so the blood has a smooth flow. This is achieved because of:

> smooth flow from the capillaries

> pressure from surrounding organs (e.g. working muscles – important for cool down)

> valves to prevent backflow

> suction caused by decreasing pressure in thorax due to inhalation.

Blood flow in muscles

The rate of blood flow around the body depends on a number of variables:

> physical activity – muscles demand more O_2
> cardiac output
> circulation.

Blood pressure also changes due to:

> cardiac output
> peripheral resistance – altered by vasodilation and vasoconstriction[1], by blood viscosity (thickness), and by the changing shape and size of arterioles. Precapillary sphincters (circular tract of muscles) also control blood flow to capillaries. Messages come from the vasomotor and venomotor centres – both centres are located in the medulla oblongata and are regulated by sympathetic and parasympathetic nervous systems.

Vasomotor control

A fall in blood pressure reduces stimulation of baroreceptors. The vasomotor centre sends nerve impulses to arterioles causing them to vasoconstrict; hence an increase in blood pressure and heart rate.

An increase in blood pressure increases stimulation of baroreceptors, which causes the vasomotor centre to send out more impulses to cause vasodilation, so reducing blood pressure.

Venomotor control

Veins can alter their shape on receipt of signals from the sympathetic and parasympathetic nervous systems by altering the venomotor tone of their muscular 'coats'.

Venous return

The volume of blood leaving the heart has a direct relationship with the pumping action of the heart. Blood flow in the veins also increases. (Thus venous return.) Veins contain approximately $\frac{3}{5}$th of circulating blood at any one time. Venous return must be in excess of the rest of the blood in the body in order to maintain steady blood flow. During exercise, the working muscles squeeze the veins, thus increasing venal return (muscle pump). During inspiration (breathing in), the reduction in pressure in the thorax aids venous return as the blood will move to low pressure areas (respiratory pump).

Stroke volume levels out before maximum effort is achieved.

Tissue fluid during exercise

High blood pressure at the arteriole end of the capillary bed forces fluid through the capillary wall into the cell spaces. Tissue cells extract O_2 + glucose; they excrete CO_2, etc. where blood pressure is lowest at the venous end of the capillary bed.

> **Exercise increases systolic blood pressure**
> ▼
> **thus increasing tissue fluid production**
> ▼
> **thus more nutrients are available for tissue respiration.**

1 Ability of blood vessels, particularly capillaries, to increase (vasodilation) or decrease (vasoconstriction) in diameter under nervous or hormonal control. When you are at risk of overheating, vasodllation of capillaries in the skin allows more blood to flow to the surface of the body, where heat can be lost by radiation. When cold, vasoconstriction prevents blood from flowing near the body surface, and heat is conserved deeper in the body.

Blood flow

Blood flow at rest

Total blood flow: 25 litres/minute

- Bone marrow: 5%
- Brain: 18%
- Heart: 5%
- Liver and gut: 25%
- Kidneys: 20%
- Skeletal muscle: 20%
- Skin: 7%

0 10 20 30 40 50 60 70 80 90
% blood flow to various organs

Blood flow during exercise

Total blood flow: 25 litres/minute

- Bone marrow: 1%
- Brain: 3%
- Heart: 4%
- Liver and gut: 2%
- Kidneys: 1%
- Skeletal muscle: 87%
- Skin: 2%

0 10 20 30 40 50 60 70 80 90
% blood flow to various organs

The mechanics of breathing

> *How the body causes movement of air in and out of the lungs.*

Inspiration and expiration

Inspiration and expiration are caused by the changes in air pressure inside the lungs (i.e. intra-pulmonary). This is relative to atmospheric pressure. The changes in pressure are caused by muscular action of the intercostal muscles and diaphragm. (This has implications for high- and low-pressure training and physical activity.)

Inspiration occurs as a result of changes in the size of the thorax, due to muscular action that reduces pressure inside the pleural membranes. This reduction is enough to cause air to rush into the low-pressure area of the lungs. Expiration is caused by an increase of pressure on the pleural membrane from the falling ribs and returning diaphragm. Also the alveoli, which have been stretched during inspiration, recoil – forcing air out of the lungs.

The respiratory muscles

1 Primary

> 11 pairs of intercostal muscles between the 12 pairs of ribs, arranged in two layers (internal and external).

> Internal muscle fibres attach from the lower margin of the rib above the upper margin of the rib below. The upper attachment is nearer the sternum.

> External fibres lie on top of internal fibres and point in the opposite direction.

As the first rib is fixed when the external fibres contract, the ribs can move towards the fixed rib (i.e. an upward and outward movement), thus causing the thoracic cage to expand. During quiet breathing, gravity returns the cage to its normal position, thus causing *expiration*. (Intercostal nerves originate in the medulla oblongata.)

Diaphragm: sheet of muscle that forms the floor of the thoracic cavity. It attaches to the vertebrae column, ribs and sternum, and radiates from a central tendon. The diaphragm is innervated by phrenic nerves. When contracting, the central tendon is pulled down, thus enlarging the thoracic cavity (reducing pressure) – causing *inhalation*.

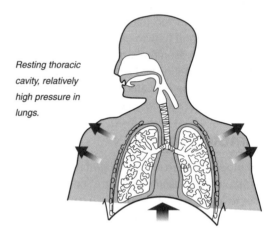

Resting thoracic cavity, relatively high pressure in lungs.

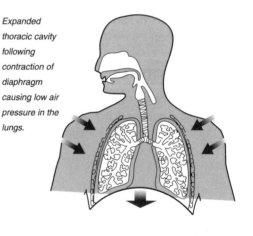

Expanded thoracic cavity following contraction of diaphragm causing low air pressure in the lungs.

2 Secondary (during exercise only)

At rest, when air requirements are low, there is no need for violent breathing movements. Heavier demands (e.g. during exercise) require contraction of the external intercostal muscles (see right).

Abdominal muscles force air out of the lungs during expiration and the internal intercostal muscles aid gravity by contracting, reducing the thorax dimensions.

Scaleni + Sternocleidomastoids contract
▼
raising first rib and sternum.
Trapezius + Back and Neck Extensors also contract
▼
increase in size of thorax.

Chemical and nervous regulation of the breathing mechanism

Breathing rates are controlled subconsciously by the medulla oblongata. The **apneustic centre** controls inspiration and the **pneumotaxic centre** controls expiration. Inspiration occurs due to an increased rate of firing of the inspiratory neurones and the recruitment of new motor units. Expiration is initiated by the abrupt cessation of the neurones firing.

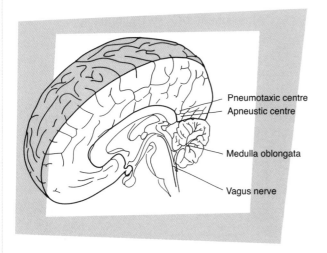

Pneumotaxic centre
Apneustic centre

Medulla oblongata

Vagus nerve

Excess inspiration is limited by the activation of stretch receptors in the bronchioles and bronchi which, when stimulated, send impulses via the vagus nerve to the medulla oblongata. These impulses either cause inspiration to be inhibited and or expiration to be stimulated. This is known as the **Hering–Breuer Reflex.**

1   Hg = chemical symbol for mercury; air pressure is measured on instruments using mercury (e.g. barometer).

Chemical controls

Peripheral chemoreceptors in the carotid arteries and the aorta respond to chemical changes in the blood – by sending impulses to the respiratory centres in the medulla oblongata.

Oxygen (O_2)

If partial pressure of O_2 falls below a certain level (60 mm Hg[1]), there is a marked increase in ventilation. This is because at 60 mm Hg **haemoglobin** is 90% saturated and transportation is still efficient, below this threshold oxygen transport is severely affected.

> **Haemoglobin:** protein composed of 4 chains, each of which contains a single atom of iron. It is with the iron atom that a molecule of O_2 combines; so each haemoglobin molecule can combine with 4 molecules of O_2. When all the iron atoms in a group of haemoglobin molecules are combined with O_2, the haemoglobin is said to be saturated (100%).

Carbon dioxide (CO_2)

Increases in CO_2 in the arteries results in an increase of carbonic acid in blood. Bicarbonate[2] buffering occurs and hydrogen (H^+) ions are formed. Increased hydrogen ion concentration stimulates increased ventilation; decreased concentrations inhibit ventilation.

Hydrogen ion concentration

When this occurs for reasons other than increased CO_2 level in blood (e.g. accumulation of lactic acid during exercise), this induces **hyperventilation.** The rate of excretion of CO_2 is increased, thus lower arterial levels of CO_2 and hydrogen ions.

2   Bicarbonate is the traditional name for hydrogencarbonate (acid salt of carbonic acid in which only one of the hydrogen atoms has been replaced).

How much air do you breathe?

> Tidal volume (TV): volume of air you breathe in (or out) with each breath.

> Respiratory rate (RR): number of breaths you take per minute.

> Minute volume (MV): volume of air you breathe in per minute.

> All three increase during exercise.

MV = TV × RR

For a typical 18-year-old		
	At rest	*During exercise*
TV (litres)	0.5	2.5
RR (breaths/min.)	12	30
MV (litres/min.)	6	75

Gas exchange in lungs

> *Getting oxygen from the atmosphere to the body's tissues.*

How air changes in your lungs

Air in

> about 21% oxygen

> about 79% nitrogen

> a tiny amount of carbon dioxide

> a little water vapour

Air out

> about 17% oxygen

> about 79% nitrogen

> 3% carbon dioxide

> a lot of water vapour

The respiration system works in conjunction with the vascular (blood transport) system in the process of gas exchange. Oxygen is transported from the lung alveoli to the working tissue cells (ultimate destination the mitochondria), whilst CO_2 travels in the opposite direction within the blood.

During inspiration, atmospheric air rushes into the lungs to equalise the pressures. It fills the alveoli sacs. Surrounding some of these sacs is a dense network of capillaries rich in blood. The air enters these sacs at rest. During exercise, there is a greater amount of air inspired; some must go to alveoli poorly supplied with blood, therefore O_2 is under-utilised. However, exercise induces an increase in the density of the capillaries within the lungs (and muscles) which effectively increases the surface area for O_2 exchange – thus more O_2 is utilised.

Gas moves in and out of the circulatory system by the process of **diffusion** (molecules move from areas of high concentration [pressure] to areas of low concentration [pressure] across the thin membrane separating alveoli and capillaries). In the capillaries about 98.5% of the O_2 combines with haemoglobin (Hb) for transportation. Diffusion is aided because the red corpuscles of blood are squeezed flatter in the tiny capillaries, thus increasing their surface area.

Partial pressure oxygen (pO_2)

Atmospheric air is a mixture of gases. At sea level the total pressure of the molecules of these gases is 760 mm Hg. Approximately 21% of air is oxygen, thus the amount of pressure applied by O_2 is 760 × 0.21 = 159.9 mm Hg (160 mm Hg). This is called the partial pressure of oxygen ($pO2$). Because the molecules in air are so far apart they do not influence each other.

Partial pressure oxygen (pO_2)

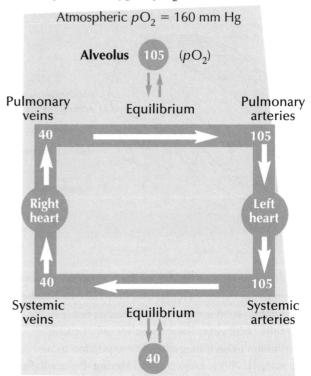

At each inspiration about 350 ml of air enters the lungs, to be added to the 2500 ml already contained there. The oxygen concentration is therefore diluted, thus alveoli O_2 has a partial pressure of about 105 mm Hg. Alveoli partial pressure remains fairly constant as inspiration raises pO_2 but decreases CO_2 – the amounts of change are insignificant as the amounts of air are relatively small compared with the air already held in the lungs.

The most important factor controlling the O_2 saturation of Hb is the partial pressure of O_2 in blood plasma (the concentration of dissolved O_2).

> As plasma oxygen increases, Hb saturation increases. In venous blood, pO_2 is 40 mm Hg and Hb is 75% saturated. In arterial blood, pO_2 is 105 mm Hg and Hb is 98% saturated.

> When the partial pressure of O_2 in the plasma is 60 mm Hg, the haemoglobin is 90% saturated. This means that even if the partial pressure of O_2 drops from its normal value of 100% down to 60%, the amount of O_2 carried by the haemoglobin would decrease by only 10%. This provides a safety factor that guarantees a constant supply of oxygen to the tissues. For this reason, certain respiratory and circulatory diseases that result in a lower alveolar ventilation do not have a significant effect on the delivery of oxygen to the tissues.

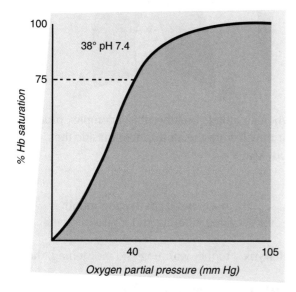

NOTE: pH = acidity

> As acidity increases, less oxygen combines with Hb.

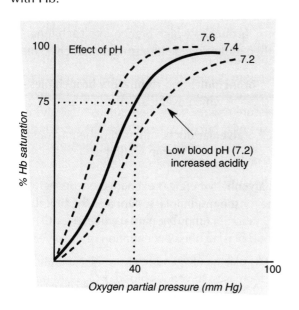

> As temperature increases, less O_2 combines with Hb.

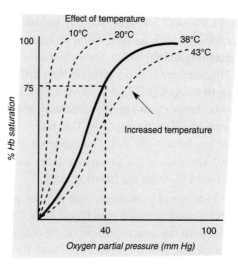

The pO_2 in capillary blood is approximately 40 mm Hg. Thus O_2 diffuses across the alveoli-capillary membrane to equalise concentrations (i.e. pO_2 on both sides of the membrane are identical at 105 mm Hg).

As the blood is then pumped to the tissue sites where O_2 is required to produce energy, a partial pressure gradient occurs between blood at 105 mm Hg and tissue cells at 40 mm Hg. Thus O_2 diffuses into the tissue cells until an equilibrium is achieved when venous blood is at 40 mm Hg. Venous blood returns to the lungs.

Gas transport

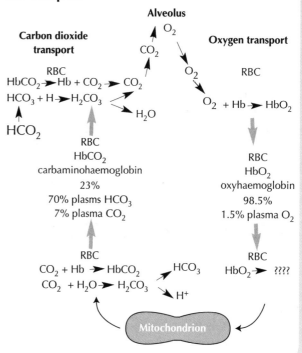

Gas exchange and reactions

> *More about how we use and move oxygen and carbon dioxide.*

More about gas exchange

1 About 98.5% of O_2 is transported by red blood cells combined with haemoglobin. This is known as **oxyhaemoglobin** (HbO_2). The extent to which O_2 + Hb combine is dependent on the partial pressure of oxygen ($pO2$). A relatively high pO_2 in the lungs causes greater diffusion across the alveoli capillary membrane. (This has implications for activity at high altitude.) A relatively low pO_2 in the tissue capillaries causes the release of O_2 from the haemoglobin.

2 Most CO_2 released from tissue cells diffuses into the blood stream, then into red blood cells. CO_2 combines with the amino portion of the protein in haemoglobin, whilst O_2 combines with the iron portion. This means that O_2 and CO_2 can be transported simultaneously with no competition.

   In the red blood cells some CO_2 combines with H_2O to form carbonic acid (H_2CO_3) and some combines with haemoglobin to form **carbominohaemoglobin** ($HbCO_2$).

3 About 70% of CO_2 is transported in the blood plasma as **bicarbonate ions** (HCO_3^-). CO_2 is thus transported dissolved in the water of the plasma.

Carbonic anhydrase

This is an enzyme that catalyzes the reaction between CO_2 and H_2O. The resulting H_2CO_3 breaks up, releasing $H^- + HCO_3^-$ ions.

Bicarbonate ions (HCO_3^-) diffuse into blood plasma and are transported to the lungs where the process is reversed, releasing CO_2 to diffuse into lungs.

The Bohr effect

As we have seen, as acidity in the blood increases, haemoglobin releases O_2 more readily. Known as the Bohr effect (see Gas transport diagram –page 21), hydrogen ions exert this effect by combining with Hb and altering its molecular structure.

BPG (bisphosphoglycerate)

This is a substance formed in red blood cells during glycolysis[1]. It binds with haemoglobin, causing it to have a lower affinity with O_2. Glycolysis and BPG production increase when there is an insufficient oxygen supply to the tissues, e.g. during the early stages of intense exercise.

The respiratory system

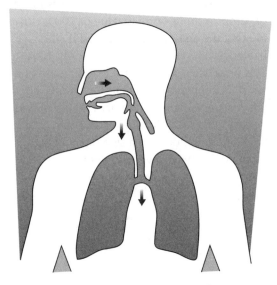

When an athlete breathes it is a complex process. Air travels from the atmosphere outside the body via:

the **nose, nasal cavity,** and **mouth** – for warming, filtering and moistening, the …

pharynx – further warming and moistening, the …

larynx – containing the epiglottis which closes during swallowing to prevent food entering the lungs; air passes from the larynx into the …

trachea – a single airway which descends and divides into …

bronchi – which branch into each lung, then further divide into smaller branches, the …

bronchioles and **respiratory bronchioles** – which eventually lead to the…

alveolar ducts – then into the millions of thin-walled …

alveoli – where gas exchange occurs between the respiratory system and the blood (in pulmonary capillaries).

1 A series of reactions in which glucose is converted. The process is anaerobic and represents the first phase in the breakdown of glucose during respiration.

Gas exchange and altitude

> *How altitude affects training and performance*

Gaseous exchange relies on the partial pressure of oxygen creating a diffusion gradient to facilitate diffusion. With increasing altitude, the partial pressure of oxygen reduces the efficiency of the respiration process.

This hypoxic condition affects performance at altitude, and the athlete's body adapts and changes to the new demands made on it. The athlete's production of EPO (erythropoietin) is stimulated, which increases the production of red blood cells and enhances the blood's oxygen-carrying capacity.

In theory, following a period exposed to conditions at altitude, an athlete returning to sea level should enjoy temporarily enhanced oxygen-carrying capacity. However, this gain may be offset by the detraining effect of working at altitude, when levels of work must be reduced.

Evidence suggests that training at between 2000-3000 m above sea level, though difficult and expensive, allows for the greatest benefit.

Performance in aerobic events at high altitude decreases whenever short-lived power events not reliant on the aerobic system have enhanced performance, possibly due to reduced resistance of the air. Athletes whose normal conditions are those of sea level return to their base-level cardiac functioning quickly after they return. Athletes whose homes are at high altitude, but who train at sea-level conditions, do benefit from a more prolonged 'altitude effect'. 'Sea-level' athletes may use hypoxic chambers to stimulate the hypoxic conditions found at high levels (an ergogenic aid).

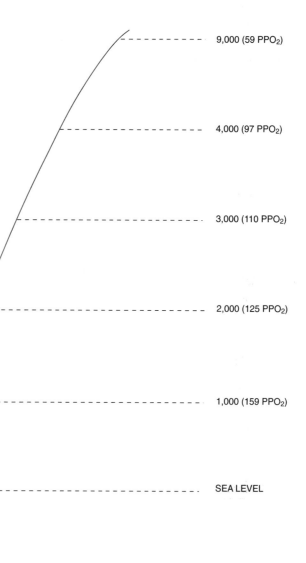

9,000 (59 PPO_2)

4,000 (97 PPO_2)

3,000 (110 PPO_2)

2,000 (125 PPO_2)

1,000 (159 PPO_2)

SEA LEVEL

Respiratory volumes

> *Adjusting volumes of air in the lungs.*

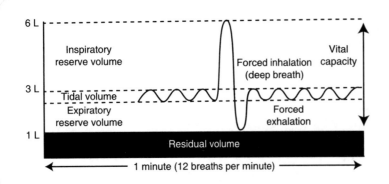

Inspiratory reserve volume = 3100 ml
Vital capacity = 4800 ml
Tidal volume = 500 ml
Total lung capacity = 6000 ml
Expiratory Reserve Volume = 1200 ml
Residual Volume = 1200 ml
Minute Volume – the volume of air inspired or expired in 1 minute: 12 × 500 = 6000 ml/min.

When you are resting, you inhale about 500 millilitres (ml) of air with each breath you take, and exhale about the same amount. You can increase the amount of air taken in by forcing your diaphragm and inspiratory intercostal muscles (see page 18) to expand further than normal. Similarly, you can increase the amount of air exhaled by contracting the intercostal expiratory muscles. Try it for yourself. Breathe in, forcing your ribcage to expand as you do so. Then breathe out, forcing as much air out of your lungs as you can. Repeat this, using the air you exhale to fill up a balloon. How big can you get the balloon with one puff?

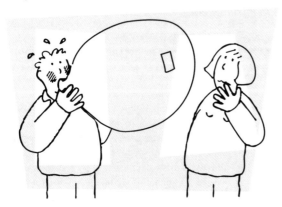

> Normally, expiration (breathing out) is a passive activity resulting from the elastic recoil of the lung tissues.

> The amount of air that enters the lungs during a normal, quiet inspiration is about 500 ml; it is called the **tidal volume**. The same volume leaves the lungs during a normal expiration.

> During forced inhalation (a deep breath), the volume of air inspired over and above the tidal volume is called the **inspiratory reserve**. This volume can be as much as 3100 ml. The inspiratory reserve can increase the normal tidal volume 6-fold.

> During forced expiration, the volume of air expired over and above the tidal volume is called the **expiratory reserve**. This volume can be as much as 1200 ml of air. It requires forceful contractions of the intercostal expiratory muscles (internal intercostals, external oblique, rectus abdominis, internal oblique and transversus abdominis).

> Even after the most forceful expiration, some air remains in the lungs. This is called the **residual volume** and equals about 1200 ml. The residual volume prevents the lungs from collapsing. Because residual air remains in the lungs at all times, newly inhaled air is always mixed with air partially depleted of oxygen that is already in the lungs. This prevents the oxygen and carbon dioxide concentrations in the lungs from fluctuating excessively with each breath.

> The vital capacity is the maximum amount of air a person can exhale after taking the deepest breath possible. It is approximately 10-times the volume of air exhaled at rest.

Vital Capacity = Tidal Volume + Inspiratory Reserve + Expiratory Reserve
4800 ml = 500 ml + 3100 ml + 1200 ml

> The vital capacity plus the residual volume equals the **total lung capacity,** which is about 6000 ml. This total varies with age, sex, and body size.

> Some of the air that enters the respiratory tract during breathing fails to reach the alveoli. This volume (about 150 ml) remains in the conducting portion of the bronchial tree (trachea, bronchi and bronchioles). Since gas exchanges do not occur through the walls of these passageways, this air is said to occupy the 'dead space' (i.e. it is non-functional for gas exchange).

Lifestyle considerations

> *The effects of modern lifestyles on the human body*

Musculoskeletal and body composition effects

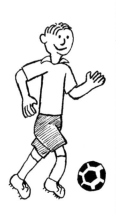

During childhood, as bones and muscles grow, appropriate physical activity is important. Strength and endurance in muscles plays a key role in achieving good posture. Overtraining is important to avoid excess on growth plate (epiphysis) , and to avoid conditions such as Osgood-Schlatters disease and other injuries, such as tennis elbow and tendonitis.

Health experts recommend that adults maintain a healthy and active lifestyle established during childhood. Moderate activity at regular intervals helps maintain strong muscles and bones, avoiding problems of poor posture. Balancing energy intake and energy expenditure also avoids problems associated with obesity and diabetes, and in particular coronary heart disease, which is associated with a lack of exercise.

A lack of regular exercise, especially in later years, can lead to two conditions commonly associated with old age.

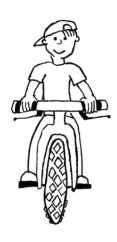

> **Osteoporosis** is a condition that occurs when bone density diminishes, leading to increased incidence of bone breaking. Regular moderate exercise can alleviate this condition.
> **Osteoarthritis** and joint instability is linked to the overuse of joint surfaces. It is particularly associated with sudden impacts, such as those in games like rugby or football. Health experts recommend learning skills in a range of activities such as swimming, golf and tennis as a way of alleviating this condition.

In the developed world, today's societies are characterised by an aging population. Technological advances mean that the population is more sedentary (they do less exercise), leading to increased occurrences of 'lifestyle diseases': high blood cholesterol levels, clogged arteries, high blood pressure, coronary heart disease (heart attacks and angina), and so on. These diseases can often be avoided by adopting a healthy, active lifestyle that includes moderate daily exercise and strengthening activities.

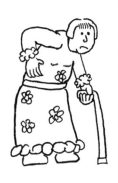

The link between healthy lifestyles and healthy cardiovascular respiratory systems

Several common modern day 'lifestyle conditions' can be linked to the functioning of the cardiac and respiratory system.

Cardiac

The link between exercise and improved efficiency of the cardiac system are well documented. **Bradycardia**, or the lowering of the heart rate, is associated with exercise, which enlarges the heart and increases strength in the muscle wall. The net effect of exercise is to lessen the strain on the heart, improving the quality of a person's life for longer. However, it is possible to have too big a heart, and lowering the heart rate to very low levels (>40 bp/m) may lead to low blood pressure, causing fainting and longer ventricular pauses, which may become arrhythmic.

Vascular

Lack of exercise is associated with a number of vascular conditions, where the transportation of blood and associated gases in the body is affected.

> **Hypertension** – prolonged high blood pressure. Symptoms include blood pressure ranges of 130/139 to 210/120. The increased heart workload involved in hypertension can lead to increased risk of atherosclerosis, arteriosclerosis, stroke and congestive heart failure.
> **Arteriosclerosis** – loss of the elasticity of the walls of the arteries, associated with thickening. The major contributing factor is smoking.
> **Atherosclerosis** – high levels of cholesterol and fat deposits accumulating within the arteries, forming a fatty plaque. This narrows the lumen, increasing the chance of blood clots forming.

Respiratory

> **Smoking** – cigarette smoking is known to contribute to arteriosclerosis but it has an even more direct impact of the transportation of oxygen for working muscles. Carbon monoxide is a by-product of cigarettes. This has a higher affinity for haemoglobin – when oxygen is inhaled the carbon monoxide reduces the carrying capacity of the blood for oxygen thus reducing the amount of oxygen available for working muscles.
> **Asthma** – associated with a number of 'modern day triggers' such as car exhaust fumes, dust and pollens. This leads to inflamed bronchus resulting in bronchi constriction.

Abilities and skills

> *The foundation of skilled performance.*

Abilities

These are the qualities that you have which make it possible for you to do something.

These abilities underpin the performance of skills.

> Abilities are stable, enduring characteristics.
> They are genetically determined.
> They can be wholly perceptual, wholly motor, or a combination – psychomotor.

Abilities have been classified in the following ways, based on the belief they can be assessed and have relevance to PE:

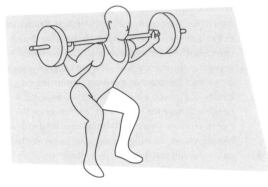

Muscular power and endurance

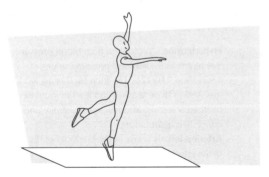

Flexibility

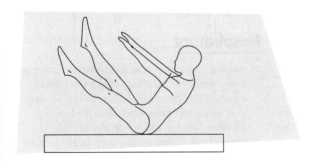

Balance

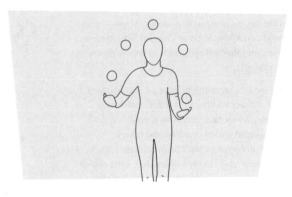

Co-ordination

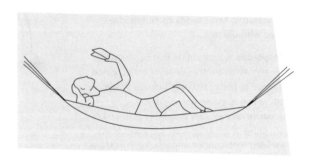

Differential relaxation

Other researchers have produced similar lists:

> Explosive strength
> Dynamic strength
> Trunk strength
> Stamina

> Extent flexibility
> Dynamic flexibility
> Gross body equilibrium
> Gross body co-ordination

Others may include:
> Reaction time
> Speed
> Agility

Skills

These are the knowledge and ability that enable you to do something – such as a job, game or sport – very well. Many skills found in a wide range of sports are underpinned by relatively few innate abilities. Talented sports people who appear to be very skilful in a range of sports may be so because they have well-developed abilities which are common to all sports.

> Skills are learnt.

> They are permanent changes in behaviour.

> They have a goal.

> Learning is revealed by changes in consistency of performance, which becomes economic and efficient.

Skills can be wholly perceptual, wholly motor or a combination of both – psychomotor (the ability to process information regarding movements and then put decisions into actions).

Skills have been classified on a variety of continuum (two opposing ends with gradual changes in characteristics between).

Snooker shot   Tennis serve   Shot putt

Fine   *Gross*
Precision of the movement.

Running   Triple jump   Badminton serve

Continuous   *Serial*   *Discrete*
Is there a definite beginning and end?

Tennis serve   Return of tennis serve

Internal pace   *External pace*
Who controls the timing of the movement?

Hockey pass:
in game   in practice

Open   *Closed*
Does the environment affect the skill?

Skill learning

If a performer is faced with a particular situation (stimulus) they must find a particular solution (response) to that situation. If the solution works, they are likely to be rewarded and they will do it again.

Coaches like performers to repeat winning or correct solutions. They therefore try to strengthen the connection between the correct response and a particular stimulus.

Some of the many theories associated with the art of learning skills are explained on the next page.

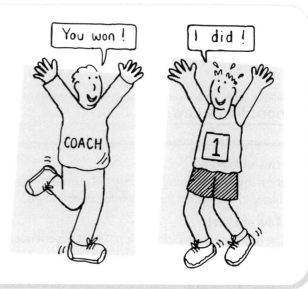

Theories of skill learning

> *How learning takes place.*

Classical conditioning (Pavlov)

This is difficult to show in a sporting context – but situations are set up to connect one response to one stimulus. In sport if the referee blows the whistle, all play stops.

This becomes a conditional response. In training, you practise a drill or routine over and over again so that you will know what to do without really thinking about it – the action becomes conditioned. Can you think of any other examples?

Ivan Pavlov (1849–1936)
Russian physiologist who studied conditional reflexes in animals. At mealtimes, he rang a bell before presenting food to his dogs. After a while, the dogs started salivating whenever they heard the bell, regardless of whether food was presented. This is known as a 'conditional reflex'.

> **Reinforcement** – any action that increases the likelihood of a response occurring again.

> **Positive reinforcement** – reward or praise. The performer is likely to repeat performance in order to be praised again.

> **Negative reinforcement** – removal of praise or reward for incorrect performance. The performer will avoid this response in order not to lose reward.

> **Punishment** – an action that decreases the likelihood of the response occurring again (e.g. 20 press-ups for every basket missed).

Thorndike's Laws

There are three of these:

1 Law of Exercise
Rehearsing the stimulus response (SR) connections is likely to strengthen them. Reinforcement helps.

2 Law of Effect
If the response is followed by a pleasant experience, then the SR bond is strengthened. If it is followed by an unpleasant experience, then the bond is weakened.

3 Law of Readiness
The performer must be mentally and physically competent to perform the task efficiently.

Operant conditioning (Skinner)

This occurs when a performer chooses or achieves the correct response from a range of actions – this is then rewarded by the coach. The performer's behaviour is shaped by the coach. The performer need not understand why he or she is performing in this way but only that he or she will be rewarded.

For example, giving a tennis server a particular target to aim for in the court (perhaps half of a service box), then reduce target area to one corner. Rewarding accurate serves strengthens the link.

B.F. Skinner (1904–1990)
American psychologist who studied operant conditioning. This involved looking closely at behaviour patterns developed by reward or punishment. Skinner held that behaviour is shaped and maintained by its consequences.

Trial and error learning

The situation occurs where a range of responses is presented and the performer works through them all until he or she finds the most effective way. This takes time.

An example would be allowing a pupil to discover as many ways as possible of scoring a basket in basketball, then refining the task, asking them to select the most efficient method, e.g. shooting from half-way versus a lay-up shot.

Problem solving (insight learning)

With this idea, learning is based on the intellectual ability of the individual. The person needs to see the whole problem and produce an appropriate solution.

Theories put forward by the **Gestaltists** support this. Learning is based on past experiences.

Feedback

This is the use of information that is available during and after a performance to alter and hopefully improve performance.

Intrinsic feedback

This occurs during the performance. The athlete can feel things in the performance which help them judge the success of the performance. This is also known as continuous feedback or kinaesthesis.

Note: Performers can become dependent on feedback. If feedback is suddenly withdrawn performance may deteriorate particularly if the performer is only doing those actions to receive positive feedback.

Extrinsic feedback

This usually occurs after a performance is completed and is provided by external sources. It is known as terminal feedback or augmented feedback. Extrinsic feedback can be further subdivided into two categories.

a) Knowledge of results (KR)
This is information about the consequences of an action, e.g. did I score a goal or miss? Feedback from a coach about the result, or evidence from a video of performance?

b) Knowledge of performance (KP)
Information about the execution of the action, e.g. coaching points from a coach or a video recording of the action.

This links to the formation of schema especially recognition schema.

Feedback can be...

Motivating

Information about the success of a performance or even a part of a performance can enhance motivation.

E.g. *"You hit all of your forehands today as winners, well done!"*

Failure can also act as a motivator.

E.g. *"You know you can hit better serves than you did today, let's go and work on that in practice."*

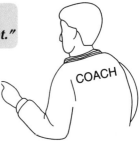

Reinforcing

Thorndike's Law of Effect (refer to page 26) states that rewarded behaviour will be repeated. Rewards may take the form of praise from a coach or from an observed improvement of performance (K.R.).

E.g. *"Great shot. That's exactly what we want."*

Informational

Feedback that points out errors and provides information to correct those faults.

E.g. *"Ok, but let's work on the angle of approach. Try to come in at a sharper angle."*

Motor programmes and schema theory

> *Putting thought into action.*

Motor programme theories

These theories deal with how the brain controls movement.

Open loop theory

This explains fast ballistic movements very well. It is concerned with the sending of information or commands.

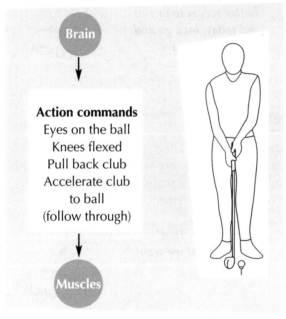

Brain

↓

Action commands
Eyes on the ball
Knees flexed
Pull back club
Accelerate club
to ball
(follow through)

↓

Muscles

1 Decision is made in the brain.

2 All information sent in one chunk.

3 Information received by muscles and they perform the action.

4 Feedback may be available but it does not control the action.

> This theory claims we have one motor programme for every action.
> How does the brain store and retrieve these quickly?
> This theory does not account for slow movements where repositioning can take place.

Closed loop theory

This theory explains slow positioning movements very well. Feedback is of prime importance in this theory.

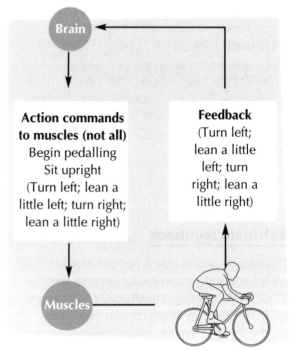

Brain

↓

Action commands to muscles (not all)
Begin pedalling
Sit upright
(Turn left; lean a little left; turn right; lean a little right)

Feedback
(Turn left; lean a little left; turn right; lean a little right)

↓

Muscles

1 Decision made in the brain.

2 Some, but not all, of the information is sent to initiate muscle action.

3 Information is received by the muscles and the movement is initiated.

4 Feedback is available and is used to alter initial movements according to the new needs.

> This theory claims we have one motor programme for each movement.
> How does the brain store and retrieve these quickly?
> Cycling requires constant adjustment of balance. Information comes from feedback to achieve this. How is the motor programme for each new balance stored?

Schema theory

The idea that individual motor programmes contain all the information needed for movement, which are difficult to store and retrieve, was challenged by R.A. Schmidt in 1977.

Schmidt suggested that motor programmes can be clustered and can be adapted to new situations.

The larger the generalised motor programme achieved through variable practice, the more likely it is that it can be adapted to new situations.

A **schema** is all of the information required to make a movement decision. It is stored in long-term memory in the brain.

Recall schema (before movement)

The performer needs to know the following to form a schema.

Initial conditions

1 Where is the:
> goal
> opposition
> team mates?

2 What is the environment like?
> grass pitch
> astro turf
> wet or dry
> wind directions

3 What condition are they in?
> fresh
> tired
> injured

Response specification

> How fast do I need to go?
> How hard shall I pass the ball?
> Where do I shoot to?
> Which technique is best?

Recognition schema (after moving)

The performer needs to know the following to correct a response.

Movement outcomes

Knowledge of results
> was it a success?
> was it a failure?

Sensory consequence

Knowledge of performance
> how did it look (extrinsic feedback)?
> how did it feel (intrinsic feedback – kinaesthesis[1])?

1 Kinaesthesis – sense of muscular effort that accompanies a voluntary motion of the body.

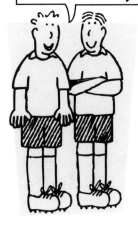

He could be good......if his responses were a bit quicker.

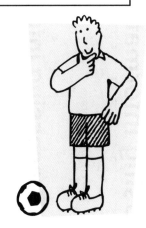

Using information

> The computer brain.

Processing information

This is how skilled performers make decisions that result in successful and efficient actions:

Stimuli
Input information
Display

(This model is closely related to Open Loop Theory – see page 28.)

Processing
Decisions made

Output
Action
Muscular response

The introduction of 'feedback' adds to the model to form this:

(This model is closely related to Closed Loop Theory – see page 28.)

Input from display

Sight
Sound
Feel
Smell
Taste

Sense organs selectively attend to relevant information

Perceptual mechanism using selective attention memory
A decision is made

Effector mechanism (a motor programme)

Muscles respond to create the desired effect

Resultant action
Performance
Success
Failure

Intrinsic feedback – Kinaesthesis/knowledge of performance

Extrinsic feedback – Knowledge of results, praise, criticism

Storing information

> *Memories are made of this …*

Memory

Information processing is aided by the memory, or experience, of a performer. It is a highly complicated process, but can be represented simply. The processes are not fully understood.

Stimuli

Sight
Sound
Feel
Smell
Taste

Short-Term Sensory Store (STSS)

> Information is constantly bombarding the senses.
> It is stored here for up to 1 second and filtered (**selective attention**).
> Relevant information only is allowed to enter the next stage.
> Irrelevant information is discarded (forgotten).

Filtering and encoding

Short-Term Memory (STM)

> Also known as the 'work space' or 'working memory'.
> This is where information is used to make decisions.
> Only a limited storage capacity. 7+/– items stored for approximately 30 seconds (e.g. Kim's Game).
> Chunking information helps in retention.
> Practice or rehearsal also helps.

Important information is then further encoded and passed to next stage. Decisions are made more quickly if previous experience stored in **LTM** is compared with current information. Response time is shortened, speeding actions up. (See Schema theory on page 29.)

Encoding
Repetition
Association
Meaningfulness
Novelty

Long-Term Memory (LTM)

This store has a seemingly unlimited capacity and can hold information for a very long time (e.g. 'You never forget how to ride a bike.'). Storage or information is achieved by:

> Repetition (practice) – strengthens motor programmes
> Association – link to already stored information
> Meaningfulness – achieved through understanding the information
> Novelty – Von Restorff Effect

There are thought to be 3 main areas of storage:

1 Procedural – how to do things, motor programmes stored here.
2 Semantic – knowledge (e.g. Paris is the capital of France).
3 Episodic – personal experiences (e.g. 'Last time I did this, this happened and it was successful. I will do it again.').

Decoding

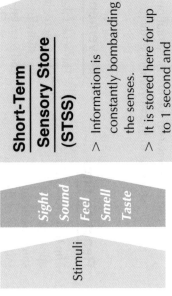

See page 30 — Input — Sense organs — Perceptual mechanism — *Encoding* — Decision making — *Decoding* — Action

Responding to information

> *How to do things more quickly.*

Response time (Reaction time)

Information processing is closely linked to a person's ability to make decisions quickly (reaction time) and then transfer them into action (movement time), together known as response time. This is important in all sports.

Response time

The time between the first presentation of stimulus to the movement ending.

Reaction time

The time from the first appearance of the stimulus to the initiation of the first movement. For example, the moment a tennis player is aware of the opponent sending the ball over the net to a particular area of the court, a decision being made to hit a forehand and the first movement to that part of the court.

Movement time

The time taken for the movement, initiated by the stimulus, to begin and then be completed. For example, in tennis the moment that the receiver begins to move into position to hit a forehand shot, including backswing, until the moment that the player comes back (after impact) into a ready position to prepare for the next shot.

Response time is affected by:

1 Number of stimuli presented – Hick's Law

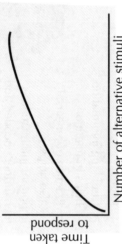

Time taken to respond

Number of alternative stimuli

2 Age

Reaction time is quicker to an optimum age, then deteriorates.

3 Presentation of stimuli in rapid succession Psychological refractory

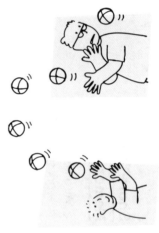

period – underpinned by single-channel hypothesis which is how a fake or dummy works. It takes time for a defender to initiate a response to a fake, which he or she must then stop and restart with their response to the actual movement.

4 Sex

Males have quicker reactions than females, but this also deteriorates more quickly.

5 Stimulus – Response compatibility

If the stimulus was expected, then reaction time will be quicker. If it is not, then reactions will be slower. For example, if a bouncer is bowled in cricket as the last ball of the over then reactions will be quicker than if a slower delivery is bowled.

6 Experience

Using memory to select the correct response speeds up response time.

7 Stimulus intensity

The stronger the stimulus, the faster the reaction, as selective attention is more easily focused on correct stimuli.

8 Anticipation

This can set in readiness the movements required by a stimulus before they are needed – known as spatial anticipation. Predicting an event of a set of stimuli is called temporal anticipation.

Phases of learning

> *Differentiating performers.*

Researchers have identified three phases or stages of learning that all performers go through:

1 **Cognitive or Understanding Phase**
2 **Associative or Verbal Motor Phase**
3 **Autonomous or Motor Phase**

"Learning may be considered to be the more or less permanent change in performance associated with experience." *Knapp (1973)*

"Performance can be seen as the amount of learning that has occurred for the process of learning must be inferred by the observed changes in performance." *Singer (1975)*

Cognitive or Understanding Phase

> Performances in this stage are inconsistent. They lack fluency and success is not guaranteed.
> Attention is all on the skill and cannot be directed elsewhere – relevant cues must be highlighted by the coach.
> Learning occurs through trial and error.
> Correct performances must be reinforced through feedback. Information is best given through demonstration – visual guidance – or through manual guidance, if appropriate.
> "The performer is getting to know what needs to be done."
> Success rate: 2 or 3 out of 10.

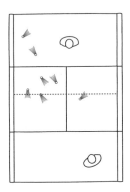

Associative or Verbal Motor Phase

> Performances in this stage are beginning to become more consistent (motor programmes are forming) though still error prone.
> Some of the simpler elements are well learnt; they look fluent; and some of the spare attention is focused elsewhere on more complex or subtle cues and actions.
> The performer can associate their movements with the mental picture they have of the skill.
> Feedback should encourage the performer to 'feel' what a good performance is like – kinaesthesis.
> The performer should begin to detect and correct errors.
> Some never progress beyond this level in some activities.
> Success rate: 5–7 out of 10.

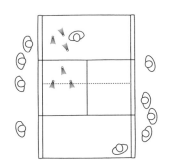

Autonomous or Motor Phase

> Performances in the final stage are skilled, fluent, consistent and aesthetically pleasing.
> Motor programmes are well learnt and stored in long-term memory; therefore reaction time is shorter.
> Skills appear to be automatic as attention is focused elsewhere (e.g. on opponents, tactics, the next move or pass or shot and on employing disguise or fakes to fool the opposition).
> Performers judge their own performances and make changes without external feedback from a coach.
> To remain in this phase constant practice is required to keep reinforcing the motor programmes.
> Success rate: 9 out of 10.

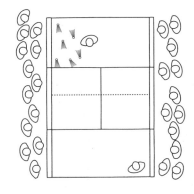

Transfer of skills

This is where the learning, or performance, of one skill influences the learning, or performance, of another skill.

Positive transfer

This occurs when the performance of one skill aids the performance of another skill. It usually occurs when the skills are similar.

"A skilled tennis player may find hitting a smash in badminton is easier because of his ability to serve in tennis."

Coaches can use 'transfer' by ensuring:

> the basic skills are over-learnt, thereby increasing the likelihood of positive transfer

> that the performer understands basic principles common to both sports.

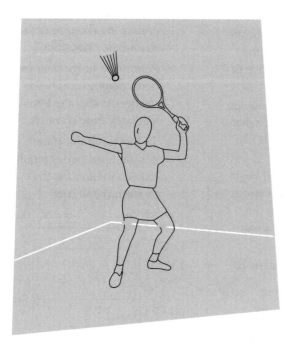

Negative transfer

This occurs when the performance of one skill hinders the performance of another skill.

Negative transfer can occur when a new action is required to a stimulus associated with another skill.

"A squash player who takes up tennis may find the playing of ground strokes difficult initially because in squash a flexible wrist is required, but in tennis a firm wrist is beneficial."

Negative transfer can be avoided:

> if the coach can make the performer aware that transfer is likely

> by ensuring that the practice situation closely resembles the 'match situation' in order to create a large, generalised motor programme.

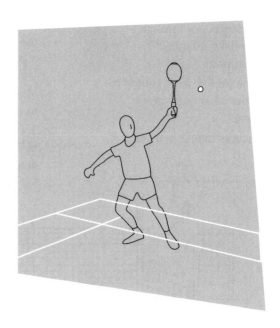

Proactive transfer

This occurs when skills already learnt affect those to be learnt in the future.

Retroactive transfer

This occurs when skills being learnt now affect those already learnt.

Zero

This form of transfer is experienced when previously learned skills do not affect the learning of new skills.

"Well learned rugby skills are unlikely to affect a person's ability to learn to rock climb."

Researchers have identified six categories of transfer:

1 Transfer between skills (e.g. badminton smash/tennis serve)

2 Practice to performance (e.g. lineout practice at training/same moves used in a match)

3 Abilities linked to skills (e.g. hand-eye coordination/catching in cricket)

4 Limb to limb (bi-lateral) (e.g. hitting tennis shots right handed/hitting tennis shots left handed)

5 Principle to skill (e.g. defensive play in soccer/defensive play in hockey)

6 Stages of learning – skills learned in cognitive phase are built upon in associative phase.

Stimulus generalisation

Is a performer transferring previously learned skills to a new situation in a general way rather than producing a special response to these stimuli?

For example, "A performer learns to catch a ball in cricket. Whenever a ball or object is projected towards that performer they catch it in the same way."

This may not be beneficial as it may not be wise to catch a thrown shot putt, etc.

Response generalisation

Once a specific response is connected to a given stimulus (i.e. well learnt) then the performer begins to adapt the response to vary it. For example, once a forehand return is well learnt the performer will adapt it to the same stimulus by adding spin, cross court, down the line, lob variations.

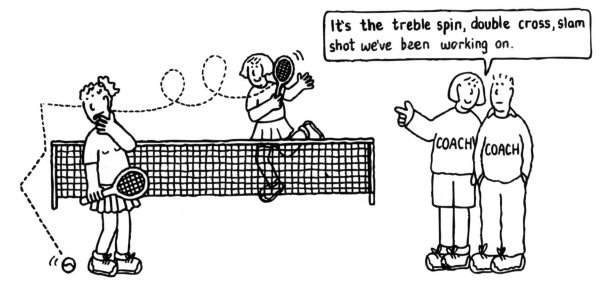

It's the treble spin, double cross, slam shot we've been working on.

Teaching – practice and methods

> *The organisation of experiences to ensure an efficient learning situation.*

Teaching

When teaching a skill, guidance is needed from the teacher, coach or friend. There are four elements to the process:

To ensure that pupils learn effectively, a teacher or coach will often manipulate the way in which new skills are demonstrated and then practised. The methods used have advantages and disadvantages depending upon the skills being taught.

1 Instructing

> May be verbal or written, or contained on a worksheet.
> Teacher ensures the pupil understands the task, knows what the targets are and can begin to practise.

2 Demonstrating

> The teacher may perform or it may be appropriate for a peer to demonstrate the skill.
> The pupil must have a model in his/her memory to work from (mental rehearsal). It must be a good demonstration.

4 Confirming

> Need to give intrinsic feedback.
> Need to provide information.
> This is a feedback process. You need to test to find out what the learner has learned. This informs the teacher, helps him/her to set new targets (above) and allows the performer to evaluate his/her performance.

3 Applying

> The pupil must practise the skill in a well-planned situation, that helps him/her to transfer information from practice to a 'real' situation.
> Need to practise skills:
  – opposed   – unopposed
  – whole   – part-whole
  – progressive; part, fixed, massed, variable, distributed.

Types of practice

Fixed practice (drills)

Particularly useful for closed, discrete skills (e.g. basketball free throw). Allows repetition of the performance to strengthen motor programme. Ideally, the skill should be 'over learnt'[1] to allow attention to be focused elsewhere.

[1]Over learning is the practice time spent beyond the time it takes to perfect the skill.

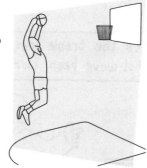

Variable practice

Particularly useful for open skills (e.g. shooting at goal in hockey). Allows repetition of skill but from many different positions and situations. This helps to build up schema to draw upon in a game situation. It can also maintain interest in training and improve motivation.

Massed practice

(No rest intervals between attempts)

Suitable for:

> simple skills (e.g. forehand drives)
> practices designed to simulate fatigued situation late in games
> short training sessions
> the fit learner.

Distributed practice

(rest intervals to mentally rehearse skills)

Most suited to:

> dangerous skills or skills that cause considerable fatigue (e.g. weight training)
> young pupils with short attention spans
> lowly motivated performers
> complex and new skills.

Negative transfer may be a problem!!

Methods

Whole method

The action is demonstrated and then practised as a whole by the pupils. Fast ballistic movements are best taught this way as all parts of the skill interact very closely (e.g. golf swing).

The performer also gets a 'feel' for the skill (kinaesthesis).

Advantages

> Learner appreciates end product.
> Learner gets a feel for the timing.
> Learner understands relationship between subroutines.

Disadvantages

> Unsuitable for complex skills.
> High attention demands; difficult for beginners.
> Not good for dangerous skills.

Part method

The sub-routines of the skill are demonstrated and practised in isolation. Useful if skills are complex with high attention demands, or if skills are dangerous. Success is achieved and motivation maintained. Serial skills are particularly suited to this method. However, transferring learning into whole skill is the key.

Advantages

> Useful for complex skills where performer can cope only with small parts of skill.
> Teacher can focus on specific elements.
> Motivation is maintained through continued success.

Disadvantages

> Transfer from part to whole may not be effective.
> Not useful for highly organised skills.
> Reduces kinaesthetic awareness.
> Lack of continuity.

Whole-part-whole

The whole action is demonstrated and practised. The individual elements are identified and improved before returning skill to whole (e.g. front crawl). Pupil tries whole stroke, weak elements are identified and then practised in isolation (e.g. using a float to practise leg kick).

If skill is very complex 'mini skills' can be taught (e.g. mini tennis instead of full game).

Advantages

> Performer gets a feel for whole skill then practises elements of it.
> Success is continual if weak elements are practised.
> Practices can be focused very carefully.

Disadvantages

> Transfer from part to whole may be difficult.

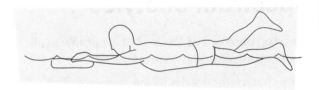

Progressive part method

Also known as **chaining method**. Skill is broken into sub-routines, which are practised in isolation and well learnt.

Part one is well learnt, so is part two; then the two are joined together; part three is then learned in isolation and then added to parts one and two. Particularly effective for serial skills (e.g. gymnastics sequences or triple jump).

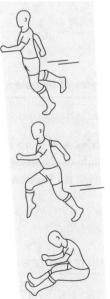

Advantages

> Weaknesses are targeted, then practised and improved.
> Performer understands the relationships of sub-routines.

Disadvantages

> Takes time to get to full skill.

Teaching – styles and guidance

> *The organisation of experience to ensure an efficient learning situation.*

Teaching styles

This is the way a coach or teacher decides to handle the learning situation.

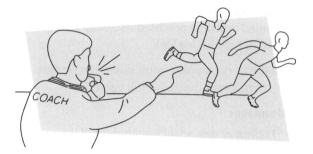

The method chosen will depend upon:
> the teacher's personality and ability
> the activity being taught – more dangerous activities will need a more authoritarian approach
> learner's ability – beginner may need more teacher input than more experienced pupils
> pupils' motivation
> age range of pupils
> learning environment.

Mosston and Ashworth spectrum of styles

Based on observed PE lessons but applicable to all teaching. Mosston and Ashworth, 1986.

They characterised styles by the degree of decision making by teacher and pupils.

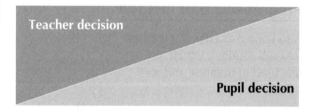

Teacher decision

Pupil decision

Styles of teaching

A   B   C   D   E   F   G   H   I   J

Styles A + B are characterised by lots of teacher-made decisions (e.g. command style, practice style). All learners do the same thing.

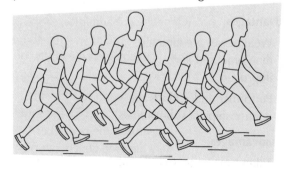

Styles C + D have the pupils making some decisions about what they do (e.g. reciprocal style).

All learners following the same basic progressions but with some ability to change practices.

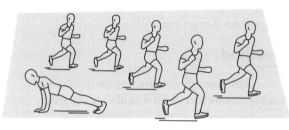

Styles E + F + G are democratic styles involving negotiation between teacher and pupils (e.g. self-check, guided discovery style).

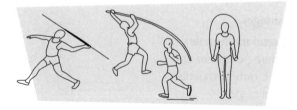

Styles H + I + J are pupil-centred discovery styles where pupils make most of the decisions: (e.g. problem solving, discovery style).

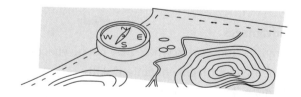

Guidance

The way in which a teacher transmits information to the learner. Learners receive information using all their senses, so a combination of approaches is usually best.

Visual guidance

Demonstration – to help create a mental picture of skill. This is closely linked to Albert Bandura's 1977 research on modelling. The 'model' must be as close to perfect as possible as the learner has to imitate it. It must be realistic (e.g. do not try to teach pupils who are around 157 cm tall to slam dunk.

Often used in conjuction with verbal guidance to highlight key points.

Visual aids:
photographs, charts and diagrams tend to be too static. Video playback in slow motion can be very effective.

Modification of display:
teacher enhances the perception of the pupil by highlighting particular aspects of the surroundings (e.g. coloured targets on court to aim at; fluorescent golf balls).

Verbal guidance

Often linked with demonstration. Not so useful by itself.

Points to note:
> Does the performer understand the language being used?

> Can the performer remember everything that has been said?

> Can the performer translate instructions into actions?

Verbal guidance highlights cues (e.g. 'Wave goodbye to the ball' when shooting in basketball; 'Clean palm, dirty neck' in shot putt).

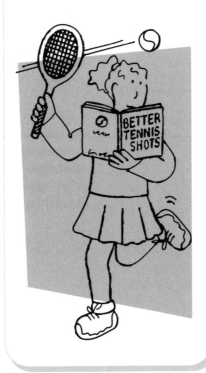

Manual guidance

Physical restriction – a person, or more commonly an object, confines the movement of the learner (e.g. 'somersault belt' in trampoline; a 'tight rope' in climbing; 'waterwings' on a young swimmer).

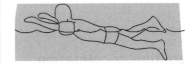

> Gives the performer confidence.

> Helps to increase safety in dangerous situations.

> Allows the performer to work out timings of the skill.

Forced response:
The performer is guided manually through the shot to be learned (e.g. badminton short serve – the teacher extends the arm by pushing on the elbow of the player).

> Gives a supported kinaesthetic feel for the shot. If overused the performer may become dependent on help or may lose motivation as hey are a passive learner.

Learning and performance

Learning

a more or less permanent change in performance as a result of experience or practice

Performance

a one-off execution of a motor skill or series of motor skills

To establish if learning has taken place, it is necessary to chart changes in performance over time. Graphs plotting changes show different patterns.

Linear

equal amounts of improvement for each unit of time.

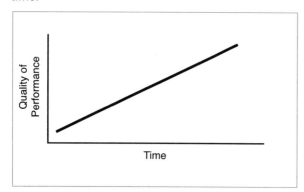

Negative acceleration

initially large amounts of improvement, then it slows

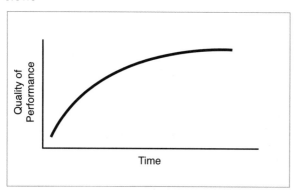

Positive acceleration

slow early improvement, and then it accelerates

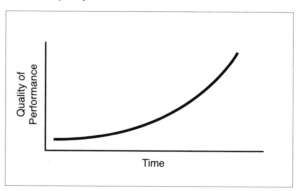

S-shaped curve

the normal learning curve, where learning starts slowly, accelerates and then slows

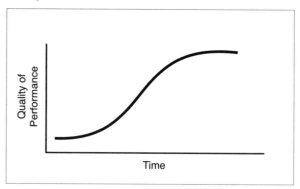

All these are theoretical – real learning is more varied than this. However, one common feature is the **plateau**, where there is no further improvement. This is caused by:
> psychological factors , e.g. anxiety, lack of motivation
> lack of fitness
> poor technique.

A coach can overcome a plateau by:
> explaining the cause
> setting appropriate goals
> structuring training
> giving feedback
> teaching new technique.

Key ideas – key definitions

> *Our field of study outlining issues and concepts.*

Historical

What was it like in the past?

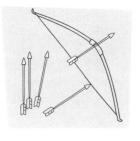

A contemporary socio-cultural view

The performer in society.

We must:
> consider issues that arise...
- excellence
- discrimination
- mass participation
- outdoor recreation
> think about other perspectives of the activity and performer...

Comparative

What is it like in other countries?

> Globalisation

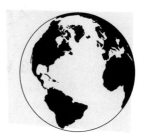

Classification of activities

Within our field of study, physical performance can be classified into **five main groups** with unique features.

Main groups

1 Combat

(e.g. fencing)

involves beating an opponent in a stylized war game

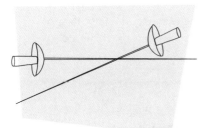

2 Outdoor pursuits/conquest

(e.g. sailing)

challenge against nature or with a physical/ psychological objective

3 Aesthetic

(e.g. gymnastics)

visual, competition criteria

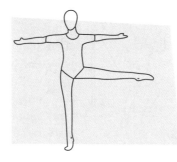

4 Individual

(e.g. swimming)
athletic, aquatic, competing on own, physical challenge, self-fulfilling, recreation, physical education or sport

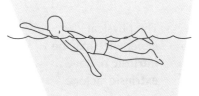

5 Games

contrived structured competitive experiences, existing in own time and space, can be partner or team

> **Invasion**

(e.g. hockey) attack by entering an opponent's territory to score in their goal

> **Target/striking**

(e.g. cricket) hit to score, opposition field to limit scoring

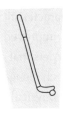

> **Court**

(e.g. tennis) non contact, score in opponent's court area

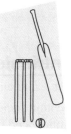

Key ideas – key definitions (cont.)

When studying socio-cultural issues we must consider three questions:

1 What do we mean by…?

> This deals with definitions.

2 How do we know?

> Here we need to consider authoritative back-up.

3 What does this tell us?

> The influence of the past on what it is like now.

Main concepts

We can also see **four main categories** or **concepts.** Most activities can exist in each category depending on the attitude of the performer and the level and organisation of the performance. Thus, as examples, football or swimming, can be undertaken for:

> play
> physical recreation
> sport, or
> physical education.

These concepts have some shared characteristics:

> improved health
> personal development
> challenge or competition
> physical endeavour.

1 Play

spontaneous, often child-like, physical activity

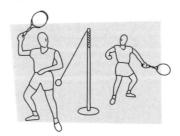

2 Physical recreation

physical activity with limited organisational structure

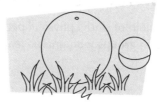

3 Physical education

formal learning of knowledge and values through physical activities

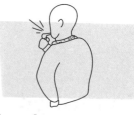

4 Sport

structured physical activity requiring a high degree of commitment

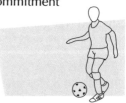

Intrinsic

An experience complete in itself.

Within society the *performer* is influenced by:

> what the activity is
> why they are doing it
> how they are doing it
> where they are doing it
> with whom they are doing it
> for whom they are performing.

Physical performance is a dynamic experience

The physical experience may be **intrinsic** or have **extrinsic** factors.

Extrinsic

The main extrinsic factors which influence the *physical situation* are:

> geographical location
> social
> political
> economic.

These factors can be influenced by local, regional, national and international influence.

Concepts of physical activity

> *The characteristics of the concepts of play, physical recreation, physical education and sport. Activities can be placed on the continuum from play to sport.*

Unorganised

('Paidia' – child's fun)
play

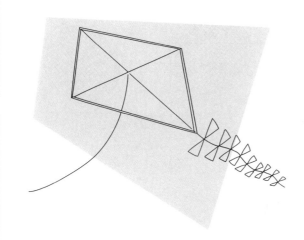

Play

Characteristics

> enjoyable
> spontaneous, voluntary
> without pre-determined rules
> child-like
> intrinsic
> self-fulfilling
> time and space – may be limited and may be changed by agreement

Refer to classical theories of play – Huizinga, Piaget, Callois and Ellis. It has been suggested that all sports have their origin in play. Callois suggested that play is a **reflection of society**.

Features of play

> biological – instinctive part of learning process in developing skills
> psychological – learning about self
> sociological – to practise social roles
> children play – to learn about life
> adults play – to escape the stresses of everyday life

"to play" – do the activity
"fair play" – the morality of sport

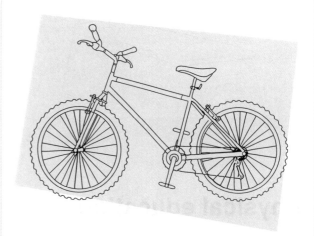

Physical recreation

Can be considered as 'constructive or active **LEISURE'** taken in the time left after work, duty and bodily needs have been met. This implies there is an **economic factor.**

Characteristics of physical recreation

> relaxation (physical recovery)
> recuperation (recover from stress)
> recreation (be creative)
> time and space decided by participant
> limited organisation
> participant chooses
> intrinsic rewards
> physical enjoyment
> spiritual well-being
> social
> mental pleasure
> non-productive

Outdoor recreation

> in the natural environment
> can be physically challenging but not necessarily competitive

Concepts of physical activity (cont.)

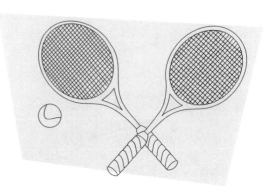

Organised

('Ludus' – organised sport)
display

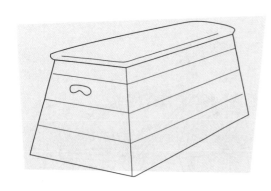

Physical education

Features of physical education

> to impart knowledge and values through physical activities concerning bodily movement
> usually in an institution
> structured lessons
> develops practical skills to be able to participate in activities
> develops social skills to work with others as part of a team, develop co-operation and leadership
> develop lifestyle activities
> extra curricular activities out of formal lesson times
> national curriculum for PE to bring uniformity
> examinations (GCSE, A-level, degree) raised the profile of PE and encouraged career development
> develops values – social, instrumental, humanistic

Outdoor education

> using the environment as a resource for learning physical activities
> challenges self
> develops awareness and respect for the environment
> learn to work with and depend on others
> provides sense of danger/adventure

Sport

Features of sport

> competitive
> highly organised
> time and space designated
> formal rules
> requires higher level of skill
> develop sportsmanship
> requires commitment
> intrinsic rewards (own achievement, satisfaction)
> extrinsic rewards (cups, money, titles, etc.)
> the 'letter' of playing the game – by the rules
> the 'spirit' of playing the game – fair play, high morals

can be functional or dysfunctional
(Refer to Nash's model)

functional – high – played in the spirit of the game – abide by the rules, even if no referee decision given

dysfunctional – low – breaking of rules, aggression towards others, 'sending off'

Sport and culture

> *Sport exists in all societies, past and present. We can look at how it is used by developing countries.*

> **Society is a community of people coming together and relating to each other.**
> **Culture is a product of this relationship – often represented by a society's customs, religion, art, etc.**
> **Sport is a part of culture... and a reflection of society.**

Sport exists within society and is a part of social life. It reflects the ideas and beliefs of the community which draws up its rules and laws and defines acceptable behaviour.

Looking at different societies in historical context we see how sports developed through the needs of the culture and society.

Ancient societies

(those civilisations that don't exist today)

Ideology – suited to their beliefs

Evidence of sports pursued by ancient societies show a relationship between ideology of the civilisation and the sports pursued.

Functional

Some sports had a functional basis:
> keeping soldiers fit for defence
> practising the skills of hunting
> keeping the masses occupied e.g. slaves watching Roman gladiators.

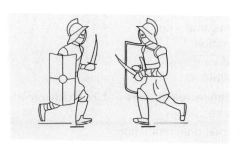

Ritual

Other sports were related to ritual:
> symbolic of life stages
> representing religious beliefs
> a ceremony or festival.

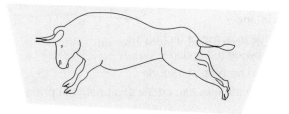

Tribal societies

(those that are lacking in sophistication, often with a 'primitive' god/man belief)

Ritual

> sports may reflect the relationship between god and man and could be used as a ritual to appease the Gods
> in ball games the ball may have represented the sun
> in some cases the heads of defeated enemies were used as the ball in a display of victory and strength
> tests of strength such as wrestling matches were used to prepare warriors or elect chiefs.

Survival

> some sports such as running and spear throwing were physical preparation for basic survival (Zulus and Indians)
> skills needed to be learnt for finding food and defence.

Natural

> learning how to adapt within the natural environment.

Some rituals survived colonisation. After colonisation sports were **ADAPTED** or **ADOPTED** by countries.

Sport and culture (cont.)

Emergent societies

(countries that are less developed economically and have a low level of technology – largely found in Africa, the Far East and South America)

> Sport is often used as a means to achieve political strategies and develop emergent countries. Sport is an area where emergent societies can emulate and compete with advanced societies.

Sport can be used as a method of creating **STABILITY** by means of:

Nation building

> increasing internal national identity
> increasing **international identity** – sport as a 'shop window' for a society
> facilitating international representation.

Integration

> encouraging multi-ethnic sporting activities and **relieving racial tensions**
> bringing the nation together to support an individual or team and so **appeasing the population** and **diverting attention** from other problems.

Health

> mass participation is encouraged to develop a more health conscious society
> increased general health produces a fit fighting force.

Defence

> creating a high profile defence to protect the country
> the military is often the organiser of sport and creates opportunities to participate.

Some emerging nations have striven for excellence in a limited range of sports, channelling money into a small elite. This may bring attention to the country and set up the champions as role models. However the disproportionate funding of one sport to achieve excellence may be at the expense of other goals (e.g. overcoming poverty).

Examples of what sport... and why?

Initially, emergent countries tend to use one dominant sport. Once established, the country can develop other sports.

Indonesia – badminton

> minority sport which suits country
> Olympic sport – thus seen by the world
> easy to administer
> non-contact – non-aggressive
> small-sided game – small population
> requires small physical stature, dexterity and quick reactions
> little equipment or space needed
> slow pace – and ideal for playing in the tropics.

The West Indies – cricket

> traditional and established game
> brought islands and races together in common purpose
> team game – co-operation
> outdoor game – healthy
> Commonwealth sport – able to play other nations
> international reputation
> income to islands.

Kenya – middle and long distance running

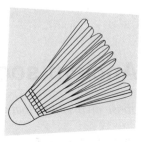

> Olympic sport – high profile
> suited to lifestyle – used to running long distances
> little expense or technical knowledge needed
> good training at altitude
> a few athletes can create great national pride.

Physical education, sport and sub-cultures

> Inequalities exist in physical education and sport. Minority groups are often disadvantaged; we can look at this in terms of opportunity, provision and esteem.

Inequalities still occur in advanced western societies and are reflected in sport, often due to cultural and historical influences.

One section of the community – minority groups – may be disadvantaged and discriminated against in physical education and sport. Also damaging is the fact that sports myths and stereotypes have developed around minority groups.

Opportunity

Race

> parental expectations
> non-acceptance in clubs may be a barrier
> may be affected by religious beliefs (e.g. muslim girls)
> lack of finance means little choice (many low paid)
> cultures may not rate PE and sport highly
> 'staking' – assumption that you play in a particular position in the team ('brawn not brain' stereotype)
> lack of career opportunities – majority of coaches (and the decision makers) are white

Disability

> some sports may not cater for disability – therefore restricted choice of activities
> few disabled sports clubs and restricted membership to others
> few disabled coaches so poor career prospects
> overall, fewer opportunities to achieve excellence

Gender

> looking after family – less leisure time
> certain religious restrictions
> fewer female coaches, managers and administrators therefore limited career opportunities
> some clubs have membership restrictions – although law is changing
> lack of competition opportunity
> restricted choice of activities and those choices may favour males – school, National Curriculum (team game bias)
> considered incapable and not aggressive enough for coaching

Age

> young – too early with hard training can 'burn out'
> young – reliant on parental attitude and finances
> participation of 50+ age group restricted, few veterans' clubs and teams
> age restrictions in some clubs
> curriculum and extra curricular opportunities dependent on schools – relies on PE staff enthusiasm

Class

> 'working class' – little leisure time, lack of finance, difficult to work and compete at a high level
> restricted access to certain clubs
> 'middle class' – more leisure time and wealth to choose activities

Provision

> associated with a particular sport, e.g. Asians playing cricket and Afro Caribbean youths boxing... therefore little provision in other sports
> lack of single sex lessons
> lack of changing facilities to cater for religious restrictions
> information not easily available
> coaches not available

> lack of specialised equipment
> poor wheelchair access to leisure centres and swimming pools
> inadequate changing facilities
> few activities provided at leisure centres
> transport to activities may not be possible
> cost of special provision may be prohibitive

> lack of creche facilities
> few females on governing bodies and little input in decision-making
> few female coaches
> lower pay and prize money
> may lack money to spend on sport if not working
> lack of transport
> competitions may be restricted to single sex
> clubs may restrict playing times or provide inferior changing facilities

> facilities dependant on geographical location
> few activity sessions specifically for older people or teenagers
> transport may be reliant on goodwill of family and friends
> fees may be prohibitive

> 'working class' may experience limited facilities and coaches – reliant on sponsorship for funding
> wealthy individuals have the ability to pay a coach, buy equipment and clothing and to travel to training and competition

Esteem

> lack of role models to give hope to achieve
> poorly paid or menial job add to low self esteem
> lack of coaches from same ethnic group
> media coverage of indigenous sports is low

> perceived to be not able to achieve and the assumption that they cannot do sport – a myth and stereotype
> few role models – paraplegic games and marathons poorly covered
> assumed lack of knowledge
> perceived as not interesting or exciting enough for media coverage, spectators or sponsorship... therefore not taken seriously

> think they can't do sport – poor self image
> lack of many role models
> media coverage poor, tends to focus on appearance instead of skill and ability – only for show portraying traditional gender role ideology (mostly golf, tennis and athletics covered)
> lack of sponsorship as competition considered not as exciting as males
> not taken seriously by spectators – considered recreational
> affected by myths – girls can't throw effectively, women will damage themselves in certain events or are not able to do others

> media coverage minimal for both elderly and very young
> few role models
> elderly perceived as only involved for recreation
> peer pressure can affect youngsters' perception of sport, particularly girls

> role models can give hope to those from deprived backgrounds – seen as way out and means to achieve wealth
> media can help promote and gain sponsorship
> less wealthy could be seen as less able or knowledgeable

The National Curriculum and initiatives

The National Curriculum

This was established in 1989 with the aim of improving standards, increasing accountability and encouraging children to adopt healthy lifestyles.

> Key Stage 1 (Years 1 and 2) : experience dance, gymnastics

> Key Stage 2 (Years 3 to 6) : experience dance, gymnastics, games – and two from athletics, swimming and adventure activities .

> Key Stage 3 (Years 7 to 9) : experience games and either dance or gymnastics, and two from athletics, swimming and adventurous activities.

> Key Stage 4 (Years 10 and 11) : experience games and one from athletics, swimming , gymnastics, dance and adventurous activities.

As individuals progress through the Key Stages, they should learn more complicated movement patterns, and develop more complex tactics. Pupils' understanding of health and fitness should also improve so by Key Stage 4 they can plan, prepare and evaluate a health-related exercise programme.

A pupil's level is assessed at each Key Stage. This provides clear goals and motivation, although it can discourage.

What is taught can be limited by:

> facilities

> time available

> funding and

> staff experiences.

Current initiatives in PE

These initiatives aim to provide greater access to sporting opportunity for groups, levels and ages.

> PE, School Sport and Club Links (PESSCL) – a national strategy aimed at increasing sporting opportunity for 5–16 year olds.

> Sports Colleges – provide high quality opportunities for their students and help develop other secondary and primary schools in their area.

> Active Sports – encourages young people to continue participating in sport at a level suited to their ability and motivation. Made up of Active Schools, Active Communities and the World Class Programme. Provides a link between club, school and national governing body development programmes.

> Sports Leaders UK – provides opportunities for the young to get the skills necessary to lead/coach sport.

> TOP programme – provides opportunities for children in school by making suitable equipment and resources available.

> Whole Sport Plans – a five-year plan that any national governing body has to produce for Sport England if it wants funding.

Active leisure facility provision

Sports facilities are provided by three sectors:

> public provision
— owned by local authority
— facilities open to all
— aims to increase health of society (physical, mental and social)
— aims to regenerate areas

— local government have tried to increase standards with an initiative called 'best value'
— cheap to use

> private clubs
— privately owned
— profit-making
— high standards

— exclusive
— managed by owners
— expensive membership fees

> voluntary sector
— owned and managed by members
— non profit-making
— financed by members fees and fundraising.

Elite sport, business and the media

World Games

These include:
> Football World Cup
> Hockey World Cup
> Olympics
> Commonwealth Games
> Paralympics
> European Athletics Championships

Characteristics

> highly competitive
> world's best performers
> nationalistic
> attractive to the media
> attractive to sponsors
> highly competitive

Impact

Performer	Spectator	Country	Business
Fame	Enjoyment	International status	Raise profile
Earnings	Excitement	Revenue	Revenue
Contracts	Relaxation	National pride	
Enjoyment	Entertainment	Political statement	
Challenge			

Organisations supporting elite sport in the UK

- UKSport – responsible for developing elite sport in the UK
- National Institutes of Sport (e.g. English Institute of Sport) – provide a nationwide network of world-class facilities, coaches, sports science and medical support.
- National Sports Councils (SportEngland, Scotland, Wales and Northern Ireland) – seek to create active nations
- National Governing Bodies (NGBs) – responsible for developing their own sport in the UK through organising competition, establishing rules, supporting clubs and developing elite and grassroots participants.
- SportsCoach UK – dedicated to developing the best coaching system in the world for every level of coach. Works alongside NGBs.
- British Olympic Association – fosters Olympic ideals, organises and coordinates British participation, assists NGBs encourages interest.

Funding

Funding comes from a variety of sources:
- Central government – funds distributed via the Department of Culture, Media and Sport, given to SportEngland and UKSport to distribute to NGBs.
- NGBs – receive funds from sponsorship, affiliation fees and donations. Some NGBs find it easier to raise money than others (compare the FA and the HA).
- National Lottery –grants money to UKSport specifically for elite performers
- Sports Aid – helps top amateurs to train full time. Self-financing, giving money to those who with real need, who are not already receiving financial support.

Business, the media and sport

Business

Sponsorship
when an organisation provides funding in return for advertising

Endorsement
actively supporting a product

Merchandising
selling goods linked to a particular sport/team

Why does business support sport?

> to raise its profile
> to increase sales
> to be linked with the best

What are the positive effects on sport?

> increases money available in sport, allowing investment in better facilities and players
> enables sports people to make money from playing
> improves the standard of sport
> puts pressure on the performer

What are the negative effects on sport?

> rules get changed to suit sponsors
> player has to conform to the sponsors' requests
> some products are unethical
> extra pressure on performers
> bad publicity for business if the performer is deviant

Market forces control how much an individual gets paid. It could be argued some get paid too much!

The media

Types

- TV
- radio
- newspapers
- internet

Effects of coverage on:

Sport

> promotes that sport
> brings money into the sport
> some rules changed to make it more exciting for spectators
> timetables altered to maximise viewing figures
> extra advertising breaks

Performer

> focus on personality rather than performance
> intrusion into private life
> development of personal wealth
> increased pressure

What are the functions of the media?

- to inform
- to educate
- to entertain
- to advertise

Deviance in sport

> *Deviance in sport*

What is deviance?

Deviance is where an individual breaks away from the expected norms in society. In PE:

negative deviance is cheating, e.g. taking drugs, game fixing
positive deviance is behaviour that tries too hard to conform, e.g. overtraining, playing when injured, rejecting other things in your life.

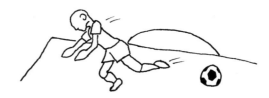

Playing fair

Gamesmanship or sportsmanship?

> **Gamesmanship** is using dubious methods, though not illegal ones; to win. Example: in football, diving in the penalty area.
> Sportsmanship is fair play – wanting to win but not at all costs. It has a positive effect on sport. Example: in netball, helping a player in the opposite team up when they slip over.

The 'contract to compete'

An unwritten contract entered into when you play sport, including:
> abide by the rules
> play to the best of your ability
> allow others to play to the best of their ability
> fair play.
The Olympic ideal grasps these features. However, financial and political pressures make it difficult for performers to stick to it.

Performance-enhancing drugs

Name	Effect	Side effects
Anabolic steroids	• athlete can work harder for longer • quicker recovery • taken by power athletes e.g. sprinters, weight lifters	• aggression • acne • tumours • menstrual disturbances • testicular atrophy
EPO (erythropoietin)	• stimulates production of red blood cells, increasing oxygen-carrying capacity • taken by endurance athletes e.g. marathon runners	• increase in blood viscosity • kidney damage
Blood transfusion	• increases the number of red blood cells • done by endurance athletes • viral hepatitis	• blood disorders • aids
Stimulants	• reduce tiredness • increase alertness • taken by 24-hour rally drivers, boxers	• increased blood pressure • addiction
Diuretics	• enable athlete to lose weight quickly • dilute urine to help mask drugs • taken by boxers, jockeys	• dehydration • cramp
Beta blockers	• decrease heart rate • decrease blood pressure • reduction in tremor	• muscle fatigue • insomnia • impotence
Painkillers	• mask pain	• highly addictive • further damage to area

How do other athletes justify drug taking?

> believe others are taking them, so they have to
> minimal cost of getting caught
> huge amounts of money and fame to be made if they win
> pressure from media, coach, nation for success
> only way of winning

What can be done to improve the situation?

> educate young people about the effects of drug taking
> closer monitoring of athletes
> put more money into testing
> impose stricter penalties

World Anti-Doping Agency (WADA)

This was set up in 1999 to coordinate the fight against performance-enhancing drugs. It is funded by the International Olympic Committee and international governments.

Hooliganism

Performers are not the only ones who can be deviant – spectators can be too. Hooliganism can be caused by:

> poor decisions by officials
> players' behaviour
> importance of the event
> alcohol
> poor facilities
> a tradition of problems.

The solutions are:
> all-seater stadia
> control of alcohol
> tough deterrents
> increased number of stewards and police.

Sport and the law

Where do these two become linked?

> negotiation of player contracts
> prosecuting players for criminal damage
> eliminating discrimination
> dealing with negative deviance

As the sums of money involved in sport increase, so there is more need for the involvement of the law.

Energy concepts

At any one time enormous numbers of chemical reactions are taking place inside a human cell. These reactions either require energy or are releasing it.

Definitions

Energy: A physical quantity that measures the capacity of a system for doing work. In other words, your capacity to perform work.
Symbol: E;
units: Calories or Joules
(1 cal = 4.2 Joules)

Work: A transfer of energy as a consequence of a force acting through a distance.
Work = Force × Distance
Symbol: W; unit: Joule (J)

Power: The rate of transfer of energy between one system and another. Measured as work performed per unit of time.
Symbol: P; unit: Watt (Joules per second)
$$\frac{Work}{Time}$$

Exothermic reaction: reaction that releases energy.

Endothermic reaction: reaction that requires an input of energy.

Enzyme: biological catalyst that brings about and speeds up specific reactions.

Metabolism: the sum of all chemical reactions in the body.

Anabolic: building up.

Catabolic: breaking down.

Basal metabolic rate (BMR): the rate (minimum energy) at which the chemical processes of the body must function in order to sustain life. Affected by: age, sex, occupation, metabolism.

Energy efficiency

To evaluate the relationship between input (energy expenditure) and resulting mechanical output in exercise, we need to assess the mechanical efficiency of human movement.

$$\% \text{ Efficiency} = \frac{\text{Useful work done}}{\text{Energy expenditure}} \times 100$$

Human range = 12–25%

For every movement made only 25% of energy consumed contributes directly to actual movement, the rest is converted into HEAT.

Note: Improvement in techniques used and overall skill levels will increase efficiency of energy used.

Respiratory exchange ratio (RER or RQ) – used to estimate energy expenditure per litre of O_2 used.

$$RER = \frac{\text{Amount of } CO_2 \text{ produced}}{\text{Amount of } O_2 \text{ used}}$$

Fats = 0.70
Protein = 0.80
Carbohydrates = 1.0
Mixture of fats and carbohydrates = 0.85
Used to estimate proportion of fats and carbohydrates being oxidised.

Forms of energy in the body

Energy in (pod) =
Energy out (work) + (heat)
Energy stored (fat)

Laws of thermodynamics

(transformation of energy by heat and work)

First Law: Energy is not destroyed or lost but passed from one form to another.

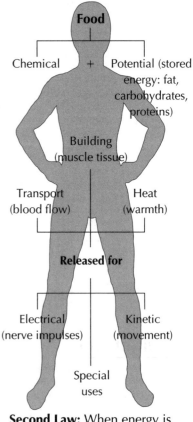

Food

Chemical + Potential (stored energy: fat, carbohydrates, proteins)

Building (muscle tissue)

Transport (blood flow)   Heat (warmth)

Released for

Electrical (nerve impulses)   Kinetic (movement)

Special uses

Second Law: When energy is exchanged, the efficiency of exchange is imperfect, and part of the energy will escape as heat.

Applying energy concepts

> *Applying energy concepts to performance.*

Constructing a training programme

> You must consider the specific energy demands of the particular sport.

> Training must mirror the demands of the sport by stressing the appropriate energy system used.

Nutrition and performance

> The right foods in right amounts at the right times can make a significant difference to a performance.

> Analysing energy expenditure of a particular activity can give valuable information on how much energy is required.

Warm up/ cool down

> It is important to do light exercise immediately before and after playing sport or doing strenuous activity.

> Increases body and muscle temperature.

> Increases enzyme activity in the metabolic reactions found in the energy systems.

> Increases blood flow by keeping capillary beds open in muscles to aid oxygen transport.

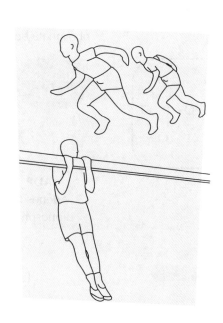

Control of body weight

> Understanding energy expenditure and energy imput will help you to maintain a constant body weight.

Input < Output
(lose weight)

Input = Output
(maintain weight)

Input > Output
(gain weight)

Maintenance of body temperature

> A large proportion of energy produced is in the form of heat.

> Understanding how heat is lost or gained through convection, conduction, radiation and evaporation will help keep your body temperature constant at 37°C.

Fatigue

> Understanding how energy is produced within the body will provide a valuable insight into what fatigue is.

> It will also show how fatigue can be reduced, or even avoided, during performance.

ATP – the energy currency

> *The body's energy wage.*

Adenosine triphosphate (ATP)

ATP is the main supplier of metabolic energy in living cells. It is a high-energy compound that is central to all that takes place during metabolism.

This part of the molecule acts like a 'handle'. Its shape can be recognised by highly specific enxymes.

This part of the molecule contains bonds (O–P) which can be hydrolysed (broken down by water) in reactions which are *exergonic* (energy yeilding) and can be coupled to *endergonic* (energy-demanding) reactions.

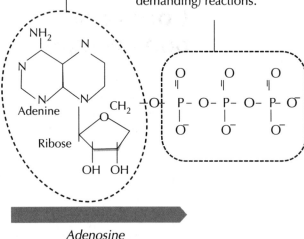

Adenosine

Adenosine triphosphate

ATP is the body's energy currency

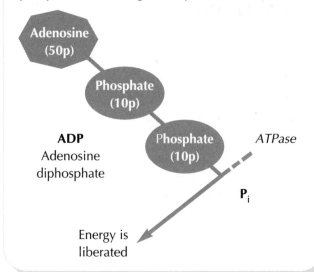

Energy is released by breaking the end high-energy phosphate bond using an enzyme called **ATPase.**

Why only enough ATP for two seconds intense work?

1 So ATP must be continually renewed.

2 To stimulate almost immediately the processes that resynthesise ATP via these systems:

Alactic   Lactic   Aerobic

ATP is stored in relatively small amounts in muscle cells.

Only enough ATP is stored to last two seconds during maximum effort (e.g. a standing long jump).

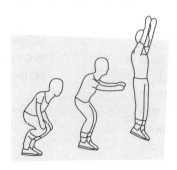

ATP provides the energy for all energy requiring processes in the body.

Nerve transmission

+

Tissue building

+

Muscle contraction

+

Circulation

$$ATP = ADP + P_i + Energy$$

The recovery process (1)

> *Paying back the energy currency spent.*

Resynthesis of ATP during and after exercise

We need ATP constantly and cannot afford to run out of it. Three sources of energy replacement ensure ATP is always available.

3 The aerobic system
overleaf

1 ATP/PC system: Phosphocreatine system Alactacid system

As maximal exercise begins, e.g. 100 m sprint/long jump, ATP stored in the muscles breaks down to ADP and energy is released. Increasing concentrations of ADP in the sacroplasm stimulates the release of the enzyme.

Creatine Kinase

This substance initiates the breakdown of **phosphocreatine** and energy is released from the bond between creatine and phosphate.

The energy released reforms the bonds between ADP and the phosphate available in the sacroplasm to form ATP, which is subsequently broken down to release energy for muscular contractions.

Phosphocreatine is a simple compound easily broken down without decay and no by-products hence it is alactacid.

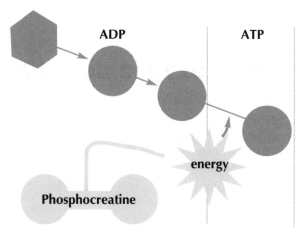

Energy restored in this way can sustain exercise for between 8–10 seconds before all PC stores are used. Source 2 is then used.

2 Lactic acid system or glycolysis

As exercise continues beyond 10 seconds another method of regenerating ADP to ATP must be found once all available PC is used up.

The second method involves converting energy from food we consume into useable energy in the body. We do this by the partial breakdown of glucose which occurs if there is insufficient O_2 to completely breakdown glucose. Glucose is stored in the muscles and liver as **glycogen** and its breakdown is called **glycolysis**.

Glycogen $(C_6H_{12}O_6)$is a complex compound that stores lots of energy in its links, when the enzyme **phosphorylase** is present it breaks down to glucose. Glucose then further breaks down when **phospho-fructokinase** (be careful how you say this!) is present and active. This occurs when concentration of phosphocreatine are low and calcium (used to stimulate Huxley's sliding filament) are high. The glucose breaks down to pyruvic acid. This further breaks down to lactic acid when O_2 is absent.

This system is not as instantaneous as the PC system as more reactions must take place, but it is still relatively fast hence high energy events, e.g. 400 m run, can be sustained.

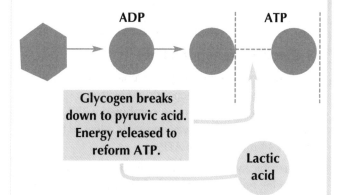

Energy restored in this way can sustain exercise for between 30 seconds to 1.00 minute depending upon the fitness level of the performer. After this time energy must be produced in a different way.

The recovery process (2)

> *The process by which the body returns to pre-exercise state.*

3 The aerobic system

Limited amounts of O_2 are stored in the muscles of the body in association with myoglobin. This is insufficient however to help produce energy efficiently with food fuels in the body hence the reliance on the anaerobic systems at the start of exercise. As exercise continues and heart rate and ventilation increase so does the amount of oxygen in the working muscles. This allows the more efficient breakdown of glucose via aerobic respiration. This leads to complete breakdown of glucose releasing vast quantities of energy for ADP resynthesis, albeit very slowly.

This occurs through 3 stages:

1 Aerobic glycolysis

Glucose is broken down to pyruvic acid and as there is sufficient O_2 available no lactic acid is produced and enough energy is released to resynthesise two molecules of ATP.

2 Krebs cycle/TCA/citric acid cycle

Pyruvic acid enters the mitochondria to be broken down to acetyl where it combines with coenzyme A (CoA) to form (acetyl–CoA).

A cyclical set of reactions takes place which leads to the release of large amounts of energy to resynthesise two molecules of ATP.

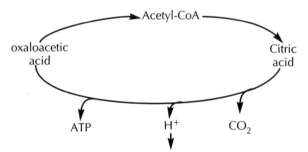

3 Electron transport chain

Hydrogen released in stage two enters the inner membranes of the mitochondria. Electrons removed from hydrogen are combined with O_2 to form water, along the way energy is released to reform 34 molecules of ATP.

The aerobic system is the most efficient method of producing energy in terms of easily disposable waste products – but it takes time due to the reactions required. ATP is therefore regenerated more slowly hence the athlete performs at a lower energy level, e.g. long distance events slower than sprints.

What changes occur in the body during exercise?

1 ATP levels decrease
2 Phosphocreatine levels decrease
3 Glycogen levels decrease
4 Triglyceride levels decrease
5 Oxygen/myoglobin levels decrease
6 Carbon dioxide levels increase
7 Lactic acid levels increase.

How does the body reverse these changes?

The body must 'work' to reverse these changes and there is a cost in energy to do this. The body does not immediately return to resting levels of heart rate or breathing rate. This increased aerobic respiration rate is used to repay the **oxygen debt.** This is the amount of oxygen consumed above resting levels for the same time period following exercise.

What is oxygen deficit?

Oxygen deficit is the amount of energy, therefore oxygen consumption, required to reform all of the phosphocreatine and glycogen used during the early stages of exercise when there was insufficient oxygen available.

Oxygen debt

Oxygen debt has two components.

Alactacid component

> This is repaid very rapidly and is used to resynthesise ATP and phosphocreatine which are depleted during exercise. Full replenishment after exercise may take 2–3 minutes and uses typically up to 4 litres of oxygen depending upon the intensity of exercise.

Games players can use this information to take rests when possible to allow replenishment of high energy stores, e.g. time outs in basketball; penalties, lineouts, scrums in rugby.

Time may not be available for full recovery but some return to resting levels of ATP and PC will occur. This will prevent further reliance on the lactic acid system.

Lactacid component

> Lactic acid accumulates in the muscle and blood during intense activity. It is removed in four ways and can take up to four hours after exercise has ceased to be completely removed.

60% of lactic acid is converted back to pyruvic acid and then used as a source of energy in the Krebs cycle. To convert this costs energy, hence increased respiration above resting values after exercise has finished. Gentle exercise or warm-down is of benefit in this process as this maintains higher respiration rate but also flushes lactic acid out of fast twitch fibres, the remaining 40% is converted to protein or muscle glycogen or it is sweated or excreted from the body.

50% of all the lactic acid is removed in the first $\frac{1}{2}$ hour after exercise and uses typically 5–8 litres of oxygen.

Myoglobin and oxygen stores

Myoglobin at rest stores oxygen within the muscles cells (it is similar to haemaglobin in the blood). During exercise it shuttles oxygen from the capillaries to the mitochondria. After intense exercise the myoglobin–oxygen stores are very depleted.

Oxygen stored in the muscle is useful because it helps to 'spare' phosphocreatine and glycogen at the beginning of exercise because the body can supply some of its needs aerobically. This store is quickly depleted. It is restored only when there is a surplus of oxygen in the system following exercise.

Elevated respiration rates following exercise means spare oxygen is available to replenish stored stock.

Glycogen stores

Only very small amounts of glycogen are stored in the body and these can become depleted very quickly when it is used for aerobic and anaerobic work. After two hours of intensive exercise, stores of glycogen will be running low.

(This is most often seen when fun runners hit 'the wall' in the marathon and they begin to lose control of their coordination.)

Glycogen is important as a source of high energy fuel, it is vital that it is spared during exercise to ensure it is there when the athlete needs it. Stores can be replaced by eating a high carbohydrate meal following exercise.

> - Athletes must learn to pace themselves during exercise to avoid crossing the 'anaerobic threshold'
> - Athletes must learn to take rests during activity to allow phosphogen and myoglobin stores to recover (this spares glycogen use)
> - Replenish stores of glycogen during exercise by taking small but regular amounts of glucose drinks.

Aerobic training allows the preferential use of fats as an energy source during sub-maximal exercise thus sparing glycogen.

The concept of an energy continuum

> *Applying energy systems to various activities.*

The three energy systems do not work independently of each other, but in unison and in response to the changing demands of the environment the body is working in.

Most sporting activities require a mix of energy – thus all three systems contribute as athletes cross the threshold (the point at which it is inefficient to produce energy via that system) of the three systems.

This is why fartlek training is so effective for games players.

We can represent the contributions made by energy systems in broad terms on a continuum.

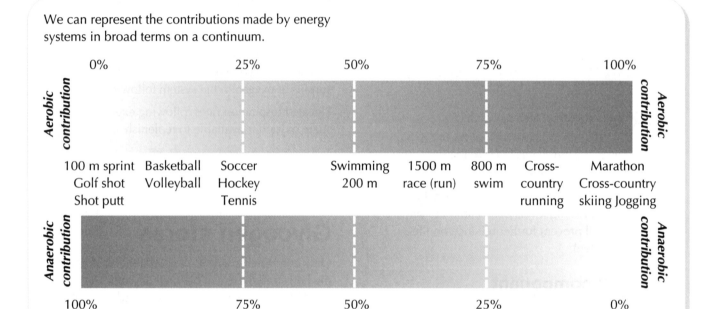

These percentages vary according to the intensity with which each activity is performed, e.g. a competitive soccer match will use more anaerobic energy than a friendly kick about in the park amongst friends.

Athlete's training regimes should take into account the requirements for energy in order to make training as specific as possible.

$\dot{V}O_2$ max

The amount of energy used during exercise is directly related to the amount of oxygen consumed.

The breakdown of glycogen and fat requires the presence of oxygen.

If we measure the amount of oxygen consumed (by comparing expired oxygen content with atmospheric air oxygen content) we can estimate the amount of energy used.

At rest we consume 0.2–0.3 litres of oxygen per minute.

$VO_2 - v$ = volume per minute,
O_2 = oxygen

During **maximal** exercise this may rise to 3–6 litres of oxygen per minute ($\dot{V}O_2$ max).

An athlete's $\dot{V}O_2$ max is determined by the efficiency of their cardiac system, respiratory system, and other physiological characteristics, e.g. muscle fibre types.

$\dot{V}O_2$ max may be improved by training – increased capillarisation, increase in red blood cells, increased cardiac output, increased myoglobin content, increase in size and number of mitochondria – by up to 20%.

Physical fitness

> *Part of fitness.*

Health components

Aerobic capacity

This is the ability of a performer to take in and use oxygen. This depends upon:

1 Respiration (external)

2 Oxygen transportation from lungs to muscles

3 Cell respiration.

> This is often referred to as **maximal oxygen consumption** (or '$\dot{V}O_2$ max') – sub-maximal activity benefits aerobic capacity (e.g. jogging, cycling, swimming).

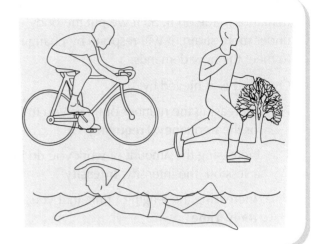

Strength

This is the amount of force a performer can exert through their muscles. Maximum strength is one single contraction. Dynamic strength or power is the ability to overcome resistance very quickly and is used in nearly all sports.

Muscular endurance is the ability to contract the muscles again and again without growing tired. This is a vital aspect of fitness for all sports people – as a match progresses fatigue sets in; the team that resists fatiguing best often wins.

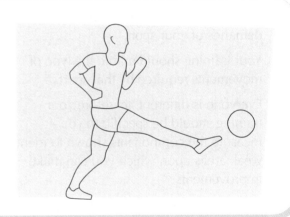

Flexibility

This is the ability to move body parts around a joint.

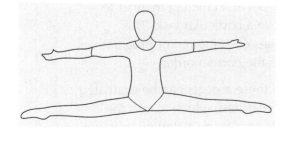

Body composition

This refers to the relative percentage of overall weight that various components of the body make up (e.g. bones, blood, muscle, organs [lean body mass] and fat).

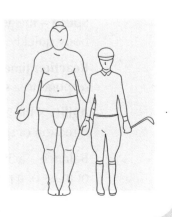

Principles of training

> Improving the training effect.

Overload

The human body is designed to adapt to new demands made on it. So if we put the body under more strain, it will respond by changing to meet the new demands.

Overload is achieved by:

F > Increasing the number of times you train or the frequency. **Frequency**

I > Increasing the amount of work you do in a session, the intensity. **Intensity**

T > Increasing the length of time that you train. **Time**

Specificity

> Fitness is made up of lots of different components. The type of fitness required by different sports is quite different. Therefore your training should reflect the demands of your sport.

> Your training should mimic the type of movements required by that sport.

> Everyone is different, therefore your training should be specific to you – measure the components shown to identify weak areas upon which you can make improvements.

> Most sports use very specific energy systems at specific times. Try to reflect these differences in your training.

Reversibility

Fitness cannot be banked to be used in the future. Any changes due to training will reverse once training is stopped.

Variance

Try to spice up your training by doing different things, using different methods to prevent boredom.

Beware: repetitive strain injuries!

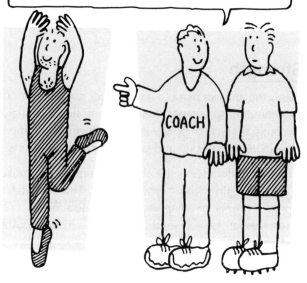

Skill components

Speed – the ability to move your body quickly.

Reaction time – the time taken to respond to a stimulus.

Agility – the ability to change direction of speed efficiently.

Balance – achieved when the centre of mass of a performer is over an area of support.

Coordination – the ability to move in a smooth and efficient manner to achieve a particular task. This involves ensuring motor programmes run in the correct order.

All of these aspects can be evaluated and measured, which allows the athlete to identify a starting point for training and to monitor improvements in each aspect.

Training programmes

> *How to improve health components of fitness.*

These must be specific to the needs of your activity and follow the principle of training. They will affect the health-related and skill-related components of your fitness.

Strength training

Strength is improved by increasing the level of resistance that a muscle group must overcome (overload). Athletes must decide very carefully what type of strength they wish to improve (see descriptions on physical fitness, page 59) and which specific muscles to work on, and the type of contraction required by their sport.

Absolute strength will be improved by working with greater resistances (more weight) and fewer repetitions per set. Muscular endurance will be improved by working with lower resistances (less weight) but more repetitions per set.

Repetition is a full contraction of a muscular group during an exercise (e.g. biceps curl and a return to its original position).

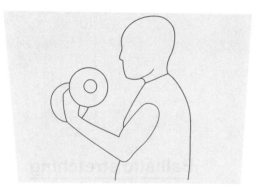

A set is a number of repetitions of a given exercise (this will depend on the type of strength being improved).

Methods to improve strength

Weight training – the use of free weights on dumbbells and bars which can allow the athlete to mimic closely some of the actions involved in his/he sport or the use of specially designed (safer) machines to work on.

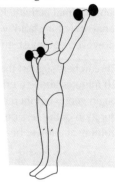

Circuit training – often using the performer's body weight on a number of exercises to improve strength, particularly good for young children (e.g. press ups, sit ups, dips, running).

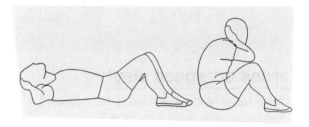

Plyometrics – muscles working eccentrically, then immediately concentrically – improve muscle strength dramatically (e.g. triple jumping, running down hill).

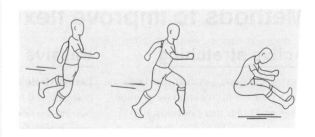

Flexibility – a performer's flexibility is limited by the structures in the joints. Bony structures cannot change, nor can the movements allowed by certain joint types. However, soft tissues – such as ligaments, tendons and muscles – can be stretched.

Improvements in flexibility can be rapid and occur to their greatest extent when the body is already warm. Too much mobility in some joints, especially in contact sports, can lead to injury. Training of this component must be very specific.

Aerobic training

Aerobic training

These are designed to increase $\dot{V}O_2$ max and will involve sub-maximal activity. Remember, working above the 'anaerobic threshold' will work only the lactacid system. However, you must still overload your system.

Researchers suggest that continuous exercise for at least 20 minutes above a critical level is necessary. You should begin gently but increase the frequency, intensity or duration of the session if you are able to perform the training at a lower heart rate than previously.

> **Methods to improve $\dot{V}O_2$ max**
> > Choose a rhythmic activity (e.g. swimming, jogging, cycling, aerobics) that uses large muscles.
> > Work in your aerobic training zone. This means at least 60% of your maximum heart rate, unless you are very fit. As you get fitter, you can move up to 75%.
> > For best results: at least 15–20 minutes at least 3 times a week.

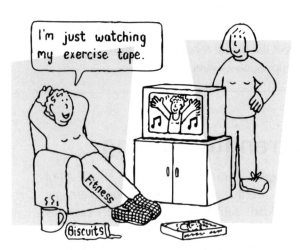

> You can use this sort of training for things like running, cycling and skiing.

> The principle is that during a continuous run, periods of more intense work are used to stress the systems, but recovery is allowed during the slower periods. This is useful as it follows the principle of variance and is good for athletes who need to 'change pace' as part of their game.

Fartlek or 'speed play'

> This is based on changes of speed. For instance, 5 minutes of gentle jogging; then 5 minutes of fast walk; then 50 m sprints every 200 m; then uphill jog with 10 fast strides every minute; and so on…

Interval training

This is training where 'work' periods are interspersed with 'rest' periods to allow recovery. It is very good for maintaining quality training, particularly in elite athletes.

Methods to improve flexibility

Active stretching

The performer moves their own body into a position just beyond the normal range and holds that position for 10 seconds. This is known as **active stretching**.

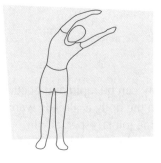

Passive stretching

Passive stretching involves the body being moved by a partner to a position beyond the normal range of movement and then being held for 10 seconds.

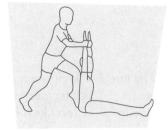

Ballistic stretching

This involves swinging/bouncing movements to take the body beyond its normal range of movement. Only athletes with a good level of flexibility should use this method.

Proprioceptive Neuro-muscular Facilitation (PNF)

The performer stretches to a point just beyond the normal range of movement. The athlete contracts the muscle, then relaxes, and then takes the stretch a little further.

Short-term effects of exercise

> *What happens during exercise.*

The human body is constantly battling with changing circumstances to maintain a stable, efficient internal condition. The responses shown below are the ways in which the body tries to maintain **homeostasis** (controlled environment within cells).

Heart

Exercise changes the chemical balance of the body:
> lactic acid increases
> $CO_2 + O_2$ levels change
> and temperature increases.

This produces stimuli for the cardiac control centre to respond to.

Nerves: the sympathetic nerve controlling the sino-atrial node (pacemaker) is stimulated to increase heart rate.
Chemical: adrenaline is released in the blood increasing heart rate even before exercise.

Cardiac output increases because the heart rate increases; venous return increases which in turn increases the amount

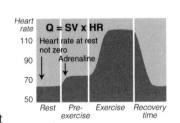

of blood entering the heart. More blood in the heart and stronger more frequent contractions leads to increased cardiac output (Q).

Lungs

Changes to the relative proportions of CO_2 and O_2 are detected in the respiratory centre, which responds by increasing minute ventilation.

Minute ventilation is a function of the number of breaths and the tidal volume. Tidal volume increases by drawing upon the spare lung capacity, known as inspiratory reserve volume and expiratory reserve volume.

The respiratory muscles, intercostals, diaphragm and scaleni become more active, especially on expiration. This increases the volume of the thoracic cavity and decreases it with greater force.

Blood

> Blood changes its constitution during exercise. This carries the messages that are detected by receptors to initiate changes in HR and ventilation.
> Blood becomes thicker during intense activity as plasma volume decreases due to sweating.
> Glucose levels begin to drop.
> Blood acidity increases due to lactic acid. This may, if not controlled, lead to a detrimental effect on muscle activity.
> Oxygen concentrations drop dramatically, thus increasing diffusion at the lungs.
> Blood pressure increases as Q increases.
> Blood flow speeds up.
> More blood is directed to the muscles and away from other areas. Vasodilation in arteries to muscles and in muscle capillaries aids blood flow here.
> Vasoconstriction around non-essential areas decreases blood flow in these areas.

Muscles

Increases in the intensity and frequency of contractions lead to a greater use of energy, thus increasing cell respiration. These changes stimulate the rest of the body to adapt.

The body's fuel energy stores are gradually depleted:
> phospho-creatine
> glycogen
> triglycerides (free fatty acids).

The myoglobin in the muscles gives up its oxygen stores for cell respiration. Thus O_2 is diffused more quickly as the partial pressure difference between cell and capillary is greater.

Carbon dioxide and lactic acid levels increase in the muscles and need to be removed by the blood.

The energy conversion in the muscle is notoriously inefficient. It is only between 14–25% efficient, with most energy being released as heat, thus increasing body temperature.

But what about the longer-term effects.... ?

Body composition

> Body composition means the proportion of the various constituents of the body bones, blood, organs, muscles and fat.

Measuring body composition

An accurate assessment of an individual's body composition can be obtained through a process called **hydrostatic weighing**. This involves the total immersion of the body in a hydrostatic weighing tank. The subject expels all the air form their lungs, then their weight is measured.

This allows you to calculate the body density, which can be further converted into the percentage for body fat using the **Siri equation:**

$$\% \text{ body fat} = 495/\text{body density} - 450$$

This measure has been used as a standard for indirect methods, such as the measurement of skinfold thickness. Here skinfold callipers are used to measure skinfolds, usually in four sites (bicep, tricep, scapular and supra iliac). The measurements are then compared with norms tables.

Body mass index (BMI) can also be calculated by dividing a person's weight by their height squared. The resulting figure is compared with norms tables.

BMI and skinfold calliper give indications only. Hydrostatic weighing gives the most accurate measurement of body composition.

Body Mass Index Table

	Normal						Overweight					Obese										Extreme Obesity														
BMI	19	20	21	22	23	24	25	26	27	28	29	30	31	32	33	34	35	36	37	38	39	40	41	42	43	44	45	46	47	48	49	50	51	52	53	54
Height (inches)																	Body Weight (pounds)																			
58	91	96	100	105	110	115	119	124	129	134	138	143	148	153	158	162	167	172	177	181	186	191	196	201	205	210	215	220	224	229	234	239	244	248	253	258
59	94	99	104	109	114	119	124	128	133	138	143	148	153	158	163	168	173	178	183	188	193	198	203	208	212	217	222	227	232	237	242	247	252	257	262	267
60	97	102	107	112	118	123	128	133	138	143	148	153	158	163	168	174	179	184	189	194	199	204	209	215	220	225	230	235	240	245	250	255	261	266	271	276
61	100	106	111	116	122	127	132	137	143	148	153	158	164	169	174	180	185	190	195	201	206	211	217	222	227	232	238	243	248	254	259	264	269	275	280	285
62	104	109	115	120	126	131	136	142	147	153	158	164	169	175	180	186	191	196	202	207	213	218	224	229	235	240	246	251	256	262	267	273	278	284	289	295
63	107	113	118	124	130	135	141	146	152	158	163	169	175	180	186	191	197	203	208	214	220	225	231	237	242	248	254	259	265	270	278	282	287	293	299	304
64	110	116	122	128	134	140	145	151	157	163	169	174	180	186	192	197	204	209	215	221	227	232	238	244	250	256	262	267	273	279	285	291	296	302	308	314
65	114	120	126	132	138	144	150	156	162	168	174	180	186	192	198	204	210	216	222	228	234	240	246	252	258	264	270	276	282	288	294	300	306	312	318	324
66	118	124	130	136	142	148	155	161	167	173	179	186	192	198	204	210	216	223	229	235	241	247	253	260	266	272	278	284	291	297	303	309	315	322	328	334
67	121	127	134	140	146	153	159	166	172	178	185	191	198	204	211	217	223	230	236	242	249	255	261	268	274	280	287	293	299	306	312	319	32	331	338	344
68	125	131	138	144	151	158	164	171	177	184	190	197	203	210	216	223	230	236	243	249	256	262	269	276	282	289	295	302	308	315	322	328	335	341	348	354
69	128	135	142	149	155	162	169	176	182	189	196	203	209	216	223	230	236	243	250	257	263	270	277	284	291	297	304	311	318	324	331	338	345	351	358	365
70	132	139	146	153	160	167	174	181	188	195	202	209	216	222	229	236	243	250	257	264	271	278	285	292	299	306	313	320	327	334	341	348	355	362	369	376
71	136	143	150	157	165	172	179	186	193	200	208	215	222	229	236	243	250	257	265	272	279	286	293	301	308	315	322	329	338	343	351	358	365	372	379	386
72	140	147	154	162	169	177	184	191	199	206	213	221	228	235	242	250	258	265	272	279	287	294	302	309	316	324	331	338	346	353	361	368	375	383	390	397
73	144	151	159	166	174	182	189	197	204	212	219	227	235	242	250	257	265	272	280	288	295	302	310	318	325	333	340	348	355	363	371	378	386	393	401	408
74	148	155	163	171	179	186	194	202	210	218	225	233	241	249	256	264	272	280	287	295	303	311	319	326	334	342	350	358	365	373	381	389	396	404	412	420
75	152	160	168	176	184	192	200	208	216	224	232	240	248	256	264	272	279	287	295	303	311	319	327	335	343	351	359	367	375	383	391	399	407	415	423	431
76	156	164	172	180	189	197	205	213	221	230	238	246	254	263	271	279	287	295	304	312	320	328	336	344	353	361	369	377	385	394	402	410	418	426	435	443

Obesity

This is a clinical term to describe the excessive accumulation of body fat. Various measures are used to determine obesity. On the BMI scale you are obese if your score is 30+; if you get a BMI of 40, you are morbidly obese. However, using BMI does not take into account an individual's body shape and so may not give a completely accurate picture. This is especially true when dealing with athletes, whose increased bone density can distort BMI results.

Long-term effects of exercise

> *Training causes long-term adaptations in body systems to cope with the new demands made.*

Aerobic changes

An improvement in an athlete's $\dot{V}O_2$ max occurs during correct aerobic exercise routines. Most of the time the athlete's muscles depend on aerobic respiration.

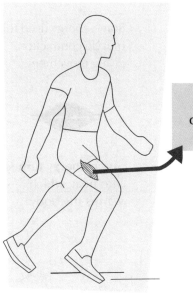

Glucose + oxygen give...

energy

Some energy used for muscle contraction, giving movement.

Some energy turned into heat, which warms the body.

Carbon dioxide: Carried away by blood and excreted through the lungs.

Water: Carried away by blood. Some excreted through the lungs and some in urine.

1 Heart

> The muscles of the heart wall (myocardium) grow in size and strength after regular exercise. This allows the heart to contract with more force, therefore ejecting more blood per heart beat.

> Increased heart size means increased stroke volume. Therefore at rest the athlete's heart has to pump less times to move the same amount of blood as an untrained heart. This results in lower resting heart rate (bradycardia).

> At maximum levels of effort, stroke volume is increased and heart rate is high. Thus more O_2 is delivered to the working muscles increasing efficiency and increasing $\dot{V}O_2$ max.

2 Lungs

> Maximum minute volume is increased.

> The respiratory muscles are stronger and more efficient, making respiration easier.

> Lung capacity improves as training increases. Capillarisation around the alveoli allows greater areas of lung to be utilized.

Anaerobic changes

During all-out effort, such as sprinting, the muscles need a lot of energy fast. Because oxygen cannot reach the muscles fast enough, **anaerobic respiration** takes over. Less energy is produced from the same amount of glucose, but it is produced much faster.

> Anaerobic training allows athletes to work harder and for longer at higher intensities.

> Muscles, particularly fibre types 2a and 2b, grow in size and therefore strength.

> Stores of ATP (see page 54) are increased.

> Phosphocreatine and glycogen are produced.

> The enzyme phosphorylase increases in concentration allowing more efficient resynthesis of ADP to ATP.

> There is an increased tolerance of lactic acid in the muscles and the recovery system for its removal also more efficient.

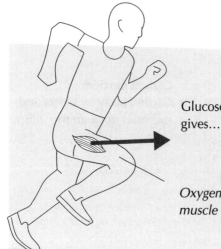

energy

Glucose gives...

Very fast

Oxygen can't reach muscle fast enough

Some energy used for muscle contraction, giving movement.

Some energy turned into heat, which warms the body.

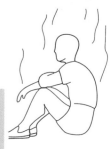

Lactic acid:
After a minute or so, lactic acid makes muscles tired and painful. All-out effort must stop or you'll collapse.

3 Blood

> Volume of blood increases, due mostly to increased plasma levels. More red blood cells are also created, allowing greater oxygen-carrying capacity.

> Acidity of the blood decreases at low level exercise as their aerobic system is more efficient.

> At maximal levels of exercise, blood acidity is higher in athletes as they have a greater tolerance of its effects.

> Arterial walls become more elastic with endurance training, allowing tolerance of changes in blood pressure. There is greater capillarisation in the lungs and muscles allowing greater diffusion of O_2.

4 Muscles

> Muscles grow larger and stronger through exercise.

> Myoglobin concentration increases.

> Mitochondria become more numerous.

> Enzymes work much more efficiently allowing greater cell respiration.

> Muscles store larger amounts of glycogen and triglycerides.

Enhancing performance

> Athletes seeking to maximise their performance can use a variety of aids to give them the edge in completion. These aids can be categorized as legal or illegal.

Legal

Dietary manipulation

Carbo-loading

This is the most common form of dietary manipulation.

> An athlete will deplete the body's store of glycogen, by heavy-training the systems that rely on glycogen for energy.
> 'Starved' of glycogen/carbohydrates, the athlete's body will super-compensate by storing increased levels of glycogen.
> The athlete then tapers their training in the lead-up to competition, and eats a carbohydrate-rich diet.

Carbo-loading is of particular benefit to endurance of aerobic athletes and to games players. Athletes may also benefit from meal immediately before a match or competition.

Possible negative side effects to carbo-loading could be:
> compromised training quality during the glycogen depletion stage
> increased water retention leading to weight gain
> increased irritability
> a lack of concentration.

Pre-match/competition meal

- Pre-competition meals can affect performance during the game/completion.
- To ensure success, the meal should be consumed 2–4 hours before the competition, ensuring that glycogen stores are high during the competition.
- For endurance athletes, ingestion of caffeine may also enhance the release of fatty acids in the bloodstream.

Post-match meals

- Ingestion of a carbohydrate-rich meal after a match will ensure quicker glycogen replacement.

Illegal

> **Human growth hormone (HGH)** The effects of an athlete using HGH include increased muscle mass (and therefore power) and possibly quicker recovery from high intensity exercise/training (this is still not fully proven). Other effects include an increased glucose concentration in the athlete's blood and quicker healing capacity.
> **Blood doping** Here the athlete will remove a quantity of their own blood and store it for several weeks, during which their body makes up for the shortfall. The athlete then injects the stored blood back into their system, increasing the red blood cell and haemoglobin levels temporarily. Useful for endurance athletes but risky, due to potential contamination problems.
> **Recombinant erythropoietin (rhEPO)** This hormone is designed to increase the red blood cell count and raise haemoglobin levels in patients with low counts, anaemia, etc. Athletes recognise the benefit of this 'medicine' and abuse it for personal gain. Endurance athletes in particular benefit from increased haemoglobin concentration.
> **Gene doping** – Gene doping involves the innovative medical technique of gene replacement, where faulty genes could be replaced with health genes. Athletes could benefit from increased production of beneficial hormones to aid performance in a wide variety of events.

As well as being illegal in many countries and leading to lengthy bans, many of these techniques produce unwanted side effects, creating potentially serious health issues.

Training aids

Training aids to increase resistance

These artificial aids are designed to increase the resistance experienced in training, overloading the athlete more quickly so that they work much harder and ensuring a quick adaptation of muscles to the new requirements.
Examples of this type of equipment include:

> parachutes attached to the athlete increasing resistance
> elastic cords, with the resistance supplied by a training partner
> 'speed ladders', mini hurdles and agility runs.

Training aids to decrease recovery time

Ice baths

Athletes usually finish their training session using traditional cool-down methods, but can enhance the effects by immersing themselves in ice baths. Lactic acid and CO_2 are removed from the muscle more quickly, diminishing pain, and the incidence of strains is reduced, as the effects of micro-tearing of muscle fibres is counteracted.

Creatine supplements

Athletes can supplement their diets with creatine-rich drinks or food to enhance the amount of stored creatine associated with phosphates to improve ATP-ADP-ATP replenishment. Sprinters and power athletes benefit the most from this.

Measuring performance – fitness testing

> *Important tools for monitoring performance changes*

Aerobic testing – VO$_2$ max

VO$_2$ Max is a measure of how fit an athlete is: it indicates the volume of oxygen a body consumes per minute. There are various ways of testing VO$_2$ max.

> **Multi-stage fitness test of 'bleep test'**– a progressive and maximum 20 m shuttle-run test. It involves running a 20 m shuttle at a pace set by a timed tape. The test progresses from an easy pace to a full sprint. Performers drop out when they can no longer keep up with the pace set. The researchers who created this test also produced score tables that are used to predict VO$_2$ max based on scores attained. This test has a limitation in that it requires maximal effort to attain an accurate score. This could prove dangerous for certain groups or individuals.
> **PWC-170 test** – an alternative assessment of VO$_2$ max for those who cannot perform maximal tests.
> **Coopers Run** – a test where participants complete a 12-minute run on a 400 m track, with 50 m intervals marked so that participants can measure they distance covered accurately. The further participants run, the greater the VO$_2$ Max. This test is not maximal but does require that the participants can pace themselves for the 12 minutes.

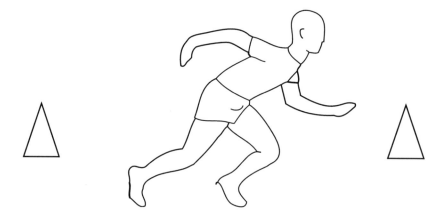

Accurately measuring VO$_2$ max requires gas analysis of expired air. This test is usually only carried out in sport science labs in universities.

Strength testing

Standard tests exist to measure three aspects of muscular strength:

> **maximal strength:** hand grip dynamometer/1 rep max using isolated muscle groups
> **elastic strength:** sergeant jumps – a two-part standing board jump.
> **strength/endurance:** national coaching foundation sit up test- the participants sit up at a pace set by pre-recorded tape which speeds up progressively.

Flexibility testing

Flexibility is the range of movement about a joint. The most common test is the 'sit and reach test', which measures hip flexibility. Other joints can be tested using specialist measures known as **goniometers,** which measure the angles of limbs affected at various joints.

Linear motion – distance, velocity and acceleration

> *Vectors or scalars? When they are the same and when they are different.*

We will start this topic by looking at 'linear motion'. What is 'linear motion'? A simple definition might be 'movement forward or backward in a generally straight line'.

Make a list in a notebook of all the sports you can think of which involve a 'linear motion'. How can we measure this motion? To start with we need to consider the following:

> **distance** – the path taken by an object moving from one point to another
> **displacement** – the shortest straight line between the starting and finishing point ('as the crow flies')
> **speed** – rate of change of position; the distance travelled by the body per unit time
> **velocity** – rate of change of position with reference to direction
> **acceleration** – rate of change in velocity.

Key points:

1 **Vector quantities** are those with both magnitude and direction. They include: displacement, velocity, acceleration and force.
2 **Scalar quantities** are those with just magnitude. They include: distance, speed and mass (amount of matter).

Distance and Displacement

It is possible to have an equal value for these measures, as is the case when considering a 100 m sprint. Here the path taken by the runner measures 100 metres. The distance from the starting point to the finish point is also 100 metres.

This is not the case in a 100 m swim (2×50 m lengths). Here, the path taken by the swimmer is 100 metres, whilst the distance from the starting point to the finish point is 0! (They start and end at the same end of the pool.)

Speed and Velocity

The difference between distance and displacement has an effect on calculations. If the swimmer covers 100 m in 60 seconds then the average speed will be:

$$\frac{\text{Distance}}{\text{Time}} = \frac{100}{60} = 1.67 \text{ ms}^{-1}$$

But the average velocity will be:

$$\frac{\text{Displacement}}{\text{Time}} = \frac{0}{60} = 0 \text{ ms}^{-1}$$

Averages

$$\text{Average speed} = \frac{\text{Distance covered (ms}^{-1})}{\text{Time taken}}$$

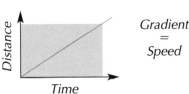

Gradient = Speed

$$\text{Average acceleration} = \frac{\text{Change in velocity (ms}^{-2})}{\text{Time taken}}$$

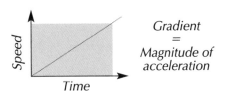

Gradient = Magnitude of acceleration

$$\text{Average velocity} = \frac{\text{Displacement (ms}^{-1})}{\text{Time taken}}$$

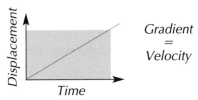

Gradient = Velocity

$$\frac{vf - vi}{t}$$

where *vf* = final velocity
vi = initial velocity
t = time interval

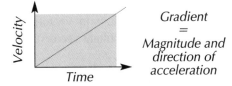

Gradient = Magnitude and direction of acceleration

Note: Displacement, velocity and acceleration are all *vector* quantities and can therefore be used together in equations. Speed and distance are *scalar* quantities and also appear together in equations. **Do NOT mix vector (those with magnitude and direction) and scalar quantities (those with only magnitude) in equations!**

Vectors

Vectors are quantities such as displacement, velocity, acceleration and force (which includes weight!) which have both *magnitude* and *direction*. We can represent a vector by a line with an arrow on the end. The length of the line represents the magnitude of the vector and the arrow indicates the direction.

Examples

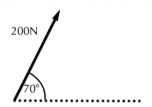

6 cm

20°

1 Using a scale of 1 cm = 1 ms⁻¹, this line
represents a velocity of 6 ms⁻¹ at an angle of 20° to the horizontal.
This principle may be used for all vectors.

200N

70°

2 Here we have a force of 200 N acting at 70° to the horizontal.

Note: Because we can represent vectors as a combination of length and angle, we can use a range of trigonometric techniques to calculate answers to problems.

Resultant vectors

When two or more vectors are combined, their overall effect is described as being their **resultant vector.** Consider the two velocities (a) and (b) below. We can combine them by making the arrows 'follow on'. The resultant is the overall effect of the two arrows 'following on' (c).

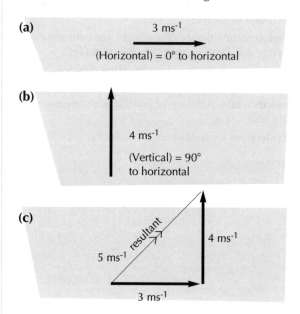

(a)   3 ms⁻¹
(Horizontal) = 0° to horizontal

(b)   4 ms⁻¹
(Vertical) = 90° to horizontal

(c)   5 ms⁻¹   resultant   4 ms⁻¹
3 ms⁻¹

The resultant vector can be measured directly with a ruler for magnitude and a protractor for direction, if velocities are drawn to scale. This is known as the construction technique. Alternatively, the results may be calculated using Pythagoras or other trigonometric rules.

(Notice how the example given is almost instantly observed as being a '3, 4, 5 triangle'!)

Component vectors

A similar technique may be used to 'dismantle' a vector into two components. This is called **resolving** into horizontal and vertical components. It involves producing horizontal and vertical 'follow on' vectors from a single vector (the reverse of resultant vectors).

Example

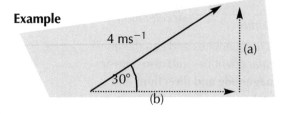

4 ms⁻¹

(a)

30°

(b)

Here the velocity of 4 ms⁻¹ has been resolved into horizontal and vertical vectors that 'follow on'. The magnitude of these vectors can be measured directly with a ruler, if drawn to scale (construction technique), but are calculated using the following rule:

> **Vector opposite angle (a) =**
> **hypotenuse sine angle = 4 sin 30° = 2**
>
> **Vector adjacent angle (b) =**
> **hypotenuse cosine angle = 4 cos 30° = 3.46 ms⁻¹**

Projectile motion

> *The interplay between horizontal and vertical components during the flight of a projectile.*

Definition

A body that is released into the air.

Examples

Throwing, striking, projecting of the body itself.

The projectile's pre-determined path of flight (parabola) is influenced by:

1 the force applied, establishing its velocity at release

2 the angle of release

3 the relative height of release.

1 Speed or velocity of release

> The greater the speed of release, the greater the range.

> The speed of release has a greater influence on the range of a projectile than the angle or relative height.

> The greater the initial vertical velocity, the greater the flight time and the greater the height reached.

> The greater the initial horizontal velocity, the greater the horizontal distance.

> The lower the angle of release, the greater the release velocity must be if the projectile is to travel the required distance.

A body projected at 30 ms^{-1} at an angle θ to the horizontal.

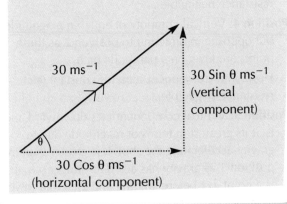

30 ms^{-1}

30 Sin θ ms^{-1} (vertical component)

θ

30 Cos θ ms^{-1} (horizontal component)

2 Angle of release

> The optimum angle at which you need to project a body in order to obtain the maximum horizontal range is **45°**. This only applies where the **release** and **landing** occur at the **same** level, and where there is no spin and no air assistance.

> In most sporting situations, the angle is almost always less than 45° => in range 35°–45°.

> If the angle of release is too high, the horizontal component of velocity is reduced, thus reducing the horizontal distance.

> If the angle of release is too low, the vertical component of velocity is reduced, thus reducing the time of flight which, in turn, reduces the horizontal distance (less **time** for horizontal component of velocity to act).

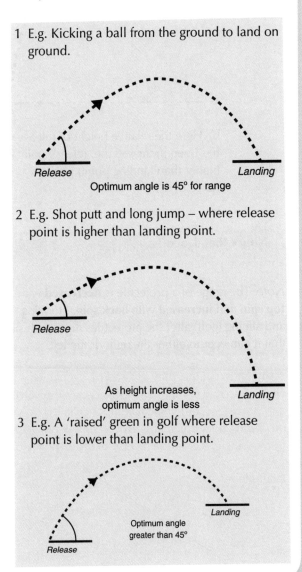

1 E.g. Kicking a ball from the ground to land on ground.

Release — Landing

Optimum angle is 45° for range

2 E.g. Shot putt and long jump – where release point is higher than landing point.

Release

As height increases, optimum angle is less — Landing

3 E.g. A 'raised' green in golf where release point is lower than landing point.

Landing

Optimum angle greater than 45°

Release

Projectile motion (cont.)

3 Relative height of release

> For a given speed and angle of release, as the relative height increases, the horizontal range increases.

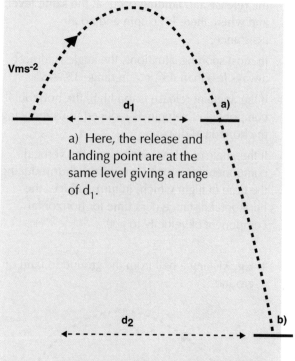

a) Here, the release and landing point are at the same level giving a range of d_1.

b) Here the relative height of release has been increased (i.e. release point higher than landing point) giving a range of d_2.

Notice that $d_2 > d_1$!

Note: The range of a projectile is **decreased** with **top spin** and **increased** with **back spin.** Hooking and slicing (golf) alter the projectiles flight path so that it can veer to either the right or the left.

The changes in the vertical and horizontal components

E.g. Shot putt

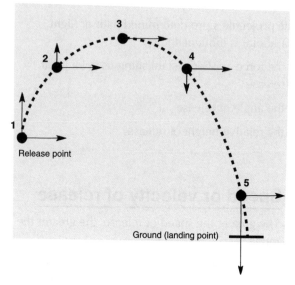

Position 1: Shot putt released with vertical and horizontal components of velocity.

Position 2: Vertical component of velocity decreases due to gravity providing resistance to **upward** motion.

Horizontal component remains unaltered under the assumption that air resistance is negligible (air resistance is the only force that **could** act horizontally to slow the shot down!).

Position 3: Shot at top of flight path therefore **no** vertical component (gravity has acted to reduce this to zero).

Horizontal component remains unaltered (air resistance negligible).

Position 4: Vertical component equal in magnitude but opposite in direction to position 2 as these points are level on a parabolic path.

Horizontal component remains constant (air resistance negligible).

Position 5: Vertical component acts downward and is at its greatest in terms of magnitude due to gravity accelerating the shot. It is greater than in position 1 as gravity has acted for longer (i.e. it is a point just before landing and therefore lower than the release point).

Horizontal component remains constant (air resistance negligible).

Linear motion – forces, Newton's Laws

> *Forces acting **on a body** and forces applied **by a body**.*

A force is a push or a pull that acts on an object in order to change its state of motion.

Forces may be **internal** (those generated by ourselves through muscular contraction) and **external** (those from outside our body such as gravity, friction, air resistance and those caused by reactions with the ground or some other external body).

Forces are *vector* quantities and therefore have magnitude and direction. They can be represented by a line of action and a point of application.

When considering forces, it is necessary to distinguish between those forces acting on the body and those applied by the body *separately*. This normally involves the consideration of external forces. This will help when analysing the interaction of two or more bodies.

Forces are measured in Newtons!

Example

In order to understand the force acting in the use of the scrummage machine we need to consider:

(a) the forces exerted **by** the rugby player(s) and forces acting on the machine

(b) the forces acting **on** the rugby player and forces exerted by the machine.

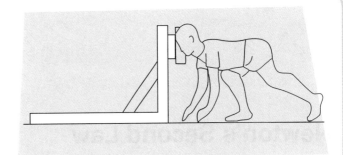

(a) Forces acting on the machine

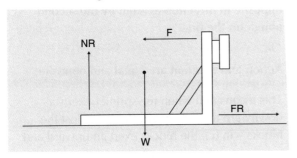

NR = Normal Reaction force from contact with ground

W = Weight of scrummage machine (acting through centre of gravity of machine)

F = Action force applied by player

FR = Friction force from ground contact opposing sliding motion of scrummage machine

(b) Forces acting on the player

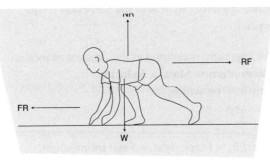

NR = Net normal reaction force from contacts with ground

W = Weight of rugby player

RF = Reaction force from scrummage machine

FR = Friction force from ground contact opposing sliding motion of feet and hands

Linear motion – forces, Newton's Laws (cont.)

Newton's Laws are the basic laws of mechanics that describe the way in which bodies move in response to forces acting on them.

Newton's First Law

> This is the law of inertia which states that:

'Every object will remain in a state of rest or uniform motion unless acted upon by an external force.'

> Also known as 'Galileo's law'.

> 'Inertia' is an object's reluctance to move. So this law is often linked to inertia. Inertia is proportional to mass and therefore more force is required to move a heavy object than a light one.

> In the sprint start, the athlete will not move unless a 'net' external force acts upon him/her. Thus a force needs to be applied to move the athlete from (a) to (b) to (c).

(a) 'On your marks'

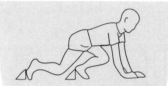

(b) 'Get set'

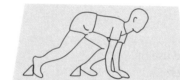

(c) 'GO!!'

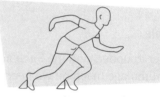

Newton's Second Law

> This law states that:

'The rate of change of momentum or acceleration of an object is proportional to the force applied and acts in the direction of the force.'

> 'Momentum' is defined as the amount of motion.
Momentum = Mass × Velocity
This may be written as:

$$F = \frac{Mvf - Mvi}{t}$$

where F = Force, Mvf = Final momentum, Mvi = Initial momentum, t = time
Rewriting gives:

$$F = \frac{M (vf - vi)}{t}$$

But!

$$\frac{vf - vi}{t} = acceleration$$

so F (force) = mass × acceleration

> In the sprint start, the athlete will accelerate more with a great net force acting.

Newton's Third Law

> This law states that:

'When one object exerts a force on another, there is a force equal in magnitude but opposite in direction exerted by the second object on the first.'
OR
Action and reaction are equal and opposite.

> This means that when the sprinter exerts a downward and backwards force against the blocks – in (c), the blocks exert an upward and forward reaction force on the sprinter.

> But if the action and reaction forces are equal and opposite, why does the sprinter move?

The answer lies with the significant differences between the mass of the sprinter and the mass of the Earth. As the blocks are *fixed* to the Earth, they become part of the Earth's mass. Therefore, the force applied by the runner is not enough to displace such a large mass. The reaction force from the blocks is enough, however, to displace the relatively small mass of the sprinter!

Linear motion – impulse

> *The relationship between impulse, force and acceleration.*

Impulse is the change in linear motion caused by a force. So a given impulse can be associated with a weak force over a long time, or with a strong force acting over a short time. The latter is termed an **impulsive force.**

Forces in a vertical jump

Consider the forces acting in a vertical jump.

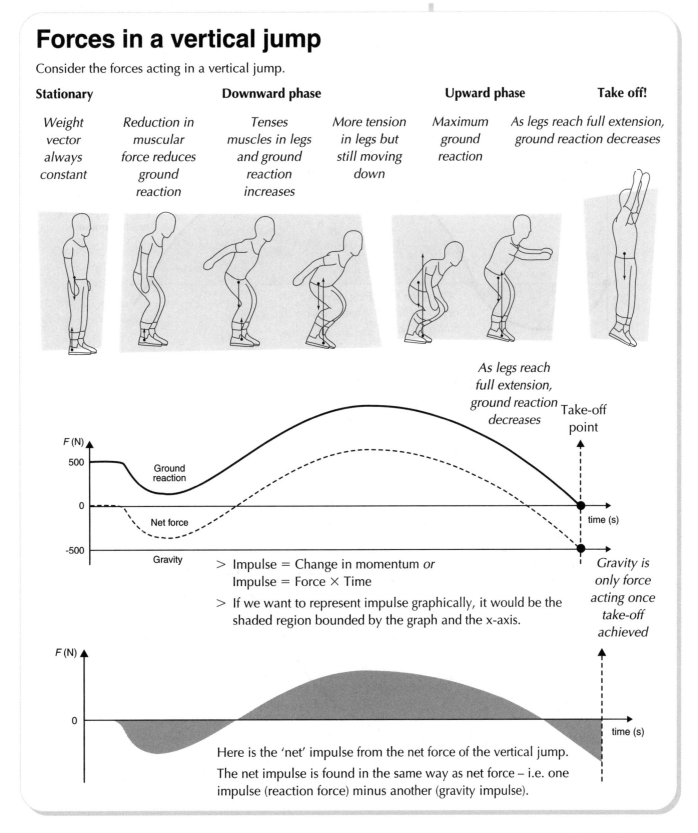

Stationary		Downward phase		Upward phase	Take off!
Weight vector always constant	*Reduction in muscular force reduces ground reaction*	*Tenses muscles in legs and ground reaction increases*	*More tension in legs but still moving down*	*Maximum ground reaction*	*As legs reach full extension, ground reaction decreases*

As legs reach full extension, ground reaction decreases

Take-off point

Gravity is only force acting once take-off achieved

> Impulse = Change in momentum *or*
> Impulse = Force × Time
> If we want to represent impulse graphically, it would be the shaded region bounded by the graph and the x-axis.

Here is the 'net' impulse from the net force of the vertical jump.

The net impulse is found in the same way as net force – i.e. one impulse (reaction force) minus another (gravity impulse).

Forces in a sprint start

Now consider a sprint start (100 metres).

1 Leaving the blocks

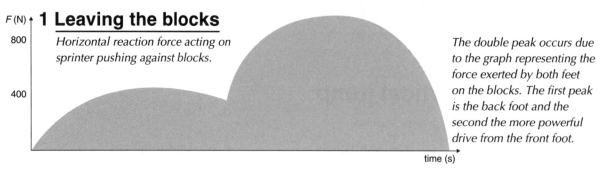

F (N)

800

400

time (s)

Horizontal reaction force acting on sprinter pushing against blocks.

The double peak occurs due to the graph representing the force exerted by both feet on the blocks. The first peak is the back foot and the second the more powerful drive from the front foot.

2 Just after leaving the blocks

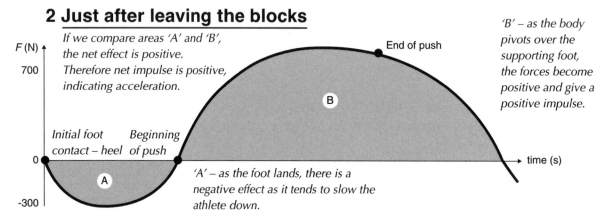

F (N)

700

0

-300

End of push

B

Initial foot contact – heel

Beginning of push

A

time (s)

If we compare areas 'A' and 'B', the net effect is positive. Therefore net impulse is positive, indicating acceleration.

'A' – as the foot lands, there is a negative effect as it tends to slow the athlete down.

'B' – as the body pivots over the supporting foot, the forces become positive and give a positive impulse.

3 A point midway through the race

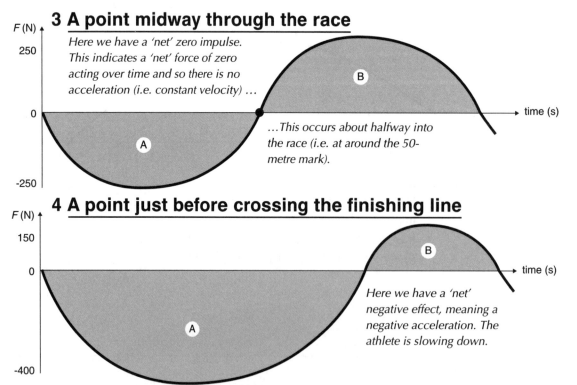

F (N)

250

0

-250

B

A

time (s)

Here we have a 'net' zero impulse. This indicates a 'net' force of zero acting over time and so there is no acceleration (i.e. constant velocity) …

…This occurs about halfway into the race (i.e. at around the 50-metre mark).

4 A point just before crossing the finishing line

F (N)

150

0

-400

B

A

time (s)

Here we have a 'net' negative effect, meaning a negative acceleration. The athlete is slowing down.

Note: some techniques in sport rely upon increasing the time a force acts, and therefore increasing impulse. For example, in javelin throwing this would occur with a longer arm extension to pull the javelin through; some shot putt techniques are rotational and therefore enable the force to be applied for longer.

Linear motion – pressure and friction

> *The interplay of forces and surfaces.*

> **Pressure** is the force per unit area applied to a surface.

> **Friction** is the force acting between two surfaces parallel to the surfaces in contact.

Pressure

> When a person stands on the floor in an upright position, the supporting area of his/her feet will experience a ground reaction force (RF). This will be equal and opposite to the weight of the person (W).

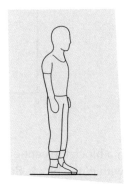

> This reaction force does not pass through a single point but is distributed over the supporting area of the feet.

> The pressure is calculated by

$$\text{Pressure} = \frac{\text{Force}}{\text{Area}} \ (\text{N/m}^2 \text{ or } \text{Nm}^{-2})$$

Fairly even distribution of pressure
Rigid sole

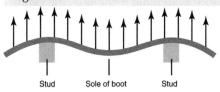

Stud   Sole of boot   Stud

Uneven distribution of pressure
Flexible sole

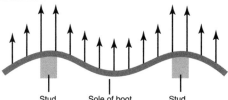

Stud   Sole of boot   Stud

Notice how pressure pays a major part in the choice of footwear.

Friction

This opposes movement or the tendency to move.

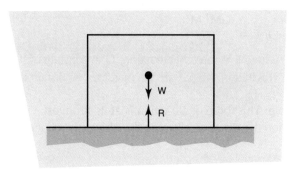

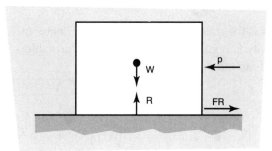

> When stationary, the forces acting on the block are W (Weight) and R (Reaction force from contact with surface).

> If a force P is applied, friction (FR) will begin to come into play to oppose any movement. (Note that until the block begins to move P = FR!)

> Frictional force has a maximum value (i.e. the value just before movement occurs [see note above]). It can be calculated by:

FR = μR

Where: FR = Friction force
μ = Coefficient of friction
R = Reaction force
Note: μ is a measure of the roughness of the two surfaces.

Linear motion – gravity and stability

> *The centre of gravity is crucial in determining stability and balance.*

Gravity

Gravity is a force that acts between two objects in order that they are pulled together. More commonly this relates to the attractive force of the Earth on all objects.

> Newton's Law of Gravitation states:
> **'All particles attract each other with a force proportional to the product of their masses and inversely proportional to the square of the distance between them.'**
>
> Or $F = \dfrac{GM^1\,M^2}{d^2}$
>
> where F = force of attraction, G = constant of gravitation, M^1/M^2 are the masses, d = distance

Note: This force of attraction is at its strongest when the distance between the objects is reduced.

Stability

This is the state of being stable. If your centre of gravity (c.o.g.) shifts, you will become unstable – liable to fall over.

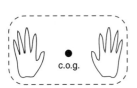 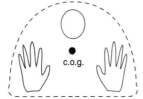

> The headstand has a larger perimeter and therefore area of support. This makes it more stable than the handstand as the centre of gravity would have to move further to be outside the base.

> Consider a rigid bar supported by a hinged base (a). Moving it through an angle of θ would result in the centre of gravity line moving outside the base. The result would be a topple forwards. (b). If we reduce the height of the bar and move it through the same angle, this does not happen.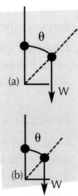

> The weight of an object will also affect stability. Think of Sumo wrestlers!

Centre of gravity

This is a single point that represents the location of concentration of mass.

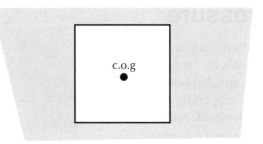

In a block the centre of gravity is 'central' and 'within' the block. But this is not always the case with humans.

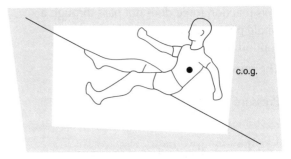

In the 'scissors' high jump technique, the centre of gravity is contained within the body and travels over the bar.

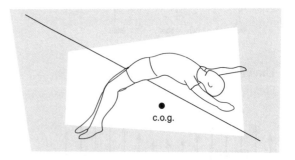

In the Fosbury Flop technique, the centre of gravity is outside the body and travels below the bar.

It is possible to move the position of the centre of gravity by changing body position.

Linear motion – work, energy and power

> *Measuring efficiency and effectiveness.*

Work

Work is a measure of force acting over a distance. It can be calculated as:

$$W = F \times d$$

where W = work, F = force and d = distance moved.

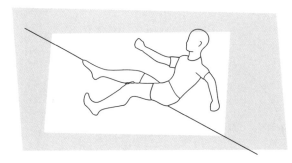

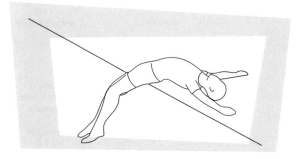

The work done when using the 'scissors' technique is more than in the 'Fosbury Flop'.

This is because in the 'scissors' technique the jumper's centre of gravity has to be moved higher (i.e. above the bar) than in the 'Fosbury Flop'. Therefore more effort and force is required. This is why the Fosbury Flop is the most commonly used technique for high jumping. It requires less work!

Work is measured in Joules (J).

Energy

This is the capacity an object has to do work.

Potential energy

The energy that comes as a result of a specific position relative to reference level. It is found by:

$$M \times g \times h$$

where M = mass, g = acceleration due to gravity (approx. 9.8 ms^{-2}) and h = height.

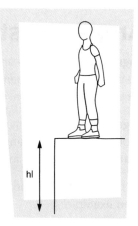

Kinetic energy

The energy that comes as a result of motion. It is found by:

$$\tfrac{1}{2} \times M \times v^2$$

where M = mass and v = velocity

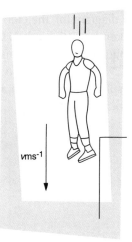

Energy is also measured in Joules (J).

Power

This is the rate of doing work.

It is measured in Joules/sec or Watts.

It is calculated by:

$$\text{Power} = \frac{\text{Work}}{\text{Time}}$$

> Work done in a short space of time would be *high power*. Work done (the same amount) in a longer period of time would be *low power*.

Angular motion – distance and displacement

> *Applying linear motion principles to define angular motion.*

The same principles apply to **angular motion** as they do with **linear motion** – except that here they are applied to rotational movement.

Angular distance and displacement

Angular distance is the angle created by a displacement or line at the point of observation.

Angular displacement is the angle through which something has rotated, or the change in the angle.

Let us take a look at the golf swing as an example.

In diagram (a), the golfer has the club at right angles to the ground.

In diagram (b), the club has been taken away through 270°. The angular distance for this movement is 270° rotation but the angular displacement is 90° in an anti-clockwise direction.

> **Angular displacement is the smallest angle between the starting and finishing position.**

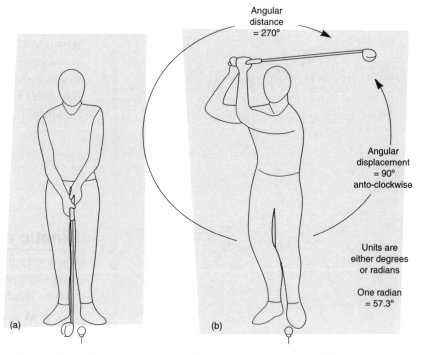

Angular distance = 270°

Angular displacement = 90° anto-clockwise

Units are either degrees or radians

One radian = 57.3°

(a) (b)

Note: when the angle between the starting position and finish position is less than 180°, angular distance and angular displacement are the same.

Angular speed and velocity

Angular speed is the time taken for the angular displacement.

$$\text{Angular speed} = \frac{\text{Angular distance}}{\text{Time}}$$

$(°s^{-1})$ or $(rad.s^{-1})$

Angular velocity is the rate of change of angular displacement, often of a rotating or revolving body (e.g. the golfer).

$$\text{Angular velocity} = \frac{\text{Angular displacement}}{\text{Time}}$$

$(°.s^{-1})$ or $(rad.^{-1})$

(Notice that 'speed' and 'distance' are together in one equation and 'velocity' and 'displacement' appear together in the other. Always keep vectors and scalars together!

Angular acceleration

This is the rate of change of angular velocity.

$$\text{Angular acceleration} = \frac{\text{Change in angular velocity}}{\text{Time}}$$

$(°s^{-2})$ or $(rad.s^{-2})$

or

$$\bar{\alpha} = \frac{wf - wi}{t}$$

where

$\bar{\alpha}$ = average angular acceleration
wf = final angular velocity
wi = initial angular velocity
t = time

Angular motion – torque, moment and levers

> *The turning effect produced by the application of a force.*

Torque/moment

The **torque/moment** may be defined as the *turning effect* of a force. The terms 'torque' and 'moment' are used synonymously because they have the same meaning.

> To calculate a torque/moment, it requires the multiplication of the *force* and the *perpendicular distance* between the line of action of the force and the axis/pivot.

> Example: if we have a force (F) acting as shown with a pivot (p), the torque/moment would be F × *d* = F*d* (Nm) clockwise.

[Nm = Newton metres]

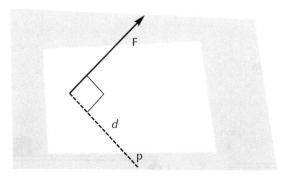

The direction of the torque/moment must be given. This may be in terms of clockwise/ anti-clockwise or positive (+) or negative (−). When using, it is usual to consider anti-clockwise as positive.

Net torque/moment

This is where two or more torques/moments are acting on a body and we are considering their combined effects.

Consider an athlete on a rowing machine.

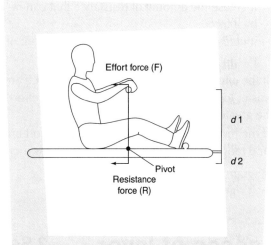

*d*1 Perpendicular distance of effort force from pivot

*d*2 Perpendicular distance of resistance from pivot

Here the 'net' torque is the combined action of the two torques. It requires a calculation. Taking anti-clockwise as positive, we have:

$$(F \times d_1) - (R \times d_2) = \text{net torque}$$
$$Fd_1 - Rd_2 = \text{net torque}$$

Angular motion – torque, moment and levers (cont.)

> *Using torques/moments to produce movement.*

A lever is a rigid structure with a pivot point (fulcrum) and two opposing forces acting at two other points.

Levers in the body system may be considered as bones (rigid structure), joints (pivot/fulcrum), effort force (muscle insertion) and resistance force (load).

> Levers are designed to:
>   – increase the amount of resistance that can be overcome by a force
>   – increase the speed and range of movement of the resistance.
> If the effort arm is greater than the resistance arm, it will be easier to move the resistance because the effort torque will be greater.
> If the resistance arm is greater than the effort arm, the speed and range of movement of the resistance is increased.

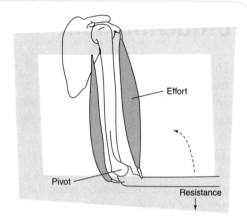

Effort arm = perpendicular distance between pivot and line of action of effort force.

Resistance arm/Load = perpendicular distance between pivot and line of action of resistance force.

Classes of lever

1 First class

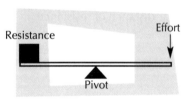

Here, the pivot is in between the resistance and effort ('seesaw' set up).

Example: nodding action of head. The neck muscles provide the effort, the skull/vertebra joint is the fulcrum/pivot and the weight of the head is the resistance.

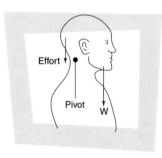

2 Second class

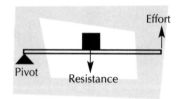

Notice that this arrangement mechanically favours effort at the expense of speed and range of movement of resistance.

Here, the pivot is at one end with the resistance in the middle (like a wheelbarrow).

Example: foot – ball of foot is fulcrum/pivot; weight of body acting through lower leg is the resistance; and the effort is the gastrocnemius (calf) acting through the Achilles tendon.

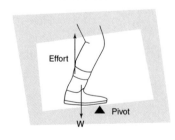

3 Third class

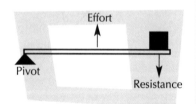

Notice that this arrangement mechanically favours resistance, but potentially we have greater speed and range of movement.

Here, the effort is in the middle and the pivot and resistance at either end.

Example: biceps acting on elbow joint. Pivot is elbow joint; effort is biceps acting through tendon; and resistance the weight of forearm. This is the most common lever system in the body.

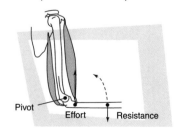

Angular motion – generating rotation

> *Adjusting the point of application of a force to produce rotation.*

> **Rotation is an angular movement; translation is a linear movement.**

Eccentric force

Consider a gymnast applying a force (*F*) to a gymnastics box in order to move it in the horizontal plane.

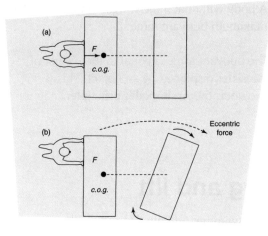

In diagram (a), because the force (*F*) is through the centre of gravity (c.o.g.) of the box, we get movement in a straight line – TRANSLATION.

In diagram (b), because the force (*F*) is 'off line' with the centre of gravity we get some linear motion (translation) and some angular motion (ROTATION).

> **Any force that causes or tends to cause translation and rotation is called an eccentric force.**

It is often the ground reaction force that acts as the force eccentric to the athlete's centre of gravity.

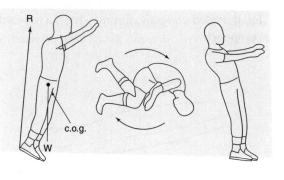

Couple

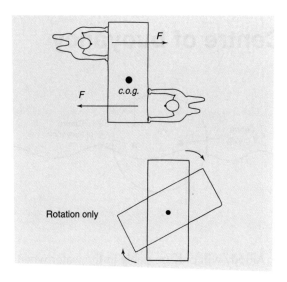

If the two gymnasts apply an equal force (*F*) an equal distance from the centre of gravity, this is known as a **couple**. This will produce rotation only.

> Therefore a couple may be defined as 'a system of two parallel, equal and opposite eccentric forces acting on an object'.

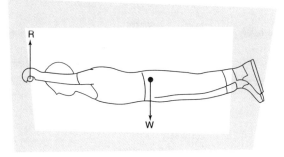

Here, the gymnast is rotating about a 'fixed' bar producing rotation only. The couple is produced by the weight force (W) and the reaction force (R) of the hand contact.

Fluid mechanics – water

We now consider what happens to a body as it moves through water.

> What forces act on it?
> How does the body float?
> How can a swimmer reduce the drag effect?

Centre of buoyancy

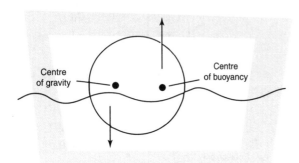

> A body will only be stable in the water when the centre of gravity is in line with the **centre of buoyancy**.

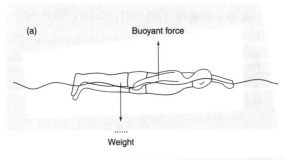

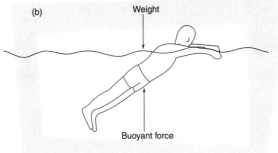

In position (a) the swimmer is unstable until the weight and the buoyant force are in line (b).

Flotation

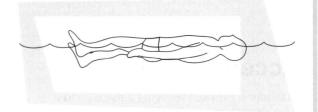

> A body will float if the weight of the body ≤ the maximum buoyant force.

The buoyant force is equal to the weight of the water displaced by an object. This is known as the **Archimedes principle.**

Drag and lift

> The swimmer will need to reduce the cross-sectional area of the body by adopting a 'flat' position in the water. This will reduce drag.
> Surface drag (skin friction) may be reduced by shaving the body or using special costumes.

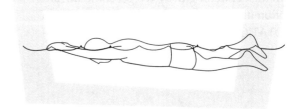

> In the same way an 'angle of attack' generates lift for a discus. Angling the hand as it moves sideways in the 'pull' phase may also generate lift. If angled correctly, this may have a forward component.

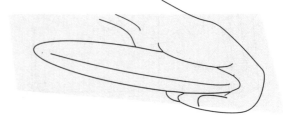

Angular analogues of Newton's Laws of Motion

> *Applying Newton's Laws of Motion to generate rotation.*

If something is an 'analogue' of something else the two things are similar to each other in some way. The following are the angular motion equivalents to the linear motion laws (see page 76).

Newton's First Law

A body will continue to rotate with constant angular momentum unless an external torque is applied.

(Notice that with angular motion we are dealing with rotational movement and not linear motion or torques).

> Here, angular momentum refers to the *amount* of angular motion.

> With linear momentum we calculate by multiplying mass by velocity.
Momentum = Mass (kg) × Velocity (ms^{-1})

> But with angular momentum we multiply the moment of inertia (distribution of mass about the axis of rotation) by the angular velocity.

Angular momentum =
Moment of inertia × Angular velocity
(kg.m^2.s^{-1})

Now let us look at the interplay of angular momentum, angular velocity and moment of inertia. Consider a gymnast performing a back somersault – flight phase only!

At the beginning ➊, the gymnast has an extended body position. This gives the gymnast a high moment of inertia (mass distributed away from axis of rotation the transverse axis passing through hips). This produces slow rotation (low angular velocity).

At ➋, the mass has been brought closest to the axis of rotation. This results in a reduction of the moment of inertia and therefore an increase in the angular velocity.

At ➌, the gymnast is 'opening' out and extending again, increasing the moment of inertia and reducing the angular velocity.

Notice that angular momentum remains constant throughout the flight as no external torque is acting due to absence of ground reaction.

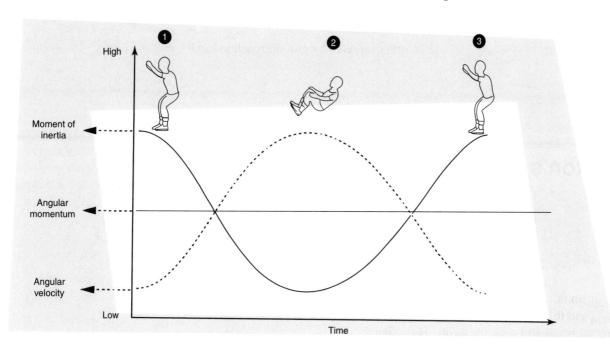

Angular analogues of Newton's Laws of Motion (cont.)

Newton's Second Law

> The rate of change of angular momentum is proportional to the external torque applied and acts in the direction of the applied torque.
>
> +
>
> The change of angular momentum is directly proportional to the length of time that the torque is applied.

This relates to angular impulse
(i.e. Angular impulse = Torque × Time).

Consider a gymnast about to perform a back somersault.

In order to get a large change of angular momentum, the torque needs to be applied for a long period of time. This requires contact with the ground for as long as possible. This is achieved by fully extending hip, knee and ankle joints prior to take off ❹.

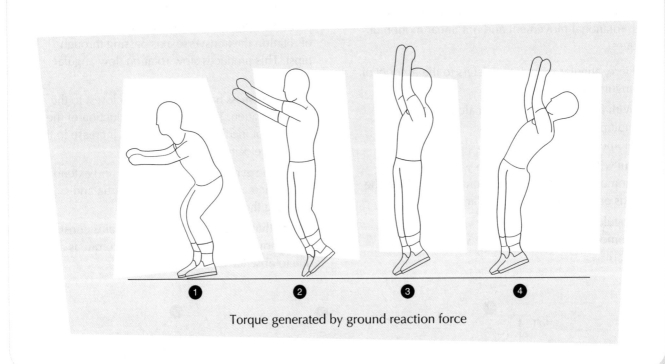

Torque generated by ground reaction force

Newton's Third Law

> For every action torque exerted by one body on another, there is an equal but opposite reaction torque.

Consider a gymnast performing a 'pike' action.

Here, an equal and opposite torque is applied to each half of the gymnast's body.

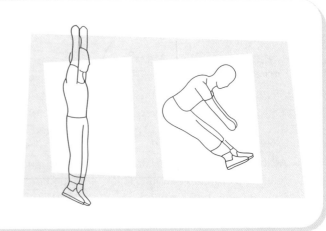

Fluid mechanics – air

> *The movement of a body through air.*

In this section we will consider what happens to a ball as it moves through the air.

> What forces act on it?
> What makes a cricket ball swing as it moves through the air after leaving the bowler's arm?

> Why do golf balls have 'dimples'?
> Why does a tennis player put 'top spin' on a tennis ball?

Air flow

Consider a ball moving through the air:

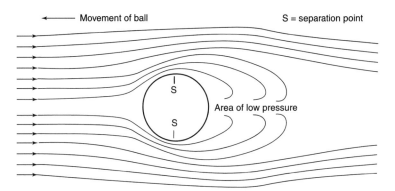

> As the flow lines of the air hit the front of the ball, those closest to the ball's surface compress and move quicker.

> Once the flow lines reach S they change from *laminar* flow to *turbulent* flow. This creates an area of low pressure behind the ball. This results in a force from front to back acting to slow the ball down. This force is known as **profile** or **form drag.**

> As the ball travels faster, the separation point S moves forward (up to a *critical velocity*). This results in greater turbulent flow behind the ball, lower pressure and therefore increased profile drag.

> A larger cross-sectional area will also produce more turbulent flow and increase form drag.

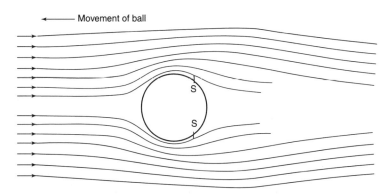

Note: the layer closest to the ball is called the **boundary layer.**

> As the ball moves faster, it reaches a critical velocity. (This changes with ball size and surface characteristics.) This results in a later separation point, less turbulence and therefore increases pressure behind the ball. This means less profile drag. (The late separation point is caused by the boundary layer becoming turbulent and 'sticking' to the surface of the ball.)

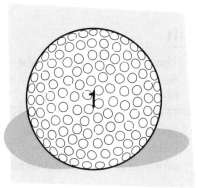

> Golf balls have dimples to 'trip' the boundary layer into turbulent flow at lower velocities therefore reducing profile drag and increasing distance.

Surface characteristics

Here we can see a cricket ball with an angled seam. When the air flow meets the seam early on (left), the boundary layer is 'tripped' into turbulent flow and 'sticks' to the ball. This pulls the other flow lines in and creates a lower pressure on the left-hand side – thus the ball will swing from right to left.

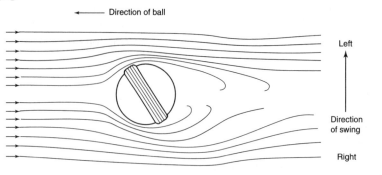

Spin

> Here we have a tennis ball hit with 'top spin'. This results in the 'compression' of flow lines below the ball. Whenever you get a compression of flow lines, the pressure is reduced (Bernoulli effect). Therefore there will be a 'net' force acting down (Magnus effect).

> The Magnus effect can also be seen in golf when the ball is 'hooked' or 'sliced'. Here, the effect is on horizontal motion.

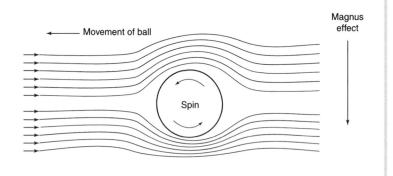

Lift

> The aerofoil makes use of the Bernoulli effect (compression of flow lines).

> Here the lines on the top of the aerofoil are compressed and produce a low pressure area. This produces a 'net' upward lift force.

This is the principle behind the design of aircraft wings!

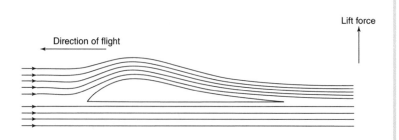

Individual differences (1)

Personality

Either
The sum total of an individual's characteristics which makes him or her unique.
Or
The overall pattern of psychological characteristics that makes each person unique.

Measuring personality

Measuring personality is thought to be useful for predicting behaviour which may help identify top-class performers from an early age. But there are problems in ensuring validity and reliability. All techniques may be time consuming and costly and the interpretation of results may cause over-generalisation, particularly if small numbers are used.

Methods include:

Interviews (e.g. Rorschach inkblot) but...
> are they reliable and valid in each case?
> are they of value in assessing a person's sporting ability?

Questionnaires (e.g. personality tests, Minnesota multiphasic personality inventory, Cattell 16 primary factors questionnaire)
> are these appropriate for the results the researcher wants?

Observation
> difficult to remain unobtrusive which will affect behaviour
> secret observation is unethical.

Personalities are formed, depending on the theory you follow.

Trait theories

Traits are relatively stable, highly consistent attributes that exert a widely generalised causal effect on behaviour (Mischel).

These are innate characteristics which can be arranged in a hierarchy, for example:
> outgoing
> aggressive
> tense
> shy
> relaxed
> sensitive

The strongest traits dominate the behaviour. Situation does not play an important part in behaviour.

Eysenck's theory

Eysenck identified two main dimensions of personality. A person can fall anywhere along the two dimensions.

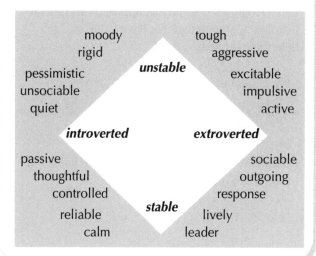

Narrow band approach

Personality seen as two contrasting types indicated by behaviour:

> **Type A** – highly strung, impatient, intolerant, high levels of stress

> **Type B** – relaxed, tolerant, low levels of personal stress

Sheldon's somatotyping personality formation

A form of trait theory (How true is this for everyone?)

Ectomorphy	tenseness (Basil Fawlty type figure)
Mesomorphy	extrovert, risk taker (sportsman figure)
Endomorphy	sociability, comfort loving (Santa Claus figure)

Lewin's interactionist approach

This recognises that the trait approach and social learning approach together have value in determining behaviour

B = f (P . E)
Behaviour is the **F**unction of **P**ersonality and **E**nvironment

Personality characteristics predict some behaviour in some situations but not all situations.

Bandura's social learning theory

Personality is learnt by observational learning, modelling and imitating behaviour, and through experience. Psychological functioning occurs as a result of environmental determinants affecting behaviour.

Assertion/Aggression

Assertion (channelled aggression or instrumental aggression) is behaviour within the rules of the game that achieves a goal, e.g. tackling fairly but forcefully within a soccer match.

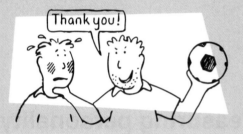

Aggression is the intention to harm another person outside the laws of a game, e.g. punching an opponent in a soccer match.

Some, not universally accepted, theories suggest that aggression occurs as a result of:

> **natural instinct.** This theory has many detractors – cultural background often disproves this and aggression is often not spontaneous.

> **frustration.** This theory states that frustration always leads to aggression; a person is blocked from their goal, they are frustrated and release the tension through aggressive action. Berkowitz (1974) maintains that this can make a person 'potentially aggressive'.

> **social learning.** People see significant others (heroes) being aggressive and imitate this behaviour in similar situations (Bandura, 1977).

Combatting aggression

A mixture of recommendations, affecting performers, coaches, administrators and others, include:

> control of arousal levels (stress management)
> avoidance of situations that cause aggression
> stopping aggressive players from further participation
> rewarding 'turning the other cheek'
> showing non-aggressive role models
> punishing aggression
> reinforcement of non-aggression (largely by significant others)
> handing responsibility to an aggressive player.

> *How we approach situations.*

Attitudes

A learned emotional and behavioural response to a stimulus or situation. Attitudes are often seen as an extension of personality.

> Attitudes are formed from:
>
> > pleasant or unpleasant experiences forming our approach to the same situation – soccer training made me ill last week; I don't like training.
> >
> > significant others (parents, teachers, friends) through encouragement, reward or punishment, or peer group pressure – soccer training is an excellent way to improve skills and all the best players do it.

Triadic Model

Attitudes are formed from three components:

cognitive	reflect your belief in information, e.g. weight training increases muscle bulk (not necessarily true)
affective	reflect your feelings or emotional response (a determined direction of behaviour), e.g. muscle bulk is good/bad
behavioral	reflect your intended behaviour, e.g. I will/will not go weight training.

> **Also note…**
>
> Attitudes do not always predict behaviour, only specific attitudes predict specific behaviours. (Fishbein, 1995)
>
> The best indicator of behaviour is an individual's behaviour intention. A positive attitude to something incorporates an intention to do that thing and therefore participation is more likely. (La Piere, 1934)

Changing attitudes

Persuasion

Three factors affect a person's ability to persuade another.

> The persuader must be of high status. He/she must be knowledgeable and appear genuine. Attractiveness and similarity to persuadee might be important.
>
> The message must be clear, concise and accurate. It may be best to put only one side of the argument, depending on the audience. The strongest argument first or last? This depends upon the proximity of expected change in behaviour.
>
> The people being persuaded must be capable of understanding the message. They may choose not to be persuaded.

Cognitive dissonance

If there is a mismatch in the Triadic Model, this will cause a dissonance (imbalance) in the mind of the person being persuaded. They must then act to reduce this imbalance by changing behaviour to meet new criteria, based on new information.

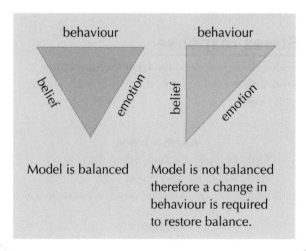

Model is balanced

Model is not balanced therefore a change in behaviour is required to restore balance.

Stress and anxiety (1)

> *Giving athletes an 'edge'.*

Stress

a stimulus resulting in arousal or a response to a specific situation.

Arousal

a state of readiness to perform that helps motivate individuals (see page 93).

Anxiety

a negative reaction of a performer to stress, often leading to over arousal.

Eustress

a positive reaction of a performer to stress, leading to optimal arousal.

Stress

Stressors

Stressors are situations that cause a stress response. In PE and sport the following are the most common:

> competition – an evaluative and comparative situation that increases anxiety

> conflict – with opponents or team mates who choose to do things differently

> frustration – can be caused if we are blocked from achieving our goals… aggression can result

> environmental conditions – extremes of heat or cold

> injury and fatigue – preventing effective performance.

Stress response

Seyle (1956) proposed the **General Adaptation Syndrome** model to explain how the body copes with stress.

Alarm reaction
Fight or flight reaction; adrenaline surge, increased heart rate, blood sugar level up.

Resistance
Body adapts to cope with new stress until it is removed or overcome.

Exhaustion
If stress is not removed the body begins to fail to cope with this stress, this may take weeks, months or even years.

Stress experience

Athletes experience psychological symptoms in addition to the physical symptoms described:

> inability to make decisions
> poor concentration
> feelings of worry
> narrowing attention.

These can lead to even more stress and the stress spiral:

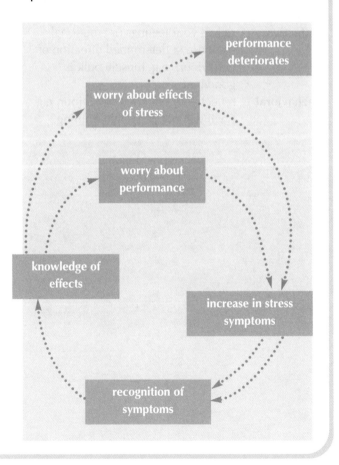

Stress and anxiety (2)

> *Our response to stress.*

Anxiety

> **Anxiety** – an emotional state, similar to fear, associated with arousal and accompanied by feelings of nervousness and apprehension.

> **State anxiety** – the athlete's emotional state at that particular time (the intensity of the response alters from time to time and situation to situation).

> **Trait anxiety** – the athlete's disposition to view any situation as threatening and to respond with heightened state anxiety levels.

Athletes with high trait anxiety levels tend to view all evaluative situations as threatening. They respond with greater intensity of state anxiety than those athletes with lower trait anxiety levels. Martens (1977) identified this trait anxiety as **competitive trait anxiety.**

Martens used a self-report questionnaire called **sports competition anxiety test** (SCAT) to find out how athletes felt prior to competitions. This has proved reliable for predicting anxiety levels in the future.

Measuring stress

This is achieved in three ways.

Self report questionnaires

Easily administered, but may not always give a truthful picture:

> Martens' sports competition anxiety test (SCAT)

> Speilberger's state trait anxiety inventory (STAI).

Physiological measurements

Often require bulky, expensive equipment and some of these measurements would be affected by exercise, before or afterwards, anyway:

> heart rates (ECG)

> temperature (thermometer)

> oxygen uptake (Douglas bag analysis)

> sweating (sudorimeter)

> skin conductivity (galvanic skin response)

> muscle tension (electromyogram).

Behavioural observation

Coaches should be able to build up a pattern of responses over an extended period, before, during and after training and competition. Changes they may see include:

> nail biting

> shaking

> rapid talking

> frequent visits to the toilet.

Stress management

Stress management skills are vital for those athletes who want to become the very best. The ability to control anxiety at crucial times is very important. Both somatic and cognitive anxiety control is essential.

Physical relaxation

Progressive muscle relaxation

The progressive tensing of muscle groups and subsequent greater relaxation of these same muscles (often coach or teacher directed) – excellent preparation for imagery exercises.

Self directed relaxation

Similar to progressive muscle relaxation but without tensing muscles first – relies on the athlete's ability to isolate muscles and then relax them (this can be improved through practice).

Deep breathing

To focus the mind only on breathing – can reduce heart and respiration rates as well as calming the mind.

Biofeedback

Immediate visual feedback of physiological measures of stress (e.g. heart rate) allows the athlete to concentrate on reducing that measurement – they get immediate feedback of their success.

Imagery

Imagery is the creation of a mental picture to relax or prepare the athlete for activity. It comes in two forms:

> external – watching yourself perform, from outside your body
> internal – seeing your performance from your body (visualisation).

Imagery for relaxation often takes the athlete to comfortable surroundings, e.g. a favourite place, or a place to relax, a tropical desert island.

Imagery to prepare for activity often involves mental rehearsal of the skills to be attempted. Explanations for the success of imagery include:

> **neuromuscular** – thinking about action produces nerve impulses that fire in correct order (a dry run)
> **cognitive** – thinking through likely scenarios the performer is ready for them when they occur
> **confidence building** – athletes gain in confidence as they know what they are going to do which reduces anxiety and increases motivation.

Goal setting

Goal setting is useful for performers in the following ways:

> attention is directed and uncertainty reduced
> learning is focused
> practices are well structured; effort is organised to fulfil all tasks correctly
> confidence is increased (success comes more quickly)
> evaluation and feedback are immediate and focused.

Goal setting will be effective if the goals:

> are appropriately challenging
  They may be just beyond the previous best performance – this generally improves motivation of the performer.
> have a long term vision
  This will be approached via short and intermediate achievements. Short term goals allow success to be gained, increasing motivation for the long term goals.
> are measurable
  Goals must be measurable to allow accurate feedback. The performer must know when they have arrived at a goal.
> suit both the coach and performer
  Negotiation is the key. The performer will have greater motivation if they feel they have ownership of the goals.

Motivation – concepts and theories

> *An internal factor that arouses and directs behaviour.*

It is suggested (Sage, 1974) that motivation is a combination of "The internal mechanisms and external stimuli which arouse and direct behaviour."

Intrinsic motivation

All suggested by Hull's 'Drive Theory'.

The performer:
> may possess the desire to overcome a particular problem or task
> develops skills or 'habits' to overcome that problem
> practises successful habits until perfected
> attains a feeling of pride, satisfaction, joy and fun in completing the task which is rewarding – motivation is enhanced
> then sets a new goal or task to continue with the drive or motivation to succeed.

The teacher/coach, to facilitate the performer's intrinsic motivation:
> aims for success with the performer
> ensures that practice and training are enjoyable
> uses a varied approach to maintain interest.

Extrinsic motivation

These are rewards that are external to the performer and fall into two categories.

Tangible rewards
> medals
> trophies
> money etc.

Intangible rewards
> praise from significant others
> recognition etc.

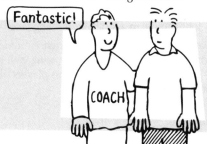

Teachers and coaches should ensure that they praise desired behaviour as this motivates individuals to repeat it. However, the use of tangible rewards, particularly with young children, should be limited as it (and not play) may become the sole reason for performance.

Goal setting

Well thought out and motivating goals must be:
S > specific
M > measurable
A > agreed
R > realistic
T > time related
E > exciting
R > recorded

Athletes require a mixture of intrinsic and extrinsic motivation, with well planned goals to achieve success.

Motivation:
> involves our inner ambition to achieve our aims
> depends upon external stressors and or rewards for our efforts
> is related to the intensity (arousal level) and direction of behaviour.

For success – these three factors must be kept in balance.

Good coaches manipulate performers' levels of motivation to maximise performance. Performance and motivation are closely linked to arousal.

Two theories explain the relationship between arousal and performance.

Arousal

Hull's Drive Theory

A linear relationship between performance and arousal (drive).

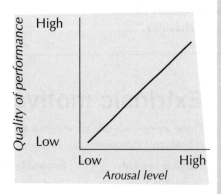

This theory helps explain *why beginners find it difficult to perform well under pressure*. Often beginners' skill level decreases if they are competing in a relay race using new skills – for example in a football dribbling race.

However it also explains *how experienced athletes perform better when under pressure* using well learned skills – for example when good tennis players play better against stronger opposition.

Performance = habit x drive

Novices have usually incorrect habits. Experts have well-learned correct habits.

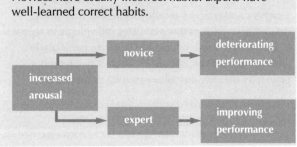

Habit is the performance that is strongest in that person (not always the correct performance) usually the one that occurs most in practice.

Yerkes Dodson or Inverted 'U' Law

An increase in arousal causes improvement in performance up to an optimal point. After this point, increased arousal leads to deteriorated performance.

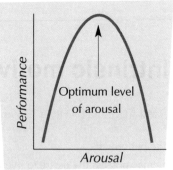

Three factors affect the application of this theory:

> **activity undertaken**
> Fine movements and complex skills (which require alot of attention) require a lower arousal level, e.g. snooker safety shots, pistol shooting.

> **skill levels**
> Highly skilled athletes, with well-learned motor programmes, have spare attention capacity to deal with excessive arousal. Beginners need all of their attention to be focused on the skill and do not cope with over arousal so well.

> **personality**
> Generally extroverts perform better with high arousal levels and introverts perform better with low arousal levels. This is linked to the brain's reticular activating system (RAS) which controls the level of arousal. Introverts have highly stimulated RAS; they avoid situations that increase their already high levels of arousal. Extroverts need high arousal situations to stimulate RAS.

Catastrophe theory

This says that an increase in cognitive arousal will improve performance (as in Inverted 'U' theory), but that if over-arousal takes place, there are two options:

> **if arousal levels drop, a performer can recover** through supportive words for a coach, and/or stress management techniques.
> **if arousal continues to increase, the performer will not recover** and catastrophe will occur.

Example: A basketball player can shoot well in practice situations but, after an argument with an opposition player, starts missing. Coach calls him off, talks to him, lowers his level of arousal, and sends him back on at an optimum level. His shots start to go in.

Attentional narrowing

During competition, performers must be able to select relevant cues and make correct decisions. If the optimum level of arousal is reached, this can happen effectively. If an individual becomes over-aroused, he or she will miss vital cues and suffer from attentional narrowing.

Motivation – personality and experience

> *Improving performances.*

What motivates the drive for achievement? Why do some people choose to undertake a particular challenge and others decline?

Three influences play major roles. They help explain why some people perform well in difficult situations (and seem to enjoy the experience) and

why some people never take up new challenges. Good coaches understand this concept.

The influence of personality

> Some people display 'approach behaviour'; they seem to thrive on challenge and possess a need to achieve (NACH).

> Others display avoidance behaviours and try to avoid challenges because they have a need to avoid failure (NAF).

These behaviours occur most readily in judgemental situations. Sport can be very judgemental, comparing two performances, thus it is said that sport attracts more 'NACH' personalities than 'NAF' personalities.

NACH personalities:

> are determined to see a task through

> work quickly at a task

> take risks

> enjoy a challenge

> take responsibility

> like to know how they have been judged.

E.g. sportsmen/women, games players, climbers

NAF personalities:

> are easily dissuaded from taking the challenge

> work at tasks slowly or not at all

> avoid situations where they or their ego is put at risk

> avoid responsibility

> prefer not to be judged and do not want to know how they have been judged.

E.g. those who play only against weaker players

Ego oriented

Athletes who view success as defeating an opponent and thus being seen as a greater player, e.g. players of games such as chess or combat sports performers.

Task oriented

Athletes who view success as an internal achievement, e.g. runners beating their personal best or climbers completing a more difficult route.

Knowing what motivates athletes helps coaches/teachers to plan training sessions for them.

The influence of self-confidence

Bandura (1977) identified a specific form of self-confidence which he called self-efficacy. Bandura claims that this type of self confidence varies from situation to situation.

Athletes will choose to participate in activities in which they have high self-efficacy and avoid situations in which they don't have high self-efficacy. Self-efficacy affects our effort in an activity and our persistence at a task.

Self-efficacy is affected by four factors:

> **Performance accomplishments**

The biggest influence on self-efficacy is the recognition of past achievements and the attributions given for successes. Controllable internal factors are likely to ensure feelings of self-confidence.

> **Vicarious experiences (modelling)**

Seeing a task successfully completed, particularly by

The influence of experience

How an athlete has performed in the past will affect how they approach the next challenge. Athletes will look for reasons for their past performances – good or bad.

event outcome – win/loss/ success/ failure

information about performance available to athlete

attribution of the causes of the performance

expectation of future performance

affective response – how you feel

decision on future participation

Weiner (1974) looked at examination performance and candidates' attitudes. He was able to make a two-dimensional model (a).

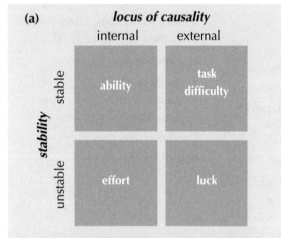

(a) *locus of causality*

	internal	external
stable	ability	task difficulty
unstable	effort	luck

stability

Learned helplessness (Dweck 1978)

This is the belief that failure is inevitable in specific situations… or in some cases in all situations. This leads to feelings of helplessness. Attribution to uncontrollable factors often leads to learned helplessness.

This is a good model for examinations but is not always applicable in sports specific situations. Roberts and Pascuzzi (1979) enhanced the model (b).

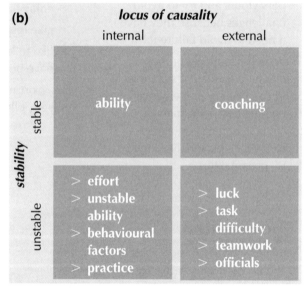

(b) *locus of causality*

	internal	external
stable	ability	coaching
unstable	> effort > unstable ability > behavioural factors > practice	> luck > task difficulty > teamwork > officials

stability

> Success is often attributed to internal causes – "I played well today and won well."
> Failure is often attributed to external factors – "He got a few lucky breaks on crucial points."

This is known as a 'self serving bias' and protects or enhances a performer's ego.

someone of a similar standard, helps raise a performers self-confidence.

> **Verbal persuasion**

  Significant others can help reluctant performers begin to believe that they can accomplish the task ahead.

> **Emotional arousal**

  If a performer feels they are in control of their arousal levels through management techniques, or due to their own ability, they will have greater self-efficacy.

In practice these factors can help athletes low in confidence to achieve. They, or their coaches, can:
> ensure success by setting achievable goals and highlighting past success
> demonstrate techniques with a peer as the model
> encourage persuasion and support from friends and others
> use relaxation techniques as a part of the athlete's training programme.

Social influences on performances

> *Watching others and learning.*

Socialisation

Socialisation is the acquisition by children of the norms of society: expected behaviours, values, rights and wrongs, and rules and status. Children acquire these qualities by observing others and imitating them. This is observational learning or modelling. Physical education plays a vital role in the socialisation of all children in all aspects of sports participation.

In physical education it is normally not possible to use powerful or famous role models in lessons.

Research (Landers & Landers, 1973) has shown that careful use of demonstration is vital if success is to be achieved. All groups observing models improved their performance compared with a control group who saw no models.

> Performances improved most when demonstration was by a **skilled teacher.**
> The least amount of improvement was by the group with an **unskilled teacher.**
> A demonstration by **unskilled peers** proved to be the second most effective model.
> **Skilled peers** produced improvements only slightly better than an unskilled teacher.

Bandura's (1961) work on modelling identified seven important considerations in the use of models relative to young people.

> Appropriate behaviour to social norms is more likely to be copied – boys will imitate assertive rugby play if it is modelled by male rugby players.
> Young people will imitate behaviour only if they see it as relevant to them – soccer players may not imitate assertive rugby play as it is not relevant to them.
> Role models who are similar to the pupils are more likely to be copied – peers who perform skills well may elicit more accurate imitation than older (professional) sportsmen.
> Encouraging and approachable models – teachers who listen to young people, who are supportive and helpful – are more likely to be copied.
> Powerful role models are more likely to be copied – a much respected performer is more likely to be imitated than a local (unknown) sportsman.
> Models whose behaviour is condoned by significant others (parents, peers, teachers) are more likely to be copied – telling a young person "I want you to go out and perform like Alan Shearer today" may encourage the young person to work hard for the team but it may also encourage them to be very assertive in their play.
> Behaviour that is consistent is more likely to be imitated – if a normally calm player shows dissent on rare occasions this is unlikely to be copied as it would be inconsistent with his normal actions.

Bandura developed his work and in 1977 established a model to demonstrate the effect of demonstration on skill learning.

acquisition				performance	
observation	**attention**	**retention**	**motor reproduction**	**motivation**	**performance**
The observer will watch the model perform skills.	The observer will pay particular attention to the cues for the skills – attractiveness and status of the model will affect this.	The observer must create a mental picture of the performance – mental rehearsal will be beneficial.	The observer must be physically capable of performing the skill and will attempt to match their performance to that of the model – the model performance must be a perfect demonstration.	The observer's motivation must be at the correct level. They must want to copy the model's performance – this may need help and reinforcement from a coach.	The observer copies what they have watched.

Questions arose from the findings…

> Do unskilled teachers inhibit learning because students don't want to show them up?

> Do unsuccessful demonstrations by unskilled teachers make students believe they will fail?

> Do unskilled peers set up a competitive standard that others try to beat?

> Should teachers only demonstrate if able to perform correctly – otherwise use peers?

Social facilitation

The influence of the presence of others on performance (Zajonc, 1965).

Alone or with others?

The presence of others creates a powerful social influence on performers due to **social evaluation** – even when this is not overt.

Performers can suffer from **evaluation apprehension** in this situation; this creates increased arousal levels, especially if the audience is made up of significant others for the performer.

In front of a crowd?

Facilitation implies performance improvement due to the presence of audience... but this is not always the case. Evidence points to a poorer performance when an audience is present in some cases.

Evidence suggests that the presence of others increases arousal level, indicated by increased palm sweating, increased heart rate, and that performance is linked to drive theory (page 93).

Four points have been raised:

> presence of audience or co-actors increases arousal or drive
> increased arousal will increase likelihood of dominant response occurring
> if the skill is well learned the response will be correct
> if the skill is not well learned the response will be incorrect.

In front of a 'home' crowd?

A 'home' crowd is more likely to contain significant others and therefore more likely to evaluate a performance. For some athletes this causes increased evaluation apprehension arousal which can lead to poorer performances depending on their skill level, personality (type 'A' persons play less well in front of an audience) and previous performances.

However, most research suggests an advantage of playing in front of friendly home support which seems to encourage adventurous attacking play and solid defence.

Can behaviour be changed?

Performers and coaches work on ways to cope with the negative effects of social facilitation.

Advice includes:
> use relaxation techniques (see page 96)
> use mental imagery to block out audience
> teach new skills in a non-evaluative way
> explain to athletes how audiences are likely to affect them
> encourage a supportive atmosphere amongst team members.

Martens (1969) found:

> in *learning* complex skills, individuals learned skills better if they were alone
> in *performing* complex skills individuals performed well learned skills better if they had an audience.

The relationship between performance and arousal is crucial and the effect of the presence of others can make control of arousal level more difficult.

Groups and teams

Definitions

> A **team** is… two or more persons interacting with one another, influencing each other (Shaw, 1976).

> A **group** has… a collective identity, sharing a common purpose, with structured communication patterns (Carron, 1980).

> **Cohesion** is… the reason why a group of people come together, and the resistance of the members of the group to its break-up.

Does cohesion facilitate improved performance?

Teams with high task cohesion have a greater potential for success than teams who are more socially cohesive. Teams in sports that require greater interaction, e.g. basketball, need greater cohesion than teams where less interaction is required, e.g. swimming or judo.

Why join a team?

Members join teams or groups for two reasons. (Although usually a combination of both motives is common.)

Either

> They want to join a successful team in order to achieve success. This is a task oriented cohesion; all members of the team have the same goal. For example, amateur soccer players leaving one club to join another more successful club at the end of each season.

Or

> People join a team because they perceive that the group has good interpersonal relationships; they appear to enjoy each others' company no matter the result of matches. For example, amateur soccer players who remain with a club despite poor results because they share similar values, attitudes and enjoy the company of the players in that club.

Group performance

How to ensure that a team of individuals produce the best team performance?

Steiner (1972) produced a model to show the relationship between the performance of the team and the individuals.

$$\text{actual productivity} = \text{best potential productivity} - \text{losses due to faulty processes}$$

'Faulty' processes fall into two categories:

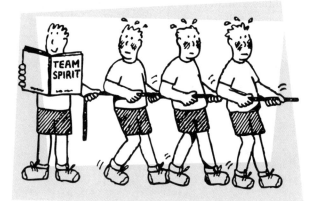

> **co-ordination problems**

Strategies and tactics involving team mates working together with good timing and co-ordination may not work because individuals do not match up with each other on the day, e.g. a mistimed pass, a fumbled ball, a poor lineout in rugby.

> **motivational problems**

Groups tend to make individuals perform below their own best potential.

> **The Ringlemann effect** – experiments have shown that teams of eight (say, tug-of-war) do not work eight times better than eight individuals; some team members lose their motivation in a team.

> **Social loafing** – team players lose motivation as they feel their contribution is not visible and therefore not valued. Records of 'assists' or passes made can counteract this… and socially cohesive teams suffer less in this respect.

Leadership

The behaviourial processes influencing individuals and groups towards set goals (Barrow, 1977). Leadership involves personal relationships and affects the motivation of individuals and groups.

Trait theory – leaders are born with leadership qualities (the 'Great Man' theory), e.g. Churchill, Alexander the Great, Caesar, etc.

Social learning theory – leaders learn to use their qualities to match the situation requirements, i.e. they treat subordinates in whatever way achieves their goals.

> **Leaders tend to occur in two ways (Carron, 1981). They either:**
> > **emerge** from within a group by consent of others or because of their talents, or
> > they are prescribed or **appointed** by an external source, e.g. manager, teacher, coach.

Leadership qualities

> ability to communicate
> enthusiasm
> high motivation
> a vision of what needs to be done
> high ability
> inspirational qualities – charisma.

Leadership styles

Two broad types of leaders occur… although most effective leaders are a mixture of both:
> **task oriented** – concerned mainly with the demands of the task
> **person oriented** – concerned mainly with interpersonal relationships within a group.

Classically the following continuum is suggested:

Authoritarian	**Democratic**	**Laissez-faire**
Task oriented, dictatorial in style, makes all decisions, commanding, direct approach.	Person oriented, values the group's view, shares decisions, shows interest in others.	Makes few decisions, gives little feedback to group members who do as they wish.

Leadership categories

(Chelladurai, 1978)

> training and behaviour – usually improves performance
> democratic behaviour – decisions made together
> autocratic behaviour – authoritarian
> social support – concern for individuals behaviour
> rewarding behaviour – giving positive feedback

Good leaders use all five behaviours as the situation demands. Effective leadership will occur when all of the demands of the situation are satisfied, i.e.

situational characteristics	member characteristics	leader characteristics
required behaviour	preferred behaviour	actual behaviour

performance satisfaction

> **The more a leader's actual behaviour matches the group's preferred behaviour – and the required behaviour of the situation – the more effective the leadership.**

Fiedler (1967) suggests that a leader's effectiveness relies upon whether they are task or person oriented and the situation.

Task oriented leaders are most effective when the situation is either *most* favourable and *least* favourable, e.g. in a very dangerous situation or in a situation where demotivation is likely due to ease of task.

Person oriented leaders are most effective in moderately favourable conditions.

Festivals... and blood sports

> *Local holidays provided time for enjoyment.*

Communal time off work with chattering, eating, drinking, singing, dancing, betting.

Parish feasts

> sometimes called wakes or revels
> celebrated around religious (e.g. patron saints, Whitsun) or seasonal events (e.g. harvest, shearing)

Rural games

> linked to seasonal work
> a chance to display skill and strength

Fairs

> once or twice a year
> linked to the farming calendar
> labourers advertised their skills
> farmers hire workers

Festival games

> **Single sticks** – winner was first to draw blood on an opponents head
> **Jingling matches** – blindfolded participants try to catch person with a bell around their neck
> **Whistling matches** – a 'Merry Andrew' pulls faces at whistlers. The winner is the participant who whistles for the longest without laughing
> **Smock racing** – women race for the prize of a dress

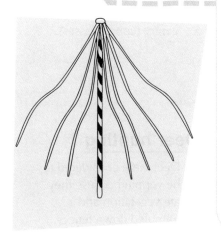

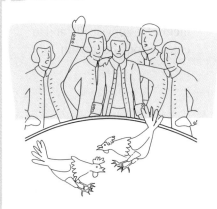

... and the blood sports

> **Cock fighting** – cocks, penned in by crowd, or in a pit, fought to the death; a big betting event.
> **Throwing at cocks** – passers-by paid to throw sticks or stones at a tethered bird; the thrower who killed it kept it.
> **Bull baiting** – bulldog attacked bull, trying to attach to its underside; the bull tossed the dogs who were caught by owners and sent back in (there was a general belief that this improved the meat).
> **Bear baiting** – dogs let loose on tethered bear causing the bear to rear up and make lots of noise (bears were not usually killed as they were expensive).
> **Dog fighting** – dogs, bred for their strength and speed, were used in noisy and viscious spectacles.

The spectators
The harsh living conditions of most people meant they had little pity when it came to the suffering of animals. Crowds were often violent, drunken and excitable. The events were a form of catharsis.

Field sports

Until relatively recently (the 1930s), the majority of the nation's population lived in the countryside. Thus field sports played an important part in their life. Hunting served two main purposes – food and recreation.

For the poor, hunting for food was a necessity, to feed the family. They were either involved in employment to feed the wealthy or in poaching (stealing animals from other people's property).

The wealthy, on the other hand, often hunted for leisure. This allowed them to show off their athleticism, to challenge themselves physically and to enjoy a social occasion.

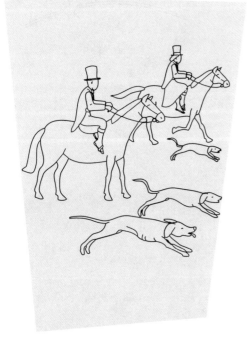

Dissenting voices

Some people did not support hunting for pleasure. One person described it as a sport "that owes its pleasure to another's pain".

Fishing

> Fishing began in the mists of time when people needed to catch fish to live. No one knows exactly how long ago it all started but bone hooks have been found that date back 50000 years.

> Also known as angling, there are three types of fishing:
> - sea fishing
> - game fishing (e.g. salmon and trout)
> - coarse fishing (e.g. roach and bream in rivers, canals and lakes).

Fox hunting

> The fox was considered as vermin and hunting it was considered an exciting way of controlling a pest.

> Leaping over ditches and hedges on horseback required a great deal of skill.

> Breeding good horses and hounds was expensive.

> The ceremony around the sport appealed to the gentry (upper classes).

Falconry

> The aristocracy spent a good deal of time and resources breeding hunting birds.

> The skill was mastering the savage nature of the birds and creating a beautiful yet deadly hunter.

> The hunt was either by foot or on horseback.

Boar hunting

> Boars were hunted to extinction in Britain.

> They were pursued by dogs, and men on foot or horseback.

Deer hunting

> Deer were considered to be vermin because they ate vegetation and trampled down fences.

> Deer were hunted with staghounds.

Ottering

> Dogs were used to track down and corner otters.

> Otters were then killed using long poles with forked ends.

> They were considered vermin because they depleted fish stocks.

Fowling

Not a nasty tackle in soccer! A fowl is a bird, especially one that is hunted or that can be eaten as food (e.g. duck or chicken). So fowling is hunting these birds, with the intention of shooting them.

Games

> *Three examples of early English games.*

Both the rich and the poor played games. The characteristics of each class were reflected in the games they played.

The rich

> Plenty of leisure time
> Etiquette
> Sophisticated
> Nice facilities
> Played to rules
> Tactics involved
> Gambling on outcome

The poor

> Played only occasionally
> often violent
> Drinking alcohol often part of the ritual
> No pitches or courts
> Few rules, easy for uneducated to understand
> Few, if any tactics
> Gambling on outcome

Cricket

> Where this game derived from has caused a great deal of debate. It is thought to be a hybrid of several games. Two of the most likely are 'cat and dog' and 'stool ball'. The first was an ancient Scottish game where the batsman guarded a hole in the ground. The latter originates from France and used a three-legged stool.

> Cricket was enjoyed by all sections of society. It could be played on the rough village wicket with a minimum of equipment, or in the fine setting of a country property.

> The gentry could play in the same team as the working class, but both sections had clearly defined roles. The former dictated tactics, the latter chased after the ball.

Tennis

> This is said to have been a game first enjoyed by the ancient Egyptians. But in the form we know it, it is derived from the French nobility.

> In the early days of 'real tennis' it was played without rackets. In France it was called 'jeu de paume' (game with the palm).

> Rackets were introduced to impart more spin and power to the ball.

> The indoor courts were a similar shape to modern courts. They were, however, expensive to build.

> The rules were complicated.

> The servants of the wealthy saw this game and derived their own version. This was often played in the courtyards of local pubs. This was convenient as it provided competitors, spectators, drink and a chance to gamble.

Mob football

> This was played all over England in various forms. Local conditions and customs gave rise to a large variety of games: Derby Mob Football, The Haxey Hood, The Halletan Bottle Game and Ashbourne Football are all examples.

> The general aim was to overcome your opponent by invading their territory or by dragging some piece of equipment into yours.

> This task was violently pursued and often caused injury.

> There were few rules. The number of competitors varied a great deal. Drinking was often part of the ritual.

> It was a game played by the lower classes and despised by the wealthy. The wealthy were worried that their property would be destroyed by the violent games.

> 'Mob football' was banned for the first time in 1314, during the reign of King Edward II. This did not stop it being played.

Combat sports

> *Modern day combat sports are boxing, karate, judo.*

> These are sports that were taken from methods of protecting yourself. Gradually, rules and regulations were laid down, allowing combatants to pit their strength and skill against one another.

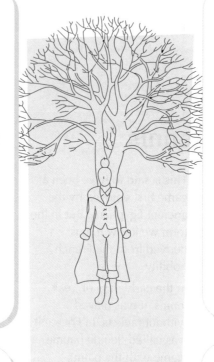

Archery

> The bow and arrow were the traditional weapon of peasants (used for hunting).

> After the Battle of Crecy (1346), when the British longbow won the day, the government decided all sports and pastimes should be stopped, except archery.

> The 17th century saw the development of firearms. Archery declined. Gradually became a refined sport for the upper and middle classes.

> It became codified with clubs, rules and ethics.

Jousting

> This appeared in various formats. It originated from the jousting tournaments of medieval knights. It was copied and from it quintain was developed. (The quintain was usually an object mounted on a post or support, set up as a mark to be tilted at with lances or poles. You could also throw darts or hoops at the quintain – as an exercise of skill.)

> The poor also had their own form on hobby horses or on small, unsteady boats.

Fencing

> The sword was the traditional weapon of the nobility.

> In the 17th century the sword was superseded by the gun. Instead, sword fighting developed into a sport and rules were drawn up for competing.

> Lower classes mimicked it with single sticks.

Wrestling

> Various types around the country. Each had its own rules and conventions (e.g. Devon and Cornwall; Cumberland and Westmoreland).

> Rural link: it was a way of demonstrating strength by local farm hands and often took place at country fairs.

Prize fighting

> Dates back to the 13th century where nobles learnt how to defend themselves.

> The nobility organised fights. For example, in 1681 the Duke of Albemarle set one up between his butcher and butler. We don't know what the prize was!

> Gradually the sport became more organised:
> 1743 James Broughton's rules
> 1857 Queensbury rules

> The former standardised fighting, but it was not until 1857 that it became more respectable and looked upon as a sport.

> Upper-class spectators; lower-class participants.

Social scene

> *How people lived.*

This is a snapshot of the social scene in Britain – as it was pre-industrial revolution. The panel provides a summary of the characteristics of popular recreation in times past.

Feudal

Gentry owned land – peasants worked for little return.

Rural

Majority of population lived and worked in the country.

Small communities

Everyone knew everyone in their community.

Literacy

Poor: mostly illiterate. Worked from a very young age.

Wealthy: generally literate.

Work

Poor: worked long hours. The work was:

> dictated by the season
> manual
> tedious
> strain on body.

Wealthy: lots of leisure time to enjoy vast wealth.

Harsh existence

Poor living conditions for the majority:

> squalid housing
> poor hygiene
> bad health
> unvaried diet.

Only the upper class lived in luxury.

Communications

Poor: stayed in village. Would only travel to local market towns, if at all. Limited knowledge of outside world.

Wealthy: likely to have a house in London or another large city. Travelled by coach. Had an appreciation of urban and rural life.

Church

Had a strong influence on daily life. Various teachings limited leisure time and controlled behaviour – not always successfully!

Puritanism: teaching strong commitment to morality. Says 'man' is basically sinful and should have no idle time in which to be sinful.

Sabbatarianism: strict observance of the Sabbath[1] – i.e. no recreation on day of rest.

Evangelism: preached against gambling, drink, idleness.

1 Since the Reformation, the 'Sabbath' is usually applied to the 'Lord's Day' i.e. the first day of the week (Sunday) observed by Christians in commemoration of the resurrection of Christ. Hebrews consider the Sabbath (or Sabbat) to be the seventh day of the week (Saturday).

A summary of popular recreation

Local coding	games developed to suit the local community.	**Ritual**	often linked to Church or seasons.
Limited rules	who could write then down?	**Wagering**	the chance to win and escape from poverty (not approved by the Church).
Rural	the population lived in the countryside so the games were rural.	**Drink**	to escape from harsh reality.
Occasional	often linked to festivals which only happened a few times a year.	**Physical force**	rather than skill required.
		Players and spectators	often little distinction between the two groups.
Violent	e.g. mob football	**Group identity**	they could be part of a team.
Cruel	e.g. blood sports. An obvious link here with the harsh existence of villagers.	**Rowdy**	most in conflict with respectable society. Often damage done to property.

Public schools – introduction

The public (now = private) schools in Great Britain played a major part in the development and organization of games and sports in the 19th century. In fact, the foundation of most of the sports played today rest in the history of the British public school.

Types of public schools

The Clarendon Schools

> The nine exclusive schools of Eton, Harrow, Rugby, Shrewsbury, St Paul's, Westminster, Charter House, Merchant Taylors, Winchester.

> Initially set up for the children of upper-class families.

> Had been around for a long time

Examples:
Winchester founded in 1382, Eton in 1440), therefore had primitive facilities.

Proprietary colleges

> These were middle-class copies of the Clarendon schools. Were generally purpose built and well equipped. Attracted the children of wealthy industrialists.

Examples:
Cheltenham, Clifton, Marlborough, Malvern.

Endowed grammar schools

> These were free schools set up in most towns around the country. Their patron was the King or Queen who had endowed it. (Names like the King Edward IV Grammar School.)

> In the mid-19th century several became fee paying and were accepted as public schools.

Denominational schools

> These were linked to the Church.

> They were predominantly small until the late-19th century when some became accepted as public schools.

Popular recreation in public schools

Home

> Boys saw different sports played at home by their parents, family friends and the locals.

Royal Tennis
Field Sports (e.g. shooting and hunting)
Combat sports
Mob games
Bathing (swimming)

School

> These sports and games were brought in from home and tailored to suit each school. They were adapted to suit the facilities that the school had to offer (e.g. courtyards, quadrangles, long corridors, buttresses, open grassy areas). As a consequence of these differences there was a great variety between the schools. For example, football might be played in a courtyard or on grass. 'Eton fives' has an upper and a lower court and a buttress.

Boys

> The pupils had lots of free time so therefore engaged themselves in playing the games they invented.

> Mostly played by the senior boys. Juniors used to collect balls or provide a minor supporting role.

> Gambling and drinking surrounded the sports.

The game of rugby is said to have originated at Rugby School in 1823. While playing football, William Webb Ellis took it on himself to pick up the ball and run towards the opposition goal. Where do you think the oval-shaped ball originated?

Public schools – developing attitudes

> *The boys' sports become more organised. Tom Brown's Schooldays is meant to depict life in the public schools.*

The enlightened headmasters

Sports and games in the 18th and 19th centuries were not developed for what they were, but how they could influence pupils' behaviour at school. What could staff do to channel all that youthful energy, to toughen up the body, and to build character?

Support

Some headmasters realised that the boys had to do something constructive with their free time. They saw the sporting activities that the boys clearly enjoyed as a way of promoting a code of ethics that could instil the sort of attitude they wanted.

Schools

From the 1830s headmasters such as Dr Arnold of Rugby School, Mr Kennedy of Shrewsbury, and Mr Moberly of Winchester began to use sport for its educational values.

Rules

As a consequence of this support the games became more formal. **Rules** were written establishing relationships between players and basic playing **techniques.** Gradually, sport began to flourish and the House system expanded to include matches between teams from different Houses.

What could be gained from sport?

Most of the sport was still run by the boys, but staff began to appear on the sidelines to encourage their House teams. The heads hoped to take away the brutal discipline that was instilled by the senior boys and replace it with activities that were not anti-social. They wanted to encourage conformity to authority with acceptable guidelines.

The effect of the 'Blues'

In the final stage of the development of public school sport we see it becoming more organised.

University

The public school boys attend university and decide to develop their games. Gradually, they adjust the rules and begin to produce hybrid games that take the best aspects of the different sports.

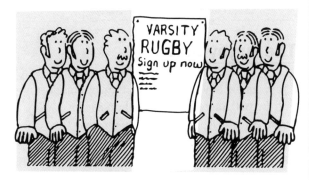

The graduates

These filter out into society taking their sports with them. Some go back to the public schools and introduce their organised games.

Sport

> The young staff become involved in coaching and running sport.
> The schools employ professional coaches.
> The standard improves; facilities improve.
> Pattern of the school day changes: lessons in the morning, games in the afternoon.

Muscular Christianity

Here we see the development of a link between **manliness** and **godliness**. The Headmasters have recognised that games can prepare their boys for adult life.

Physical endeavour	Moral Integrity
> Health	> Social cohesion
> Activity	> Respect for authority
> Move from over-studying	> Development of leadership
> Toughen up an indulgent society	> Response to leadership

Tom Brown's Schooldays
by Thomas Hughes

Several extracts from this book, first published in 1857, can be used to highlight the code of ethics that the liberal headmasters hoped to establish by allowing the introduction of sport. In the book, the school is Rugby School, and the headmaster is Thomas Arnold (Head of Rugby School, 1828–42).

The rugby match

Tom, a new boy to the school, throws himself on the ball, thereby saving his house team from defeat. He is injured in the process. The Head of House picks him up, checks he is OK and congratulates Tom on his bravery.

Technical aspects
> Rules
> Pitch
> Teams
> Supporters
> Uniforms

Moral values
> Selflessness of Tom
> Putting team before self
> Looked after by Head of House
> Support from team members

The fight

Slogger Williams, a big boy, picks on Arthur. Tom steps in to stop the fight and ends up fighting against the bully. An epic fight takes place that is watched by the rest of the boys. It stops when the headmaster arrives. He questions the Head Boy about it. Later the Head Boy encourages Tom and Slogger to make it up.

Technical aspects
> Rules
> Supporters
> Seconds
> Ring formed by crowd

Moral values
> Tom stands up for the rights of Arthur
> Authority of Headmaster
> Forgiveness
> Authority of Head Boy

The cricket match

Tom, the captain of the team and playing his last match for the school, sends Arthur in to bat at a crucial stage of the match. He realises he may not win the game but sees it as a good learning experience for Arthur. After the game Tom has tea with his form master and discusses his time at Rugby School.

Technical aspects
> Rules
> Equipment
> Uniforms
> Tactics

Moral values
> Tom identifies the needs of Arthur over the need to win
> Relationship with staff
> Respect for rest of team over Tom's captaincy

Public schools – elitism and athleticism

> *What about women?*

Elite girls schools

Women in Victorian society were seen as inferior to men. They were valued in the home for looking after children and running the house. Education was not seen as important.

Ladies' academies

> In the early 18th century several ladies' academies were established. They were for the upper classes and varied a great deal in quality and cost. Some were more expensive than the most exclusive public schools.

> They taught dancing, a form of callisthenics, sewing, singing, playing the piano, verse speaking, posture and any other graces it was felt important for a woman to have.

Girls' schools

> By the mid-19th century there was an emergence of girls' private schools (e.g. Roedean in Sussex, Malvern College in Worcestershire, Cheltenham Ladies).

> The development of their sport was influenced by what the girls had seen at home, often played by their brothers.

> As these girls' schools developed after the boys, they developed more quickly. By the 1880s tennis and cricket were being played in girls' schools. The girls wore their normal clothing and the games did not involve contact.

> Gradually the 'medical' reasons for women not participating in sport were set aside.

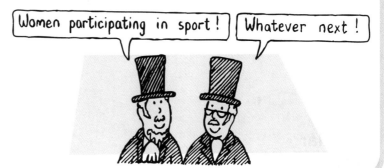

The effects of public schools on the local community

How did having a public school education have an effect on the whole of society? Boys from the public schools went into all aspects of society – from the armed forces to medicine, to the Church, to teaching, to industry and to the legal system. This promoted and developed sport in all areas of the community.

Army

As the British Empire grew, sport was taken all over the world. All ranks of soldiers and sailors were encouraged to play.

Industry

The industrialists began to see the benefits of health and attitude that sport could have on their workforce. They gradually allowed their workers time to play and provided facilities.

Church

The values of the Church were seen to be upheld in sport. This officially approved sport for all classes. The church also developed its own teams for its parishioners.

The characteristics of public school athleticism

Development of education

Prior to mid-19th century

> Classical education – learning Latin and Greek.
> Leisure time of boys mis-spent – gambling, drinking, fighting.

By mid-19th century

> Wider social and intellectual education.
> Greater variety of subjects taught, relevant to the modern world.
> The whole person looked at.
> Pupils' leisure time becomes a time for games and sport.

Ethics

> Godliness and manliness.
> Social control – responsibility, respect, morality.
> Physical endeavour – moral integrity.

Facilities

> Sponsored by old boys.
> Purpose-built buildings.
> Playing fields.

Technical development of sport

> Regularity.
> Respectability.
> Codification.
> Well organised.

Muscular Christianity

> Win gracefully.
> Lose with honour.
> Bravery.
> Brotherhood.
> Leadership.

Changing attitudes of Heads

1 Heads actively discourage games – pupils flogged.
2 Then realise games promote values: some support given to House games; not actively discouraged.
3 Finally, Heads actively promote games/sports: allowed time; provided staff and facilities.

Rational recreation

> We now see sport moving from the public schools into the community.

How did sport become an activity for all?

How did team sports spread and develop across the length and breadth of the country?

How did the 'sport of kings' become a major spectator sport that all levels of society could enjoy?

We will try to answer these questions.

Mid-18th century social attitudes leading to the development of sport

Aristocracy

(upper class)

> Privileged elite
> Used to being in control
> Exclusive pastimes that only they could afford.

Middle class

> Made rich by the industrial revolution (from mid-18th c.)
> Had a social conscience
> Liked to look after the morality of the nation
> Large pressure to conform to their high moral ground.

Acceptance of sport

> Sport was gradually seen as an appropriate way of occupying the lower classes away from drinking and gambling, and other anti-social and morally low habits.
> Gradually more free time was granted allowing more opportunity for sport.

Physical changes leading to the development of sport

Let us start by looking at Britain in the 19th century. The industrial revolution is well under way.

Urbanization

The majority of the country's population now lived in the cities, rather than the countryside. This meant large concentrations of population needed meaningful leisure time activities to divert them from gambling and drinking.

Technology

Equipment – advances in materials led to better bats and balls. They lasted longer, were fairly regular in bounce and performance, and could be mass-produced.

Sports pitches – machines were invented to maintain and prepare pitches.

Timekeeping – stopwatches were developed allowing more accurate timekeeping.

Communications

Roads – improvement of road surfaces and the introduction of coach travel.

Rail – steam power meant the growth of the railway system.

These two developments allowed teams – and supporters – to move around the country to compete against each other.

Telegraph – this meant results and information could be sent quickly from one end of the country to another.

Printed word – the development of newspapers meant people could keep in touch with results of sports matches and sporting events.

Literacy – this was promoted. More people were able to take an interest in sports by reading newspapers and the like.

Working class

> Poor
> Uneducated
> Squalid living conditions
> Subservient

Living conditions

> Squalid
> Infant mortality high
> Poor sanitation
> Disease common

Working conditions

> Low wages
> Hazardous working environment – many accidents and deaths
> Long hours of work
  – prior to 1870, 72 hour week
  – after 1870, white collar workers had a half day off on Saturday
  – after 1880, the same was granted to most semi-skilled workers
  – after 1890, the rest were given a half day off each week

National Championships start

Leagues

International matches

Governing bodies developed to co-ordinate sport

Newspapers inform people about sport

Formal condification

Church support

Development of leisure facilities for inhabitants

Continue the high moral attitude started in public schools

A summary of rational recreation

Large populations based in and around towns

Channelled aggression

A captive spectator base

Some sport kept exclusive

Better transport leading to greater access to sport

Spectatorism develops

Those with money can travel to play and watch sport

Professionalism develops

Physical education in state schools: 1902–1914/18

> *Schooling before 1900 is minimal and varied.*

So what physical education was taught in state schools in the late 19th and early 20th centuries? 'Not a lot' may be the answer. For the lower classes in state schools, few pupils if any experienced games as their physical education consisted of structured physical training.

State physical education before 1902

Legislation

Before 1870

The education of those who could not afford a private education was the responsibility of the Church. The quality and accessibility of education varied a great deal. The majority remained uneducated.

The 1870 Forster Elementary Education Act

> This was the first step towards creating a **state education system**.

> It only made recommendations, however. As a consequence of this, improvement was not as complete as it could have been.

Mundella's Education Act, 1880

> This made it compulsory for all children between the ages of 5 and 10 to attend school.

> Led to a significant increase in the number of school places.

> By 1899 the school-leaving age had been raised to 12 years.

Facilities

The majority of schools that were in towns had little space for playing fields. There were those that also had no playground. This clearly placed restrictions on the sporting activities that could be offered.

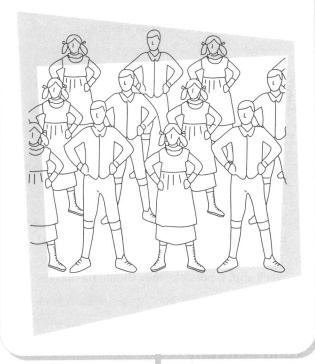

Activities

> Prior to 1870 there was a mixture of Swedish, German and English gymnastics. Archibald Buchanan was the main proponent of the latter type of gymnastics. Once again there was a great deal of variety from school to school in content and regularity.

> In the 1870s drill was developed, for boys and girls. This was taught by NCOs from the army.

> By the 1890s some of this drill was being taught by teachers.

Physical training 1902–1918

The Boer War (1899-1902)

> This war saw the British Army defeated by a band of men who were part-time soldiers. The health and fitness of the British troops was blamed, and it was felt that this was a consequence of inadequate physical training at school.

> Colonel Fox of the Army Physical Training Corps was appointed by the government to find a solution.

> Physical training remained part of the curriculum for the next fifty years.

1904 syllabus

> This identified two main areas: health and education.

> To achieve this, 109 exercise tables were drawn up. These were specific lesson plans that teachers or instructors could follow.

> It allowed for poor facilities, no equipment and the large numbers in classes.

> Three 20-minute lessons were to be held per week and, if possible, they should be outside.

1909 syllabus

> Over the year leading up to this syllabus more concern was taken over the welfare of children of working-class families.

> With this in mind, Dr Newman was appointed to the Board of Education. His influence ensured a slightly more therapeutic angle.

> The number of exercise tables was cut to 71 and some organised games were introduced. With these we see the first tentative move away from military-style PT teaching.

1902 model course

> The three main components of this course were:
  – fitness
  – familiarity with weapons
  – discipline.

> It was to be delivered by military instructors.

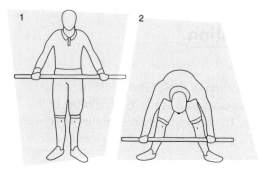

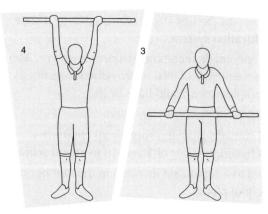

> The 1902 model course soon came under attack as it clearly did not take into account the educational aspect that should be the purpose of physical training in schools. It had children doing exercises designed for adults.

Commands

'Attention'   'Stand at ease'

'Head, turn'   'Trunk, turn'

'Marching on the spot'

'Marching, about turn'

Physical education in state schools: 1914/18–1988

> *Physical training shifts to become physical education.*

Physical training 1914–1939

The First World War

> The years 1914–1918 saw the tragedy of the first great world war. A generation of young men was almost totally wiped out. The effect this had on the education system is interesting.

> Firstly, it was recognised that a slightly more child-centred approach was needed. The authorities still wanted a disciplined and hardworking lower class, but they wanted them to show some initiative.

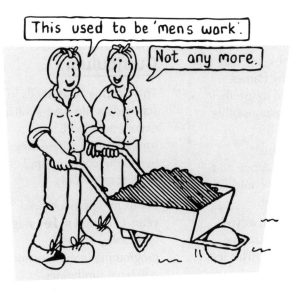

> Secondly, women had worked in munitions factories and on the land during the war. This increased their social status and afforded them more equality, as they had shown they could cope with demanding physical work.

1919 syllabus

> Dr Newman was once again involved with this.

> The syllabus allowed more freedom and individual interpretation in the use of the exercise tables.

> It also stated that during each session time should be set aside for games and dancing.

> For the older pupils therapeutic exercises were still the main emphasis.

1919–1932

This period in history was full of social upheaval. The biggest impact was from the economic depression that started in the late 1920s. This led to very poor living conditions for the less well off as they suffered even more than before. (There was no welfare state system so no unemployment benefit or family allowance.) The result was the production of the 1933 syllabus.

1933 syllabus

> This has been recognised as the best syllabus that the Board of Education in England and Wales had produced to date.

> It allowed more game play; introduced group work; but still kept some therapeutic aspects.

> At last we see a move from a teacher-centred approach to one where more choice is available and decisions can be made by pupils.

> Tables were still being produced to give teachers ideas, but they were less restrictive and more open to change.

Post Second World War physical education

The 1944 Butler Education Act

The emphasis here was on equal access to education for all, in theory.

The main points of it were:

1. Grammar schools were to be free, but selective. Pupils had to pass the 11+ exam to gain entry. Pupils from all economic backgrounds could now attend. (Those who did not pass the 11+ went to secondary modern schools.)

2. All children would leave primary school at 11, and start at the grammar or secondary modern school.

3. New schools were to be built to accommodate extra pupils.

4. The school-leaving age would be raised to 15.

5. Better forms of PE were to be devised for the older pupils.

The effect of the Second World War

> As with the First World War everyone was touched by the long, hard years of war. Due to the development of aircraft bombers and long-range missiles, the lives of everyone in Britain, including children, were affected directly. People looked to their children for hope; and we now see a further step towards child-centred learning.

> The training that had been used to create 'thinking' soldiers during the war was now adapted to suit schools. Assault course type equipment was put up in schools – ropes, benches, ladders and climbing frames. Pupils were required to use their initiative and take responsibility for each other.

> Leading educationalists introduced 'modern' dance and gymnastics. The latter could also require equipment.

> Variety and enjoyment, as well as high levels of skill learning now became important. This led to the publication of two documents by the ministry of Education:
Moving and Growing (published in 1952) and
Planning the Programme (1953).

Education Reform Act, 1988

Reinforced the position of PE in British schools, making it a compulsory subject. However, it was only in 1992 that the government decided the details of the bill. Revised in 1995 following the publication of the Dearing Report in state education.

National Curriculum

This provides that pupils in schools should have similar experiences in PE irrespective of where they live in the country. Applies to all state schools.

Pupils in different school years allocated to **key stages** (see table). The PE programme in every school will have similarities. However, every school has different facilities and equipment will vary, so there will be variations in PE up and down the country.

Key Stage	Pupil's age	Year group	Activities in PE
1	5–7 years	1–2	Games, gymnastic activities, dance
2	7–11 years	3–6	Games, gymnastic activities, dance, athletic activities, outdoor and adventurous activities, swimming. Pupils to be taught the six areas of activity
3	11–14 years	7–9	Pupils taught four of the above activities
4	14–16 years	10–11	Pupils taught a minimum of two of above activities. One must be a game

Physical education and sport

Physical education and sport

At the heart of all physical education are sporting activities. PE is a school subject.

In PE and in sport participants learn:
> how to perform in sports, e.g. swimming strokes, dribbling in hockey, ball control in soccer.
> through taking part in physical activity.

Extra-curricular activities

> These are games and sports that take place outside normal school time.

> For most children, physical education at school is their first contact with organised sport. (Although they may have learned to swim before starting school.)

> At school, children have the opportunity not only to take part in a range of physical activities during lessons, but also in organised games during lunchtime, after school and against other schools.

Interschool competition

This is considered important in developing high standards of play. However, the activities involved depend on a number of factors:

> Which activities are included in the school PE curriculum.

> Facilities available to the school.

> Interests and skills of the staff.

> Coaches and parents might be involved in PE, school teams and organised matches.

Differences between teaching PE and coaching a sport

PE teaching	Sports coaching
> time is spent on general exercise	> more time is spent on an activity
> participants are there because it is part of the curriculum	> the participants are usually there by choice
> groups are of mixed ability	> groups being coached are often of a similar ability
> the social aspect is as important as the skill acquisition	> selective

Summary

Which of the following words could be linked to the dates listed below?

1902	1909	1919	1933	1944

Teaching style	Facilities	Equipment	Educational values
Command	Classroom	Batons	Accepting authority
Discovery	Playground	Poles	Subject centred
Problem solving	Gymnasium	Ropes	Child centred
Authoritarian	Playing field	Benches	Physical skills
Formal		Climbing frames	Social skills
Informal		Boxes	Therapeutic
Progressive			
Traditional			

Games and activities

> *Sport has now become far more organised.*

Many activities and games were developed in the latter half of the 19th century and the early years of the 20th century. Below are a few which highlight the level and speed of development.

Football

This was popular with all sections of society. It is a game that began with the lower classes and was refined in the public schools.

Notable dates:

1863: Some school old boys' teams founded the Football Association (FA)

1885: Professionalism was made legal

1888: The Football League was started.

By the early 1900s there were 10000 clubs within the FA

Athletics

Athletics was initially developed in the public schools. It was copied from the ancient Greeks.

We can also see an influence from the early days of pedestrianism where the wealthy would arrange races between their footmen (servants).

Notable dates:

1860s: Gradual appearance of athletics meetings; founding of Thames Hare and Hounds cross-country club

1866: Amateur Athletics Club formed

1880: Amateur Athletics Association (AAA) born

1913: International Amateur Athletics Federation (IAAF) founded

Swimming

Public baths – these were cheap and consequently used by poorer citizens. They promoted exercise and hygiene.

Turkish baths – these were more exclusive and from these we see the development of competitive swimming. Competition swimming became popular, particularly in London, in the 19th century.

Notable dates:

1869: First organised swimming governing body (London)

1874: First national swimming championships

1884: Formation of the Amateur Swimming Association (ASA)

1905: Fédération Internationale de Natation Amateur (FINA) – world governing body – founded in London

1926: First European championship

Tennis

Lawn tennis evolved slowly. It developed from handball, an outdoor game popular in France.

This was a game for the middle classes. It was developed as a cheaper form of sport than 'real tennis'. It could be played in the garden at home but also clubs sprang up that the middle classes could join.

Cricket

This was a game participated in by all sections of society. The fact that it was non-contact and it promoted gentlemanly behaviour contributed to this.

In the late 19th century we see the development of cricket grounds as the middle class begin to support games.

Notable dates:

1864: First county championship

1873: Qualification of the sport's rules for county cricketers

1875: Modern rules drawn up by the Marylebone Cricket Club (MCC)

1877: 1 March – first 'Test' match in Melbourne, Australia

1880: Kennington Oval staged first Test match in England

Notable dates:

1871: First lawn tennis club in the world formed at Manor House Hotel, Leamington Spa

1873: First book of rules. Major Clopton Wingfield patented a 'new and improved court for playing the ancient game of tennis' – shaped like an hourglass

1876: The All-England Croquet and Lawn Tennis Club established at Wimbledon

Historical issues – amateur *v* professional

Throughout the history of sport there have been debates over what is the difference between an 'amateur' and a 'professional' in sport. In recent years there has been a growth in the number of professional sportsmen and women. Think of sports such as athletics and rugby union. Basically, there are three types of sportsperson:

> Amateurs – who take part in sport for enjoyment and do not get paid or receive prize money.

> Professionals – who are paid (some highly!) to take part in sport – playing, coaching or managing. For these people sport is their job.

> Semi-professionals – who are paid for playing, coaching or managing but also have another job. For these people, sport alone does not pay enough.

A brief history of amateur *v* professional

In the Ancient Greek Olympics athletes only received a laurel wreath for winning. There was no prize money. However, to be good enough to win, these athletes had to be able to train, eat the right food, and use the best equipment (javelins, discuses, etc.). Their normal work (usually as soldiers) would not have paid for all this. Instead they were supported by wealthy individuals, or given help by their employers. Although these athletes were amateur, they did receive some financial support.

18th and 19th centuries

The gentleman amateur
He was wealthy so could take time off to play sport. The 'gentleman amateur' competed to prove himself as a person and to test his ability. He did not train as that would make him a 'professional'. He was a respected member of the community with a good education.

The professional
He was generally from a poor background, therefore had to make money from sport. If he could not make money then he could not afford to play. The professional was perceived to be corruptible as he was controlled by money (i.e. might take a bribe to throw a game or contest).

The middle class
They could not afford time off work to play sport, but at the same time did not want to get paid to play. They admired the high cultural values of the gentleman amateur. They played in their free time.

Early professionals

1. The **prize fighter** was paid to represent the noble. All sections of society watched and wagered.
2. **Wager boats** – the river men would race each other. Spectators would place bets on the fastest crossings.
3. **Footmen** – the wealthy would match their footmen (servants) and place bets on the winners. This was the start of pedestrianism (professional running).
4. **Cricket** was one of the first truly professional games. Between 1750 and 1850 there were several professional touring teams taking part in matches in all parts of the country. Cricket coaches were employed at the large country houses to prepare wickets, coach the owners and to play for their teams. Later they worked in public schools.

Developments

> The modern Olympic Games began in 1896, with the intention that amateurs would compete against one another. There would be no prize money for the winners, only medals.

> As sports developed there was more scope for professionalism. To be a good player you needed to devote time and money to training. You needed money to attract the best players to your team in order that you could do well in the leagues and attract supporters.

> As the class system gradually eroded, the stigma of being a professional diminished.

> The abolition of the maximum wage meant players could negotiate wages and turn from tradesmen into professionals.

> In soccer the maximum wage in England was £4 in 1900. George Eastham, of Newcastle United, went on strike in 1961 over the maximum wage (£10 then). A couple of years later, Johnny Haynes of Fulham became the first £100-a-week soccer player.

Historical issues – women and sport

> *Historically, women's opportunity in sport has been far less than men's.*

The Victorian era (1837 – 1901)

> This era had the biggest single effect on limiting women's participation in sport.

> It was felt during this time that women should not exert themselves physically as it was not good for their health and it was not 'ladylike'. Dress had to completely cover their body, thus limiting their ability to move freely. Things remained like this until after the First World War (1914–1918).

> The daughters of wealthy families who received an education did so at a ladies academy, or one of the new private schools. The former concentrated on social graces. The latter gradually broadened its outlook and allowed some 'ladylike' sports (such as tennis and hockey).

> Working-class women were almost totally excluded from sport. Their only experience was in the late 1800s – with drill (see page 117).

Madame Bergman-Osterbeg

> This lady was involved with PE in London and among other achievements introduced a ladies PE College in 1895. This influenced the spread of women's sport.

> Some of her former pupils set up their own colleges, thereby encouraging more female PE teachers to enter the profession.

> Madame Bergman-Osterberg's philosophy was based around a mixture of Swedish gymnastics and team games. She advocated single sex lessons.

Female sports

Field sports – these were participated in by the upper class and were on the privacy of their own land. Women joined in with these social occasions.

Archery – this was non-contact and used no physical exertion.

Garden games – tennis, croquet and badminton were all adopted by the middle classes. They could be played at home in the privacy of their garden.

Golf – clubs allowed women to play at certain off-peak times. They were discriminated against.

Athletics – the women's AAA, formed in 1922, promoted athletics. The 1928 Olympics were the first games in which women were allowed to compete. The fact that several competitors were ill after the 800-metre race caused a real setback – a case of 'I told you so'!

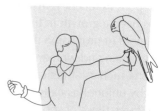

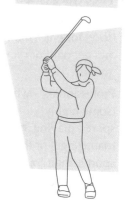

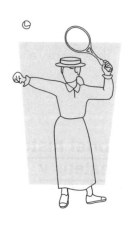

Restricted opportunity

Even today there are fewer opportunities available for women.

> They cannot compete in as many events in the Olympics as men, and in professional sports they generally get paid less.

> The media focuses on them less.

The Women's Sports Federation (WSF)

This association was founded in 1984 to help women become more involved in sport at all levels. You can find out more about WSF from their website: www.wsf.org.uk

USA (1)

> *Cultural factors which influence sport in America.*

We will begin our comparative studies by looking at games and sport – and the wider curriculum – in North America. The focus is on the United States of America (USA). In many ways the USA is a world leader: the way that sportsmen and women are treated, the facilities available, and the way major sports are funded.

History

> Native American Indians played lacrosse as Baggatoway.

> Many Native American Indians were killed by Europeans who settled on the East Coast (//[1] Australian Aborigines).

> Colonialists were pioneers migrating west. 'Frontier spirit' developed – the spirit of survival in alien territory, a sense of adventure.

> Sports reflected the origin of the colonialists in areas where they settled – hunting, horseracing, cricket, rugby: middle-class English.

> Many sports suffered from the imported Puritanism. [Many early English and Dutch settlers were Puritans, who lived according to strict moral and religious principles. They avoided physical activities such as sport.]

> The War of Independence (1777–1783) severed the links with their European past and sport reflected the emergence of an American identity:

  – from rugby came 'gridiron' (American football)

  – rowing and athletics – intercollegiate competitions

  – baseball established 1860

  – volleyball developed some time after as a pastime for exercise-seeking businessmen

  – James Naismith invented basketball in 1891 as a game to be played indoors in winter, while attending a YMCA (Young Men's Christian Association) training School.

  – Middle-class women played tennis and croquet, and cycled.

Ideology

> The **'American Dream'** – 'rags to riches'. The idea that everyone and anyone can achieve success/the pursuit of happiness. Sport is seen as a way out of the gutter (e.g. boxing).

> **Win ethic** – winning is the only thing. This is also known as the Lombardian philosophy, after Vince Lombardi, Head Coach of Green Bay Packers in 1959, who transformed them from a losing American Football team into a major power in the sport. The emphasis is on competition and rewards. Professionalism and commercialism – society only interested in winners.

> **Radical ethic** – winning is important but so also is the process – intrinsic value (the middle way).

> **Counter-culture ethic** – some Americans are trying to change the focus and suggest that it is not whether you win or lose but 'how you play the game'.

Political

> Decentralised

> Federal republic, with elected president

> 2 elected Houses – Senate and Congress

> Two-party system – Democrats and Republicans

> 51 states (// Australia) almost independent; each has own parliament and funding

> A young society 'looking for identity and forming a modern unified nation, forging their way with their 'frontier spirit'.

---

1 Symbol denotes 'parallel'. These draw out comparisons with the other comparative studies in this section.

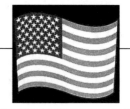

Geography

Population: 250 million

$^3/_4$ live in cities, therefore population dense in cities and sparse in other areas.

Climate: Every kind – from very cold (High Plains) to semitropical (Gulf Coast), rainy (Central Plain + Appalachians) and desert (// Australia).

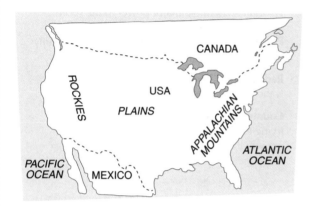

Size: 3.5 million square miles

(// Australia but population 15 times as large)

51 states: Alabama, Alaska, Arizona, Arkansas, California, Colorado, Connecticut, Delaware, District of Columbia, Florida, Georgia, Hawaii, Idaho, Illinois, Indiana, Iowa, Kansas, Kentucky, Louisiana, Maine, Maryland, Massachusetts, Michigan, Minnesota, Mississippi, Missouri, Montana, Nebraska, Nevada, New Hampshire, New Jersey, New Mexico, New York, North Carolina, North Dakota, Ohio, Oklahoma, Oregon, Pennsylvania, Rhode Island, South Carolina, South Dakota, Tennessee, Texas, Utah, Vermont, Virginia, Washington, West Virginia, Wisconsin, Wyoming.

> Each state is approximately equivalent to a European country but with less population.

3 geographical areas which are very varied:

1. highland (Appalachians to the East)
2. plains (central America)
3. mountains (Rockies to the West)

Still many wilderness areas (// Australia).

Communications

> Airlines and interstate buses (called 'Greyhounds') are heavily used.

> Transcontinental railways.

> Heavy car usage – long distances to travel.

Social/economic

> A capitalist society, where commercialism is strong; based on private enterprise.

> Material wealth is important.

> Individuals tend to identify with their state rather than nation. People are New Yorkers or Californian first; American second. Sport is a way to nationalism with the flag, oath and national anthem to remind them.

> $^3/_4$ population white; $^1/_4$ black. Last into the country tend to be at the bottom of the social ladder.

> Stacking

WASPS
Black community
Puerto Ricans
Mexicans
Vietnamese

WASPS – White Anglo-Saxon Protestants (privileged and affluent)

> Racial groups identify with specific sports (e.g. basketball 'dream team' had few whites; certain nationalities play particular positions in gridiron).

> Pluralist society – the right of every ethnic group to keep its identity.

Excellence

Win ethic

> Striving for excellence is developed through interscholastic and intercollegiate sport and sports scholarships.

> Few sports schools because all schools aim to achieve excellence. School sport generates its own funding – very big occasion covered by the media.

> Draft system – football and basketball clubs have choice of college students who are 'drafted' to professional teams.

> Commercial enterprise of collegiate football and basketball funds scholarships. Federal money is used to finance the Olympic team. Motivated to win by need to beat other superpowers.

USA (2)

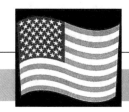

> *Thematic considerations of sport in the USA. Compare these with other countries.*

Education, PE + sport

> Predominantly free state education, plus some private schools linked to Church groups. Each state is responsible for education (states vary considerably with climate and geography, so education more relevant to own state).

> Administered by local District School Board (DSB). Policy is <u>not</u> devolved to individual schools. Kindergarten (4–5); elementary (6–12), high school (12–17). The aim of all is to pass high-school diploma.

> Physical Education is part of the curriculum – work on the physical, mental, social and emotional development of the child. High schools have fitness testing. This suits the culture – the importance of being the best, and accountability.

> Sports are more important than PE in the USA. Therefore the PE teacher has lower status and is separate from the sports coach (although they are trying to improve the importance of PE).

> Counter-culture – heuristic[1] approach conflicts with competitive ethic.

> Inter-scholastic sport is very important. Schools often have excellent facilities and are self-supporting (charging for entrance to matches etc.). It can be elitist – everything is spent on the most able. Coaches are highly paid but are expected to produce results ('hire and fire').

> Legislation to bring equality of programme and funding to boys and girls – female performer in professional sport was the cheerleader!

> Adaptive programme for children with special needs.

> Intercollegiate sport – Harvard and Yale reflected the traditions of Oxford and Cambridge but abandoned the amateurism. 2 divisions:

  1. National Association of Inter-collegiate Athletics (NAIA) responsible for the control of athletic competitions between smaller colleges.

  2. National Collegiate Athletic Association (NCAA) responsible for inter-scholastic programme at larger colleges.

> Individual sports governing bodies replaced Amateur Athletic Union (AAU).

> Sports scholarships to universities – sport is seen by coaches to be more important than academic studies increases pressure on students.

> Sport is entertainment and commercial – big business.

Mass participation

> No specific plans by the federal government.

> Programmes for adults are part of school programmes.

> For children, 'little league sport' (e.g. little league basketball) – originally set up by parents, now a business organisation catering for 8–18 year olds (senior division 13–15; big league 16–18). Attracts media coverage.

> National senior sports organisation - image of a healthy old age.

> No real private sports clubs except elitist ones (tennis and golf). Expensive. Less wealthy involved with activities at:
  – ice rinks
  – swimming pools
  – basketball courts.

> All interested in going to the game (baseball).

Outdoor education/ outdoor recreation

> Outdoor education is a tradition in USA but it is out of school. Children go every year to summer camp (// France). Programmes introduce Americans to nature but socialisation is important too. Some are privately run, others by organisations such as the YMCA.

> Pioneer/frontier spirit – to overcome alien environment. The variety of landscape gives scope for challenging and exciting experiences.

> National parks are under federal law. State parks administered by state.

> Many go to enjoy these wilderness areas. Land is classified according to isolation:
1 – close to towns; 5 – wilderness

Safety is important particularly with risky sports becoming more popular and the dangers in the wilderness areas.

1 Methods of learning which involve reasoning and part experience rather than solutions that are given to you by a teacher/coach.

Australia (1)

As a final comparative study, we will look at Australasia, with particular reference to Australia.

History

> Aboriginal culture – went through cycle of oppression. Aborigines (native Australians) seen by European settlers as sub-human and were presumed dangerous (// Native American Indians).

> When settlers wanted their territory, the Aborigines were forced inland so that the European arrivals could settle by the coast. The colonialists moved in and suggested 'white' was better.

> Missionaries and soldiers tried to destroy the Aboriginal culture.

> Australia became a British colony – the colonies becoming self-governing.

> At the end of 19th century – the Commonwealth of Australia was formed.

> Sport reflects the developments in the UK – predominantly middle class as little industrialism.

> Colonial influence was considerable and can be seen in the sports played (e.g. rugby and cricket). They still like to beat the 'old enemy' (England).

> Later took in other Europeans, South Africans and Asians.

Ideology

> 'Sun, sea and surf' (// USA; France).

> It is suggested that sport is an obsession to Aussies. Certainly the 'win ethic' is strong (// USA).

> Because of colonial influence, they adopted many of the British/Celtic ethics.

> Strong sense of survival in alien environment.

> Aboriginals at home in the natural environment.

> 'Dream time' – go walkabout to find self in nature.

> They are trying to re-establish the Aboriginal culture by claiming back land through the courts. They re-enact their culture for the tourists (// North American Indians).

Political

The 5 states all have a federal democracy.

Political parties – National Party, Labour Party, Liberal Party – mix of British and USA systems.

> Pre 1950 – predominantly British/Irish descent and some displaced Europeans.

> Post-war – there was a need (1950s) to repopulate. Encouraged British to go, then took in other Europeans e.g. Greeks, Italians, Germans.

> 1960s – middle eastern and north African immigrants.

> 1970s – Asians admitted (affected business).

> 1990s – achieved quota for new settlers – now control numbers of immigrants.

Therefore Australia is a diverse multi-cultural society, but there is a limit to the population it can support.

Social/economic

> A prosperous capitalist country based on agriculture but developing new technology (Asian influence). Rich material wealth but high unemployment.

> Young society (// USA).

> Pluralist society quickly developed (// USA).

> Pluralism – every ethnic group has a right to their own identity (// USA).

> Assimilation – ethnic groups mixed in. Acceptable if done freely (France and UK); not acceptable if done by force.

> Separatism – works if both groups are equal but the more powerful can often try to remove weak – to be discouraged.

Anglo-Celt

Greeks and Italians

South-East Asians

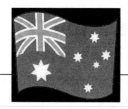

Geography

Population: Approximately 18 million

> Population density is very low. Mostly live in major cities (80% of population is urban) in the coastal areas.

> 34% of Australia is desert which is mostly unpopulated and uninhabitable – Red Centre – alien territory.

> Great Divide – mountain range to East, running north to south.

> Tourists tend to go into the Bush; Aussies stay at home and watch sport.

> Climate – southern hemisphere (North – tropical; South – temperate). Allows for seasonal sports to be played all year (e.g. skiing). Healthy outdoor philosophy (can ski and surf in same day).

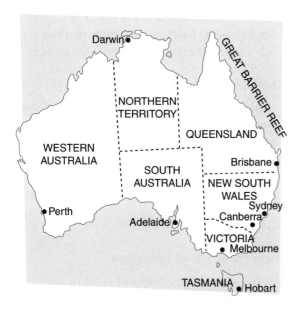

Size: Almost as big as the whole of Europe or North America.

6 states:

Western Australia (capital: Perth)
Victoria (capital: Melbourne)
Queensland (capital: Brisbane)
New South Wales (capital: Sydney)
Northern Territory (capital: Darwin)
Tasmania (capital: Hobart)

Communications: Good roads along coast and between major cities. 'Red Centre' mostly dirt tracks. Good rail and internal air services.

Mass participation

> **Aussie sport**

Programme to develop young people through sport – focus on juniors. Included are codes of behaviour. Programmes included Sportstart, Sportit and CAPS.

> **Active Australia**

To encourage participation of whole population (6–60). Achieved the need to expand the base of pyramid, which leads to 'excellence'.

Sports

> Adopted colonial sports – cricket, rugby union, horse racing.

> From immigrants – football.

> Established own sporting identity – swimming; Aussie rules.

Aussie rules

This sport developed in 1840s, as a mixture of rugby and Gaelic football. Played mainly in 4 states but with great intensity. A 40-a-side game of Aussie rules played in Melbourne in 1858 was abandoned – after 3 weeks.

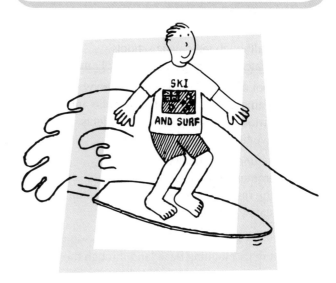

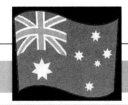

> *Thematic considerations of sport in Australia. Compare with other countries.*

Excellence

Have a desire to do well in Olympics, Commonwealth Games and cricket Test matches.

Poor performances in the 1976 Olympics led to change (// France).

> ASC (Australian Sports Commission) researched in other countries to look for the most effective method to select and train athletes. Set up the AIS (Australian Institute of Sport), an academy of sport in Canberra (where the federal government and ASC are located). Realised need for more than one institute of excellence.

> Set up more in other states – Queensland (at Brisbane); Western Australia (at Perth); South Australia (at Adelaide); Victoria (at Melbourne); New South Wales (at Sydney) – each specialised in one sport (e.g. cricket at Adelaide; rugby at Brisbane).

> Now each state devolved with centres of excellence in their main city. All part of the AIS federal system. Have programme of talent identification – Sportsleap, Sports search – run at all levels (to identify talent).

> Aussie able – provision for disabled athletes – some sports schools.

Outdoor education and outdoor recreation

> Within schools there is a programme of outdoor education that students can elect to study (not compulsory; // UK). The emphasis is on knowing about the importance of safety, conservation and recreation – *education in the outdoors*. A positive physical experience in the natural environment.

> Outward bound centres, e.g. Timbertops (// Gordonstoun in UK). There is a tendency to think of Australians as outdoor people but most live in cities.

> Outdoor recreation is associated with the beach as large cities tend to be near the coast. Therefore good water sports – yachting, windsurfing, rowing. The rest of Australia is pretty hostile.

> DASETT (Department of the Arts, the Environment, Tourism and Territories) has administrative control over the large areas of wilderness and deserts. Specific codes of behaviour.

> National parks are controlled by the local state, except for the Great Barrier Reef (popular for tourism).

Education, PE + sport

> Education is compulsory 6–15 years. Comprehensive (// USA; UK). Colonialist roots.

> Free, although fee-paying schools associated with religious bodies (// France).

> 'School of the air' is a system whereby programmes are transmitted by radio and television to outlying stations. Students receive tuition over the airwaves.

> Some funding allocated by federal government from taxes, but each state has the responsibility for education within the state (// USA).

Administered by:

DSE (Department of School Education)

Responsible for educational context of syllabus, sport and teacher training. Much has now been passed onto individual schools (// UK). PE or PASE (Physical and Sports Education) is compulsory throughout school years, but optional in Year 12 where can be taken as part of HSC (Higher School Certificate) [// A level PE in UK; Baccalaureate in France].

ACHPER (Australian Council for Health, Physical Education and Recreation)

Provides federal input, is committed to programmes and projects both commercial and educational. Its mission is to promote healthy lifestyles for all Australians. Has physical education development programme.

Questions

> The questions here are examples of the style of question that occur in the final papers. The information to answer these questions can be found in the relevant sections of this book. (For answers and guidance, see pages 134–138

Applied anatomy and physiology

1 Explain, how the Sliding Filament theory applies to muscular contraction. *(5 marks)*

2 Describe the characteristics of fast twitch and slow twitch fibres; relate the differences in function to the differences in structure. *(7 marks)*

3 (a) Describe the structure of a motor unit. *(2 marks)*

(b) Explain why not all muscle fibre in a particular muscle contract at the same time. *(2 marks)*

(c) How does the human body increase the size of the force of muscle contraction? *(4 marks)*

4 (a) Describe what happens to a student's heart rate during a lesson in which he or she completes a bleep test. *(5 marks)*

(b) Draw a graph to represent this. *(7 marks)*

5 What is the relationship between heart rate and stroke volume with respect to cardiac output? *(3 marks)*

6 How does training effect the values of these parameters? *(3 marks)*

7 Explain the electrical conduction system of the heart. *(6 marks)*

8 Explain the 'lub' and the 'dub' heart sound heard through a stethoscope during the cardiac cycle. *(4 marks)*

Acquisition of skills

9 What is ability? Give three examples of abilities. *(5 marks)*

10 Using an example from sport, explain the open loop theory of motor control. *(5 marks)*

11 Using the example of catching a cricket ball, explain the closed loop theory of motor control. *(5 marks)*

12 Feedback can do many things for a performer.

(a) How does feedback affect the motivation of a beginner? *(2 marks)*

(b) How might you change the type of feedback for a more experienced performer? *(2 marks)*

13 Explain, with practical examples, reaction time, movement time and response time. *(3 marks)*

14 There are believed to be three stages or phases of learning; name them. *(3 marks)*

15 Explain the benefits of using a distributed practice style with beginners. *(3 marks)*

16 (a) When might you use manual guidance in the teaching of skills? *(1 marks)*

(b) List the disadvantages of this approach. *(3 marks)*

Contemporary studies

17 (a) What are the four main concepts behind sport? *(1 mark)*

(b) What are the main features of one of these concepts? *(4 marks)*

18 Using one emergent country as an example, state which sport has developed there. Give reasons for the development of that sport. *(4 marks)*

19 Inequalities exist in PE and sport. Give the disadvantages that may be experienced by one minority group. *(6 marks)*

Exercise physiology

20 What does ATP stand for in terms of human movement? *(1 mark)*

21 If exercise is to continue for more than 10–12 seconds another method of ATP regeneration must be used.

(a) What is this system called?

(b) About how long can exercise be maintained using this system? *(2 marks)*

22 After completing exercise involving this system, why is it important to continue with some form of gentle exercise? *(5 marks)*

23 Define the term 'basal metabolic rate'. *(1 mark)*

24 (a) List the components of health-related fitness. *(4 marks)*

(b) List the components of skill related fitness. *(5 marks)*

Questions

Biomechanics

25 (a) Define the term 'friction'.   *(2 marks)*

(b) Give two examples from sport where players try to increase friction in order to improve performance. (Exclude examples where interactions with air or water are responsible for the friction force.)

(2 marks)

(c) Give two examples from sport where players try to decrease friction in order to improve performance. (Exclude examples where interactions with air or water are responsible for the friction force.)

(2 marks)

26 *Figure 1* shows four forces acting on a scrummaging machine immediately prior to starting to move across the surface of the pitch.

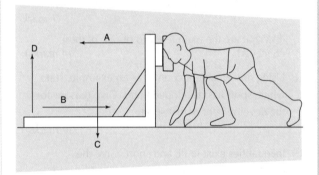

Figure 1

Match the letters A, B, C and D on the diagram with the following forces:

(a) weight of the scrummaging machine;

(b) the 'normal' force;

(c) the friction force;

(d) the applied force exerted by the player.

(4 marks)

27 State Newton's Law of Gravitation.   *(3 marks)*

28 *Figure 4* shows three positions of the jumper:

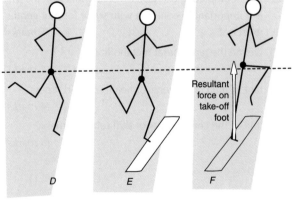

Figure 4

D – two strides away from the take-off board;

E – just before take-off, with take-off foot in contact with the board;

F – at the moment of take-off.

The large dot on the diagrams is the position of her centre of mass and the broken line is a horizontal line through the first position of the centre of mass (position of dot at D).

(a) Explain the meaning of the term 'centre of mass'.

(2 marks)

(b) Sketch a graph showing the vertical velocity of the centre of mass (y axis) against time (x axis), as the jumper moves from position D through E to position F.   *(3 marks)*

(c) Position F shows a resultant force acting on the jumper's take-off foot. Explain the meaning of the term 'resultant'.   *(1 mark)*

(d) Use your sketch graph to explain why there must be a resultant vertical force acting on the jumper between E and F.   *(4 marks)*

Psychology

29 Define personality?   *(1 mark)*

30 What possible problems can occur when researching a performer's personality?

(4 marks)

31 What is cognitive dissonance?   *(3 marks)*

32 (a) Explain the possible causes of aggression in team sports.   *(3 marks)*

(b) How might aggression be prevented from occurring in performers in a team?   *(4 marks)*

33 (a) Describe the characteristics of a person showing a NACH personality.   *(3 marks)*

(b) Describe the characteristics of a person showing NAF personality.   *(3 marks)*

History

34 Until relatively recently, field sports played an important part in people's lives in this country. Describe the main purposes that hunting served.

(2 marks)

35 Describe, for a sport of your choice, how both the rich and the poor became involved.

(2 marks)

36 How did public school boys develop games to suit their environment?   *(4 marks)*

37 Why did public school headmasters allow pupils to play games?   *(4 marks)*

38 Why did the growing middle classes want to promote sport for their factory workers?

(4 marks)

39 Describe the sporting activities that girls were expected to do in Victorian schools in Britain.

(2 marks)

40 Why did the government like the 1902 Model Course and why did educationalists dislike it?

(6 marks)

41 How did the role of the PE teacher change between 1904 and 1954? Use examples of subject content during the period to highlight your answer.

(6 marks)

Comparative studies

42 (a) What is the 'American Dream'? *(1 mark)*

(b) What is the 'win ethic'? *(1 mark)*

43 How is mass participation in sport encouraged in the USA? *(4 marks)*

44 What changes were brought in after the poor performances by Australian athletes at the 1976 Olympics? *(4 marks)*

Answers

Applied anatomy and physiology

1 The alternating bands of light and dark areas in the sarcomere give clues as to how Huxley's sliding filament theory works. When an impulse arrives at the muscle cell, this triggers the release of calcium ions. These calcium ions bind to troponin and cause the binding sites on actin to be exposed. ATP is broken down and energy is released. This energy is used to power the myosin head. The cross-bridges attach, detach and re-attach further along the actin filament – pulling the actin past the myosin. This has the effect of shortening the length of the sarcomere and so shortening the muscle.

2 *Fast twitch fibres* are bigger than slow twitch fibres and have larger motor neurones. This means they can generate force faster. However, fast twitch fibres tire more quickly than slow twitch fibres.

Slow twitch fibres contract at a rate of about 20% slower than fast twitch fibres. Because they are smaller than fast twitch fibres, slow twitch fibres generate force comparatively slowly. Slow twitch fibres do not fatigue as easily as fast twitch fibres, which makes them perfect for low-level activities. Fast twitch fibres tire more quickly, which means they are only useful for high-level activities. The Fast Twitch High Oxidative Glycolytic (FOG) type of fibres are used for longer sprint events; the Fast Twitch Glycolytic (FTG) type are used for shorter sprint events. (FOG have a greater resistance to fatigue than FTG. This is entirely due to endurance training, which encourages muscular adaptation.)

3 (a) A motor unit has a motor neurone controlling large numbers of individual fibres. The axon of the motor neurone – which runs from the spinal cord – branches as it reaches the muscle. The branches connect with a structure called the motor end plate.

(b) Each muscle fibre is served by a nerve fibre that is attached to the muscle. The nerve impulses that are carried along the nerve fibres are fired in different patterns. The stimulus may activate one motor unit to produce a twitch. Muscles will contract for longer than a fraction of a second when a stimulus occurs that activates many motor neurones.

(c) The human body increases the size of the force of muscle contraction by wave summation (i.e. by sending impulses one after the other in quick succession). The stimuli arrive so fast there is no time for any relaxation of the muscle. A state of 'absolute contraction' then occurs.

4 (a) The student's heart rate starts at the normal resting rate. There is an increase just before starting the bleep test as adrenaline is released. The rise continues as the test starts. Then there is a steep rise in heart rate as the exercise increases in intensity. A plateau occurs in the heart rate as the bleep test is reaching the higher levels. When the level 12 is reached and the student slows down the heart rate begins to fall. This drop in heart rate slows down in order for the body to clear the by-products of tissue respiration, before finally returning to normal (resting rate).

(b)

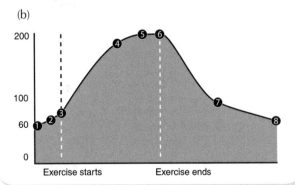

5 Heart rate x Stroke volume = Cardiac output

6 Training can improve the stroke volume (both the size of the heart and the muscle wall thickness increase), which therefore causes an increase in the cardiac output.

7 The heartbeat is initiated by electrical impulses that originate from the heart's 'pacemaker', the sino-atrial node. The impulse travels down the myocardium of the atrium until it reaches the atrio-ventricular node. A short delay then occurs, to allow atrial systole to complete. The impulse then enters specialist tissues called 'bundles of HIS' which branch through the septum as Purkinje fibres. These connect to myocardium fibres that cause the ventricles to contract (ventricular systole). This process can be seen by tracing the electrical signals in the heart using an electrocardiogram (ECG).

8 The 'lub' sound is the heart forcing blood out of the atria into the ventricles. Semi-lunar valves remain closed, but atrio-ventricular valves close after the passage of blood.

Once the blood has left the heart and the contraction ceases, the semi-lunar valves snap shut – causing the 'dub' sound heard through the stethoscope.

Acquisition of skills

9 Ability is the quality or skill that you have which makes it possible to do something.
Three possible examples:
- Ability to co-ordinate when dribbling a football.
- Flexibility when doing gymnastics.
- Using muscular power when lifting weights.

10 Using golf as an example, the open loop theory of motor control is as follows:
- The brain sends action commands to the muscles, in one chunk – eye on ball; knees flexed; pull back club; accelerate club to ball and follow through.
- Feedback may be available but it does not control the action.

11 Using catching a cricket ball as an example, the closed loop theory of motor control is as follows:
- The brain makes a decision – catch that ball!
- Some information is sent to initiate muscle action – eye on ball; move into position; hold hands ready; take catch.
- Feedback is available and is used to alter initial movements according to the new needs – the ball has bounced out of hands; keep eyes on ball; move hands to new position; try again.

12 (a) Feedback can provide motivation, especially for a beginner. For example: 'You hit nearly all of your forehands as winners. Well done!'

(b) Feedback can act as a motivator for reinforcement for an experienced player. For example: 'You know you can hit better forehands. You were hitting the ball too late. Let's go and work on that!'

13 'Reaction time' is the time from the first appearance of the stimulus to the initiation of the first movement. For example, the moment a tennis player is aware of the opponent sending the ball over the net to a particular area of the court, a decision being made to hit a forehand and the first movement to that part of the court.

'Movement time' is the time taken for the movement, initiated by the stimulus, to begin and then be completed. For example, in tennis the moment when the receiver begins to move into position to hit a forehand shot, including backswing, until the moment the player comes back (after impact) into a ready position to prepare for the next shot.

'Response time' is the time between the first presentation of stimulus to the movement ending. For example, the tennis player becomes aware of the opponent sending the ball over the net to a particular area of the court, decides to play a forehand, moves into position to hit a forehand shot, lifts the racquet back, swings through the forehand, makes impact, and moves back into a ready position to prepare for the next shot.

14 The three stages or phases of learning:
   • Cognitive or Understanding phase
   • Associative or Verbal motor phase
   • Autonomous or Motor phase

15 A distributed practice style of teaching allows beginners to take rests between practice, in which they can mentally rehearse the skills involved. It is a useful technique when teaching complex skills and for young pupils with short attention spans.

16 (a) You might use manual guidance when teaching:
   • someone to swim;
   • trampoline techniques;
   • rock climbing.
   (b) If overused the performer may become dependent on help or may lose motivation as they are a passive learner.

Contemporary studies

17 (a) play; physical recreation; physical education; sport
   (b) They might have chosen any of the following:

Play:
   • biological – instinctual part of learning process in developing skills
   • psychological – learning about self
   • sociological – to practice social roles
   • children's play – to learn about life
   • adults' play – to escape the stresses of everyday life.

Physical recreation:
   • relaxation and recuperation
   • can require limited organisation
   • participant in charge of time and place
   • personal goals (e.g. creative, spiritual) and rewards
   • mental pleasure, enjoyment, non-productive.

Physical education:
   • to impart knowledge and values through physical activities
   • structured lessons, usually in an institution
   • develops practical skills to be able to participate in activities
   • develops social skills, team working, co-operation and leadership… often within lifestyle activities
   • extra curricular activities out of formal lesson times
   • examinations (GCSE, A-level, degree) raised the profile of PE and encouraged career development
   • develops values – social, instrumental, humanistic.

Sport:
   • competitive
   • highly organised – time and space designated
   • formal rules
   • requires higher level of skill and commitment
   • develop sportsmanship
   • intrinsic rewards (own achievement, satisfaction)
   • extrinsic rewards (cups, money, titles, etc.)
   • the 'letter' of playing the game – by the rules
   • the 'spirit' of playing the game – fair play, high morals.

18 Students might choose any emergent country, but it's likely they will select one of the following:

Indonesia – badminton
   • Minority sport which suits country
   • Olympic sport – thus seen by the world
   • Easy to administer
   • Non-contact – non-aggressive
   • Small-sided game – small population
   • Requires small physique, dexterity and quick reactions
   • Little equipment or space needed
   • Slow pace – and ideal for playing in the tropics.

The Caribbean – cricket
   • Traditional and established game
   • Brought islands and people together in common purpose
   • Team game – co-operation
   • Outdoor game – healthy
   • Commonwealth sport – able to play other nations
   • International reputation
   • Income to islands.

Kenya – middle and long distance running
   • Olympic sport – high profile
   • Suited to lifestyle – used to running long distances
   • Little expense or technical knowledge needed
   • Good training at altitude
   • A few athletes can create great national pride.

19 They are asked to give the disadvantages for *one* group. They could pick any of the following:
   Race
   Opportunity:
   • Parental expectations
   • Non-acceptance in clubs may be a barrier
   • May be affected by religious beliefs (e.g. muslim girls)
   • Lack of finance means little choice (many low paid)
   • Cultures may not rate PE/sport highly
   • 'staking' – assumption that you play in a particular position in the team
   • lack of career opportunities – majority of coaches are white
   Provision:
   • associated with a particular sport (e.g. Asians playing cricket)…therefore little provision in other sports
   • lack of single sex lessons
   • lack of changing facilities to cater for religious restrictions
   • information not easily available
   • coaches not available
   Esteem:
   • Lack of role models to give hope to achieve
   • Poorly paid jobs add to low self-esteem
   • Media coverage of indigenous sports is low
   Disability
   Opportunity:
   • Some sports may not cater for disability – therefore restricted choice
   • Few disabled sports clubs and restricted membership to others
   • Few coaches so poor prospects
   • Fewer opportunities to achieve excellence
   Provision:
   • Lack of specialist equipment
   • Poor wheelchair access to leisure centres and swimming pools
   • Inadequate changing facilities
   • Transport to activities may not be possible
   • Cost of special provision may be prohibitive

Answers

Esteem:
- Perceived to be not able to achieve and the assumption that they cannot do sport – a myth and stereotype
- Few role models – paraplegic games and marathons only beginning to be given media coverage
- Assumed lack of knowledge
- Perceived as not interesting or exciting enough …therefore not taken seriously.

Gender

Opportunity:
- Looking after family – less leisure time
- certain religious restrictions
- fewer female coaches, managers and administrators therefore limited career opportunities
- some clubs have membership restrictions – although law is changing
- lack of competition opportunity
- restricted choice of activities and those choices may favour males
- considered incapable and not aggressive enough

Provision:
- lack of creche facilities
- few females on governing bodies and little input in decision making
- few female coaches
- lower pay and prize money
- may lack money to spend on sport if not working
- lack of transport
- competitions may be restricted to single sex
- clubs may restrict playing times or provide inferior changing facilities

Esteem:
- think they can't do sport – poor self-image
- lack of many role models
- media coverage poor
- lack of sponsorship
- not taken seriously by spectators
- affected by myths

Age

Opportunity:
- young – too early with hard training can 'burn out'
- young – reliant on parental attitude and finances
- participation of 50+ age group restricted, few veterans' clubs and teams
- age restrictions in some clubs
- curriculum and extra curricular opportunities dependent on schools – relies on PE staff enthusiasm

Provision:
- facilities dependant on geographical location
- few activity sessions specifically for older people or teenagers
- transport may be reliant on goodwill of family and friends
- fees may be prohibitive

Esteem:
- media coverage minimal for elderly and very young
- few role models
- elderly perceived as only involved for recreation
- peer pressure can affect youngsters' perception of sport, particularly girls

Class

Opportunity:
- 'working class' – little leisure time, lack of finance, difficult to work and compete at a high level
- restricted access to certain clubs
- 'middle class' – more leisure time and wealth to choose activities

Provision:
- 'working class' may experience limited facilities and coaches – reliant on sponsorship for funding
- wealthy individuals have the ability to pay a coach, buy equipment and clothing and to travel to training and competition

Esteem:
- role models can give hope to those from deprived backgrounds – seen as way out and means to achieve wealth
- Media can help promote and gain sponsorship
- Less wealthy could be seen as less able or knowledgeable

Exercise physiology

20 Adenosine triphosphate – the main supplier of metabolic energy in all living cells.
21 (a) Lactic acid system, or glycolysis.
    (b) Exercise can be sustained using this system for between 30 seconds and 1 minute.
22 Gentle exercise, or warm-down, after training involving the lactic acid system is important as this maintains higher respiration rate and flushes lactic acid out of fast twitch fibres.
23 Basal metabolic rate (BMR) is the energy you need just to be alive, awake and comfortably warm.
24 (a) Health-related fitness components:
    - aerobic capacity
    - strength
    - flexibility
    - body composition
    (b) Skill-related fitness components:
    - speed
    - reaction time
    - agility
    - balance
    - coordination

Biomechanics

25 (a) Friction is the force that acts between two surfaces to oppose motion.
    (b) Studded boots in football; the use of magnesium carbonate in gymnastics to aid grip on high bar. (c)Waxing skis to aid sliding movement; brushing ice in curling to aid sliding movement.
26 (a) C; (b) D; (c) B; (d) A
27 Any two bodies attract each other with a force proportional to the product of their masses and universally proportional to the square of the distance between them.
28 (a) A single point that represents the concentration of the body's mass.
    (b)

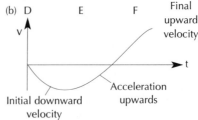

    (c) The resultant is the overall/sum vector of all the forces acting.
    (d) The upward slope between E and F means upward acceleration. With F = Ma, this means a net (resultant) upward force as Force is proportional to Acceleration.

Psychology

29 Personality is *either* 'The sum total of an individual's characteristics which makes him or her unique' *or* 'The overall pattern of psychological characteristics that makes each person unique'.

30 There are problems in ensuring validity and reliability. All techniques may be time consuming and costly. The interpretation of results may cause over-generalization, particularly if small numbers are used.

31 Cognitive dissonance is a mismatch in the Triadic Model. This causes an imbalance in the mind of the person being persuaded. You must act to reduce this imbalance by changing behaviour to meet new criteria, based on new information.

32 (a) Possible causes:
- natural instinct – cultural background often disproves this and aggression is often not spontaneous
- frustration – a person is blocked, they are frustrated and release the tension through aggressive action
- social learning – people see others being aggressive and imitate this behaviour.

(b) Combatting aggression:
- Control of arousal levels (stress management)
- Avoidance of situations that cause aggression
- Stopping aggressive players from further participation
- Rewarding 'turning the other cheek'
- Showing non-aggressive role models
- Punishing aggression
- Reinforcement of non-aggression (largely by significant others)
- Handling responsibility to an aggressive player.

33 (a) NACH personality:
- determined to see a task through
- work quickly at a task
- take risks
- enjoy a challenge
- take responsibility
- like to know how they have been judged.

(b) NAF personality:
- easily persuaded from taking the challenge
- work at tasks slowly or not at all
- avoid situations where they or their ego is put at risk
- avoid responsibility
- prefer not to be judged and do not want to know how they have been judged.

History

34 Hunting served two main purposes – food and recreation. For the poor, hunting for food was a necessity, to feed the family. They were either involved in employment to feed the wealthy or in poaching (stealing animals from other people's property). The wealthy, on the other hand, often hunted for leisure. This allowed them to show off their athleticism, to challenge themselves physically and to enjoy a social occasion.

35 The answer will depend on the sport chosen by the student. The following are possible answers:

Cricket
- Cricket was enjoyed by all sections of society. It could be played on the rough village wicket with a minimum of equipment, or in the fine setting of a country property.
- The gentry could play in the same team as the working class, but both sections had clearly defined roles. The former dictated tactics, the latter chased after the ball.

Tennis
- The servants of the wealthy saw this game and derived their own version. This was often played in the courtyards of local pubs. This was convenient as it provided both competitors and spectators.

Mob football
- It was a game played by the lower classes and despised by the wealthy. The wealthy were worried that their property would be destroyed by the violent games.

36
- Games changed to suit available playing space.
- Different sports played at different times of the year to suit conditions.
- Rules were developed.
- Inter-house competitions allowed the sport to become regular and competitive.

37 Games:
- encouraged their moral development
- developed leadership
- developed courage
- pupils learnt to put team before self
- usefully occupied free time.

38 For factory workers sport:
- meaningfully occupied free time
- improved health
- boosted morale
- created worker loyalty
- showed the benefits that they themselves had gained from participating while at school.

39 In ladies' academies they taught dancing, a form of callisthenics, sewing, singing, playing the piano, verse speaking, posture and any other graces it was felt important for a woman to have.
By the 1880s tennis and cricket were being played in girls' schools. The girls wore their normal clothing to be worn and the games did not involve contact.

40 The 1902 Model course:

Government:
- disciplined
- created young soldiers
- promoted health
- provided a scapegoat for recent failures in the Boer War.

Educationalists:
- treated children as adults
- limited educational value
- no differentiation between girls and boys.

41 Role of the PE teacher:
- Developed from a trainer who taught exercise-related drill to an educationalist who taught skills, games and gymnastics.
- The teaching style moved from being autocratic where there was a one-way flow of commands (e.g. 'attention', 'about turn') to a mixed style that varied from autocratic to self-discovery lesson whose content was more varied.
- Initially the process was more important than the pupils. This changed and the needs of pupils were taken into consideration. Enjoyment, skill development and social development became more important than just obedience.

Answers

Comparative studies

42 (a) The 'American Dream' is the 'rags to riches' story. It is the idea that everyone and anyone can achieve success/the pursuit of happiness. Sport is seen as a way out of the gutter (e.g. boxing).

(b) The 'win ethic' means winning is the only thing. This is also known as the Lombardian philosophy, after Vince Lombardi, Head Coach of Green Bay Packers in 1959, who transformed them from a losing baseball team into a major power in the sport. The emphasis is on competition and rewards.

43 Mass participation:
- No specific plans by the federal government.
- Programmes for adults are part of school programmes.
- For children, 'little league sport' (e.g. little league basketball) – originally set up by parents, now a business organisation catering for 8–18 year olds (senior division 13–15; big league 16–18). Attracts media coverage.
- National senior sports organisation – image of a healthy old age.
- No real private sports clubs except elitist ones (tennis and golf). Expensive. Less wealthy involved with activities at:
  - ice rinks
  - swimming pools
  - basketball courts.
- All interested in going to the game (baseball).

44 Poor performances in the 1976 Olympics led to changes:
- ASC (Australian Sports Commission) researched in other countries to look for most effective method to select and train athletes. Set up the AIS (Australian Institute of Sport), an academy of sport in Canberra (where federal government and ASC located). Realised need for more than one institute of excellence.
- Set up more in other states – Queensland (at Brisbane); Western Australia (at Perth); South Australia (at Adelaide); Victoria (at Melbourne); New South Wales (at Sydney) – each specialised in one sport (e.g. cricket at Adelaide; rugby at Brisbane).
- Now each state devolved with centres of excellence in their main city. All part of AIS federal system. Have programme of talent identification – Sportsleap, Sports search – run at all levels (to identify talent).
- Aussie able – provision for disabled athletes – some sports schools.

Index